STONEHILL COLLEGE

"Securing the Vision"
The Campaign for
Stonehill's Future

Women's Health

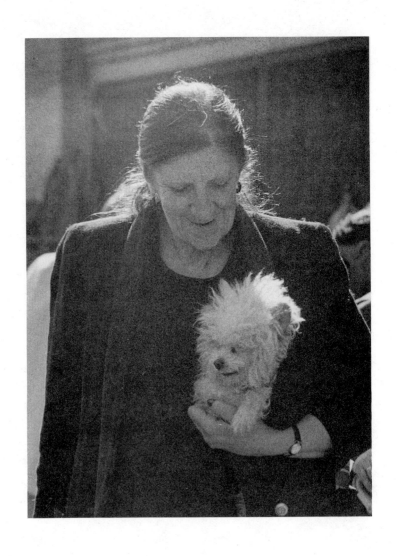

Women's Health

A Relational Perspective across the Life Cycle

Judith A. Lewis, PhD, RNC, FAAN
Associate Professor and Chair
Maternal Child Nursing
Virginia Commonwealth University
Richmond, Virginia

Judith Bernstein, PhD, RNC
National Policy and Resource Center on Women and Aging
Brandeis University
Waltham, Massachusetts

Jones and Bartlett Publishers
Sudbury, Massachusetts

Boston　　London　　Singapore

Editorial, Sales, and Customer Service Offices
Jones and Bartlett Publishers
40 Tall Pine Drive
Sudbury, MA 01776
508-443-5000
info@jbpub.com
http://www.jbpub.com

Jones and Bartlett Publishers International
Barb House, Barb Mews
London W6 7PA
UK

Library of Congress Cataloging-in-Publication Data

Lewis, Judith A., 1945–
    Women's health : a relational perspective across the life cycle /
Judith A. Lewis, Judith Bernstein.
        p.   cm.
    Includes bibliographical references and index.
    ISBN 0-86720-485-0
    1. Women—Health and hygiene—Sociological aspects. 2. Women's
health services. 3. Women—Health and hygiene. 4. Life cycle,
Human. I. Bernstein, Judith, 1944–   . II. Title.
    RA564.85.L49   1996
    613'.04244—dc20   95-33320
                                                                              CIP

Acquisitions Editor: Jan Wall
Associate Production Editor: Nadine Fitzwilliam
Senior Manufacturing Buyer: Dana L. Cerrito
Typesetting: UltraGraphics
Cover Design: Mimi Ahmed
Printing and Binding: Malloy Lithographing, Inc.
Cover Printing: New England Book Components, Inc.

Photographs by Mariah Bowen

Printed in the United States of America
00 99 98 97   10 9 8 7 6 5 4 3 2

Contributors

Ruth M. Barnard, PhD, RN
  Associate Professor
  School of Nursing
  University of Michigan
  Ann Arbor, Michigan

Judith Bernstein, PhD, RNC
  National Policy and Resource
    Center on Women and Aging
  Brandeis University
  Waltham, Massachusetts

Bernardine A. Clarke, MS,
    CPNP, FAAN
  Associate Professor Emeritus
  School of Nursing
  Virginia Commonwealth University
  Richmond, Virginia

Molly Dougherty, RN, PhD
  Professor
  College of Nursing
  University of Florida
  Gainesville, Florida

Andrew D. Lacatell, M.I.S.
  Center for Environmental Studies
  Virginia Commonwealth University
  Richmond, Virginia

Judith A. Lewis, PhD, RNC, FAAN
  Associate Professor
  School of Nursing
  Virginia Commonwealth University
  Richmond, Virginia

Debra E. Lyon, RN, MS
  Doctoral Student
  School of Nursing
  Virginia Commonwealth University
  Richmond, Virginia

Catherine Malloy, DrPH, RN, FAAN
  Professor
  College of Nursing and
    Health Science
  George Mason University
  Fairfax, Virginia

Snowy Molonsankwe
  Doctoral Student
  Brandeis University
  Waltham, MA
  Researcher, Department of Health
    and Social Services
  Mmbatho, South Africa

Allen F. Moore
  Student
  University of Virginia
  Charlottesville, Virginia

Ellen Olshansky, DNSc, RNC
  Associate Professor
  School of Nursing
  University of Washington
  Seattle, Washington

Amelia Marquez de Perez
  Professor
  Faculty of Public Administration
  University of Panama
  Cuidad Panama, Panama

Susan Pfister, PhD, RN,C
  Assistant Professor
  School of Nursing
  Washburn University
  Topeka, Kansas

Nancy E. Reame, PhD, RN, FAAN
  Director
  Center for Nursing Research
  University of Michigan
  Ann Arbor, Michigan

Evelyn Slaght, PhD
  Associate Professor
  College of Nursing and Health Science
  George Mason University
  Fairfax, Virginia

Martha Neff Smith, PhD, RNC
  Associate Professor
  School of Nursing
  Virginia Commonwealth University
  Richmond, Virginia

Sarah S. Strauss, PhD, RN
  Associate Professor
  School of Nursing
  Virginia Commonwealth University
  Richmond, Virginia

Ruth E. Zambrana, PhD
  Professor and Enochs Chair
  College of Nursing and Health Science
  George Mason University
  Fairfax, Virginia

Table of Contents

Introduction

Women's Health : A Relational Perspective across the Life Cycle provides an integrated, multidisciplinary approach to women's health. Designed for use in women's studies or nursing, the material integrates historical, sociocultural, biophysiological, and psychosocial aspects of women's development in a way that provides a multi-lens, woman-centered perspective on the health of women.

We decided to write this book because we could find no available resource that provided such a perspective. There are several excellent books in print which address women's health and illness problems from a medical perspective. These books discuss the diagnosis and treatment of conditions affecting women. There are also several excellent books in print which address women's growth and development. What was lacking was a book that provided a marriage between these two perspectives. This book is intended to fill this void.

Part One provides the theoretical framework for the rest of the book. We set the social context and provide the historical perspective underlying the modern health care system. The traditional model of women's growth and development is analyzed in terms of its deficiencies in adequately explaining women's strengths. Relational psychology is used as a framework for reframing the strengths of women, and women's ways of knowing and communicating are used to describe the female voice. Finally, we examine the interaction of gender, class, and race to expose some of the stereotyped roles and expectations that interfere with health and affect the treatment of illness.

Part Two looks at the maturation of women across the life cycle. Adolescence, the reproductive years, perimenopause, and aging are the broad categories under which physical and psychosocial growth and development are reviewed. Common health issues are addressed, and the major threats to health are discussed. The emphasis is on maintaining health and wellness, while identifying those conditions that may pose hazards to women as they progress through the life cycle.

Part Three focuses on the complexity of women's roles. Women are viewed as individuals, in all the diversity of their achievements and challenges. At the same time we recognize the integral relationship between individual women and the family, as well as community contexts that contribute to both health and illness. The global context of women's health care is presented, including case studies of women's conditions in Panama and South Africa. We conclude with the development of a contextual new model for the care of women.

This book is suitable for graduate-level courses in women's studies and nursing as well as for selected upper-level undergraduate courses. We also believe that it will be interesting and thought-provoking for the general reader interested in a woman-centered approach to women's health. Finally, we think that it will stimulate further study in the field. Our hope is that our work has raised more questions than it has answered.

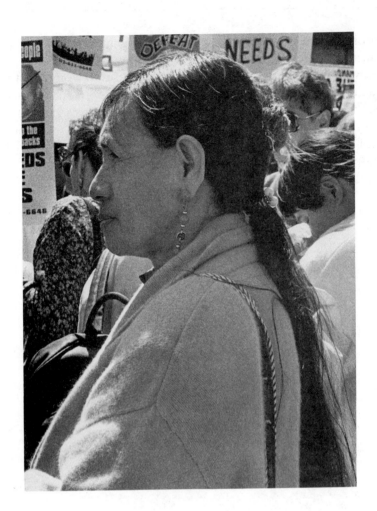

Part One

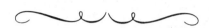

Women's Experience as Basis for a Theoretical Framework for Health

1

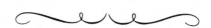

The Modern Health Care System and Gender Bias

The Historical and Ideological Context

Judith Bernstein
Judith A. Lewis

*One must have health! You may banish money,
banish sofas, banish wine!—Banish health and
you banish all the world!*
Anne Crawford Flexner (1875–1955)

Introduction

Throughout history, the most salient factor affecting the health of women has been their position in society. Recent discoveries and interpretations of prehistory suggest that the earliest human cultures may have been either matriarchal and matrilineal or forms of partnership organization, with men and women assigned roles that were equally respected and valued (Eisler, 1988). These early societies worshipped goddesses as well as gods (Stone, 1976), and ascribed considerable powers to women, who were not just fertility emblems but the spinners of destiny, associated with justice, wisdom and intelligence, and the arts as well as reproduction (Frymer-Krensky, 1992). Assisted by a relatively abundant food supply and favorable environmental conditions, a high level of civilization developed, graced by agriculture, trade, religious art, and the development of writing. In this world, which continued through at least 20,000 years of human history down into the Mesopotamian and Greek eras, health was defined in the very broadest of senses, encompassing emotional, spiritual, and physical well-being, and thought to be achieved through harmony among individuals, society, and the natural world. Women were assigned responsibility for the health of their families and their communities (Colliere, 1986). This was the golden time described by Hesiod. It was surely not a perfect time—there were still conflicts and cruelties, inadequacies and want—but overall, life was more collective, and the position of women relatively favorable. Women were as likely as men to be buried with valuable artifacts, an indication of equal status, and they had considerable authority as inventors of cultivation and distributors of food (Lorber, 1994).

Then a major social revolution occurred. The devastation of Minoan culture 3000 years ago was one of the final episodes in a protracted war between this partnership system, and a patriarchal or patrilinear form of social organization. In Assyria, Doria, and Canaan, hierarchical warrior cultures set out to conquer the world, and the male gods of war became dominant. As humankind became less nomadic and acquired property, property rights and inheritance became a major concern, and women and children became property as well. Women were subjugated, relegated to a reproductive role, no longer valued for their knowledge, and far removed from the sources of governance and power (Goldenberg, 1979). Large numbers of women were enslaved, and the practice of female sacrifice became commonplace. Warriors were often buried with several wives or concubines (Eisler, 1988). Women had previously held political power; many of the ancient Egyptian tombs initially ascribed to kings were later found to have been the resting places of powerful and wealthy queens (Stone, 1976). They had also held great symbolic authority under a system of religious beliefs based on ancient origin myths that gave women the responsibility of ritual action to stave off elemental chaos (Grahn, 1993). In the new world, however, women were reduced to property, as noted by Anati (1963) in *Palestine Before the Hebrews*, "men bringing with them their goods and donkeys, wives and children" (p. 389).

In service of this ideology, new patriarchal religions were founded, which developed into the three main Western religions: Judaism,

Christianity, and Islam. These religious traditions shared a common thread—the empowerment of men over women. Over time, worship of the goddesses was suppressed, and temples, ritual objects, statuary, and writings destroyed. Religious worship was denigrated as "cult," and *qadishtu*, or sacred women of the temples, as "ritual prostitutes." The Old Testament, for example, does not even have a word for goddess (Stone, 1976). When observant Jewish males today perform the morning ritual of putting on *tefillim,* and say as part of a blessing, "Thank God I am not a woman," they speak, in spirit, for the Judeo-Christian/Islamic world (French, 1992). This shift in authority and power for women, both temporal and spiritual, has had profound consequences for health.

As long as health remained a cottage industry, largely a private, familial matter, remnants of knowledge and authority from the ancient female domain of healing could persist and exist alongside the fledgling science of medicine. Over the last 150 years, however, with the expansion of the health care industry into the marketplace, the patriarchal world view has been tightly consolidated into the conceptual framework of modern health care delivery systems. Health definitions and roles have been transferred from female to male responsibility, as the old network of women's remedies, "witch"-healers, and granny-midwives (Ehrenreich & English, 1973) gave way to the medical academy and the hegemony of male physicians (Scutt, 1990).

The origins of the female science of gynecology, for example, reflect a very direct historical bias against women. J. Marion Sims, revered as the father of gynecology, learned to perform surgery through multiple experimental operations (as many as 30 in 2 years' time) on four black female slaves whom he addicted to opium and kept in a hut in his backyard. And in 1883, the year of Sims's death, it was written that surgeons could "apply their knives at will to the whole range of woman's being, reduced as it was to sex" (Barker-Benfield, 1976, p. 119). This legacy persists in recent times in the form of unnecessary hysterectomies and caesarian sections performed for physician convenience, memorably described by Mary Daly (1990) in *Gyn/Ecology* as the Sado-Ritual System.

Even if such abuses were to be set aside, the norms and power relations inherent in medical practice have still had a negative impact on women's health. The emergence of the medical model brought dramatic changes in outlook, because the physician's knowledge base is organized around treatment of physical symptoms and disease, and is oriented toward illness, rather than health. The perspective is that of the immediate medical crisis, as defined by the requirements of diagnosis and treatment, and the larger picture of health maintenance throughout the life span receives only token consideration (Cohen, Schwartz, Bromet, & Parkinson, 1991). The whole person attended to by the lay midwife or traditional healer has become an interesting collection of inadequately functioning body parts.

Nursing, as a traditional occupation for women, became the repository for caring in the health care field. As Reverby (1987) describes, once nursing became professionalized, an ethic of caring was enforced, often at high cost to the individual nurse. The job of caring was closely tied to tasks of housekeeping for the sick, and women's work was accorded low status in the authoritarian, hierarchical hospital system. Eventually, the demands of technological development drove up the requirements for entry to nursing, however, and there was less and less time for caring. The tension created by the gap between ideal and real conditions has been partially resolved by co-optation of nurses into the medical model. Nurses, especially those in extended and advanced practice roles, allied themselves with the medical model in pursuit of the promise of professionalism and increased wages, at the cost of alliance with patients for a jointly shared vision of health promotion (Ashley, 1976).

Under our present specialized health care system, physical attributes are split off from each other and from other dimensions of humanity. Pathophysiology, information about physical disease processes, is characterized as *real* or *hard* science. Psychology and sociology, the sciences of human interaction, are characterized as *imprecise* or *soft*. Talk of the power to heal or the importance of therapeutic touch creates discomfort in both medical and nonacademic nursing circles. Under the influence of highly developed technology, the human body has itself been fragmented into a myriad of specialty realms. Personal agency and responsibility have been lost, and the objectives of health care have been redefined toward curing illness, with little or no participation from the recipient. The discipline of medical sociology (Freund & McGuire, 1991) characterizes the medical model by its adherence to three central principles: mind-body dualism (separation of physical and mental domains), physical reductionism (the exclusion of social, psychological, and behavioral dimensions of health and illness), and the doctrine of specific etiology (one disease, one cause).

With this perspective as context, health promotion and preventive medicine are considered to be interesting ideas, but luxuries for which there is no available funding. Prevention is expensive—approximately $58,000 for each year of life saved by mammography screening, for example. Within the health care reform debate, cost effectiveness weighs more heavily than improvements in quality of life (Brown, 1992; Mushlin & Fintor, 1992), and most prevention measures, contrary to common belief, carry a high price tag. The Center for Risk Analysis at the Harvard School of Public Health prices annual cervical cancer screening for women beginning at age 20 at $233, $620 for each year of life saved.

In keeping with this world view, medical students report financial motivation to far outweigh a sense of altruism in the choice to become a doctor (Binder, 1992). Nursing has attempted to introduce concepts of wellness and holism but, as a predominantly women's profession, has had little influence or authority (Agan, 1987). The experience of medical care, for female patients and, to a lesser degree, for practitioners as well, is an object lesson in powerlessness and unmet expectations. Health care for women has been characterized by "indifference and fatalism toward the diseases of women" (Rich, 1976, p. x).

We are beginning to see some changes. Recent pressure from women's advocacy groups and advocates of change within medicine has resulted in an Office of Women's Affairs within the National Institutes of Health (NIH), a change of policy requiring that women be included in research whenever possible, and funding for the Women's Health Initiative, an extensive longitudinal research project. In 1991, Medicare began to cover mammography screening once every two years. A few departments in medical schools now have women as chairs, and a large multi-center project is underway to introduce women's issues into medical school curricula.

Change comes slowly. Despite the NIH directive to include women as research subjects, the number of women so designated has increased only slightly. The Women's Health Initiative has been criticized by many groups, including the Institute of Medicine, for poor research design and ethical questions. Medicare, in the first year of benefits for mammography screening, paid only 670,000 claims despite the fact that 19 million women were estimated to be eligible for Medicare-paid mammography screening (General Accounting Office Report, 1993).

Health Care for Women: Definitions

The World Health Organization defines health as "a state of complete physical, mental and social well-being, and not just the absence of disease or infirmity" (World Health Organization, 1946). Factors contributing to health can be categorized in five main groups: adequate nutrition and shelter; sanitary, safe, unpolluted living and working conditions; exercise, rest, and lifestyle considerations; preventive, curative, and rehabilitative personal medical services; and nonmedical personal support services (Ethics Committee, Society for Academic Emergency Medicine, 1992). Although the medical model accepts as its health mission only curative and rehabilitative personal medical services, the wider definition of health care, which includes psychosocial concerns and public health issues, is a far better standard for describing health needs and evaluating care.

Access to Care

Women in the United States, as receivers of care, and as lower-level workers in the health care system, have suffered from the hierarchical, impersonal, disconnected, and constricted perspective of the medical model. As patients they face restricted access to care for themselves and their families because of gender-related economic discrimination (Googins & Burden, 1987). Although women are now a major segment of the permanent work force, their share of higher paying professional jobs has not increased substantially from 34 percent in the 1900s, to 48 percent in the 1980s (Amott & Matthaei, 1991); these numbers, of course, include professions such as teaching that have relatively low pay and even lower status. Even though law and medicine have opened up considerably in the last decade, the number of women in the nontraditional occupations has remained about the same at 9 percent, and two thirds of minimum wage workers are women (Matteo, 1993). Despite an active advertising campaign to convince society that women have "come a long way, baby," women in the work force are paid 64 cents for every dollar earned by males (Rosenberg, 1992). From the mid 1960s to the mid 1970s, the number of poor adult males declined, while the number of poor in households headed by women increased by 100,000 per year. Although two thirds of women work outside the home, they are more likely than men to work for small companies or as part-time employees and therefore not be covered by employer-mandated health insurance (McBarnette, 1988). Low wages for women are maintained by job segregation by sex; hierarchies of power in production; segmentation of the labor market based on racial, ethnic, and citizenship status; and playing workers off against each other (Hansen & Philipson, 1990). Economic barriers to health care are the direct result.

More than one-fifth of women are currently raising families alone, and of those, 40 percent of Whites and 60 percent of African Americans are below the poverty line. The typical homeless woman, today, is 27 years old and the mother of two, not the 65-year-old "bag lady" of popular stereotype (Bassuk, 1992). She is more likely to have acute and chronic medical problems, be at risk for violence and sexual abuse, and have a high incidence of unwanted pregnancy, sexually transmitted diseases, substance abuse problems, and depression, and a "startling deficit of social support" (Ovrebo, Ryan, Jackson, & Hutchinson, 1994).

Under the guise of welfare reform, the safety net of the Aid to Families With Dependent Children (AFDC) assistance program will be changed, over the next few years, to a mandatory work program that will have neither regulatory teeth nor funding to provide adequate training for existing jobs, does not create permanent jobs, and does not provide child care or other supports necessary to a working mother (Abramovitz, 1992). It appears likely that a limit will also be imposed of no more than 2 years of federal/state assistance, and that women who have another pregnancy while receiving support will be disqualified. While reform may be necessary and the goal of independence for women and their families is admirable, the types of change currently under discussion will not provide real jobs, real child care, or real reform. The economic position of the most vulnerable women is likely to worsen, with a negative effect on their health and their children's.

Life expectancies for minority women are significantly lower than for white women, a reflection of reduced access to medical care (Hale, 1992). Substance abuse treatment facilities for pregnant women are woefully inadequate; waiting lists for the nonpregnant woman are interminable (Amaro, 1993). Women with coronary disease are less likely than men to receive surgical intervention or other advanced technologies (Wenger et al., 1990). Undesired teen pregnancy is a major health problem, and a large number of pregnant women never receive prenatal care. New state laws designed to limit abortion impose undue hardship, and there is a shortage of trained practitioners. Information about abortion has been difficult to obtain, and access to the procedure has been restricted by cost. For some women, safe contraception has not been readily available; others have experienced coerced sterilization (Rodrique, 1990). Psychosocial problems that affect women's health—battering and family violence, rape, homelessness, and eating disorders, for example—have finally been identified as serious health problems, but rates of detection and referral for treatment fall far behind prevalence. In every aspect of medical care for women there are serious problems of access to appropriate care.

Quality of Care

Even when there is access to care, high quality care is often not available. As a result of social attitudes based on gender, research and treatment dollars have been inequitably allocated. For the older woman, the lesbian, and the woman of color, gender issues are intensified by ageism, homophobia, racism, and ethnic discrimination. The attributes of subordinates, as defined by social psychology, fit the health behaviors of women very well. The female patient is expected to be passive, receptive, and nondemanding, and to work hard at being a "good" patient in order to be eligible to receive treatment. Jean Miller, in *Toward a New Psychology of Women* (1986), describes well what women have had to do: study and internalize the dominant culture, disguise themselves, learn indirect ways of acting and relating, and appease those in power. These efforts have not won for women the health care that they need.

There is profound scientific ignorance about basic female physiology (Greer, 1971). Despite the obvious fact that more than half of the population will eventually experience menopause, the metabolic mechanism for hot flashes has not been identified; even though breast cancer is the most common cancer in women, the normal physiology of the breast has yet to be described. Pregnancy and delivery have been medicalized into a disease state, and efforts to develop women-respectful birth options are scattered and slow to be implemented (Martin, 1987; Boston Women's Health Collective, 1992). Women have generally not been included in clinical drug trials, limiting understanding of physiology, pathology, and effective treatment of major disease entities (Corea, 1992; Angell, 1993; LaRosa & Pinn, 1993). Research in diseases primarily affecting women—breast cancer and osteoporotic hip fracture, for example—have been drastically underfunded (Love & Linsey, 1990). In the absence of specific information about both normal physiology and disease states specific to or experienced differently by women, many pharmaceuticals are overprescribed. Many research studies document, for example, the propensity of physicians to give psychotropics to women and disease-specific drugs to men

or the same set of symptoms (Bernstein & Kane, 1985). The estro-
;en diethylstilbestrol (DES), touted as a miracle drug, was given for
 decade to pregnant women who were asymptomatic to ensure a
'quality pregnancy," resulting in vaginal cancer and fertility problems
n female offspring (McDowell, 1991).

   Illnesses to which minority groups are more susceptible have received
ven less scientific attention. The incidence of HIV infection in women
s rising rapidly, and is currently the fastest growing source of new cases,
et definitions on which access to treatment are based did not, until
ecently, include the forms in which AIDS presents in women (Vol-
)erding & Jacobsen, 1992). Entry to drug treatment programs that
)rovide AZT and other experimental therapies has, until recently, been
:ategorically restricted for women on the grounds that they might
)ossibly be pregnant; yet recent research suggests that taken during
)regnancy, AZT may actually reduce the likelihood of transmission of
:he virus to the fetus.

   Women who are members of minority groups are at greater risk
 or serious disease; a 2.6 times higher rate has been described for mor-
:ality from cervical cancer (Centers for Disease Control and Preven-
:ion [CDC], 1990a) and 1.8 times higher from ectopic pregnancy
(CDC, 1990b). Infertility, a problem of concern to a large number of
women, is not covered by most insurance; treatment is restrictively
expensive, prevention largely ignored, and research prohibited, until
recently, by governmental restrictions against including women of
reproductive age in clinical trials (Blackwell et al., 1987). Health needs
of lesbian women have largely been ignored by the mainstream health
system (Bem, 1993). Factors involved in violence against women are
now being highlighted, but a large number of the primary care physicians, obstetricians and gynecologists, and gynecologists and emergency
department physicians who treat battered women have inadequate detection skills and knowledge of referral resources and appropriate standards for safe discharge (American Medical Association [AMA], 1992).
The U.S. spends 14 percent of its gross national product (GNP) on
health care (National Leadership Commission on Health Care, U.S.,
1989; Aaron, 1991)—the highest rate among developed nations—but
ranks 16th in perinatal mortality, a sensitive indicator for success in
health care delivery (Schieber, Poullier, & Greenwald, 1991). Women
wait longer for treatment of chronic pain, and are more likely than men
to receive minor tranquilizers in place of pain therapy (Lack, 1982).
Within the health care industry itself, women are at greatest risk for
occupational injury; the majority of needle sticks and back strains happen to women hospital workers (McCray, 1986).

The record for women in the field of mental health is no better. On the one hand, there is often a failure to recognize psychosocial factors precipitating illness, resulting in inappropriate diagnosis and treatment. On the other hand, women are often labelled depressive, and overmedicated with psychotropics (Chesler, 1989). Women are much more likely than men to receive a psychiatric diagnosis of depression, and twice as likely to receive a prescription for a tranquilizer (McDowell, 1991). Cumulative doses of mood altering drugs are also higher for women, even though their weights are lower than those of men. Imprisonment of women in institutions on totally unsubstantiated psychiatric charges has been well documented (McBride, 1987). As late as 1945, women were still being castrated for psychological disorders, overeating, and masturbation as a form of social control (Levy, 1992).

Major transitions in women's lives have not been adequately studied to provide health professionals with standards to judge psychological health or illness. For example, norms for adolescent development of identity, abstract thinking, and moral reasoning have until very recently been available only for men (Gilligan, 1982; Gilligan, Lyons, & Hanmer, 1990; Brown & Gilligan, 1992). Assumptions are made about emotional effects of major physiological events, such as menarche and menopause, but scientific data are not available to sum up the lived experience of women of different classes and ethnic and racial backgrounds. What percentage of women experience depression as a result of an "empty nest" syndrome? How many perceive menopause as a period of grievous losses, and how many mark cessation of menses as entry into a new world of increased freedom and self-development? What are the effects of these transitions on psychological state? We cannot say that we know.

In the absence of adequate social supports such as affordable day care or respite care, women assume multiple roles with substantial unpaid responsibilities; the additional physical and emotional stress that results carries an uncomputed toll (McBride, 1988). Women are also expected to care for ailing parents, as part of the feminine image of woman as fountain of nurture (Gomes, Given, & Given, 1992). Instead of society at large paying the bill for health and survival care for elders, women who work, mother their children, and at the same time provide daily personal care for dependent parents are paying with their own health (Young & Kahana, 1989). And as women age, having provided for others all their lives, they are likely to be alone, poor, and vulnerable to institutionalization, when, for example, they break an osteoporotic hip in a preventable fall.

The needs of women of all ages are not being adequately met. It is clear that many women lack food and shelter, and sanitary, unpolluted living and working conditions. Personal safety is a major issue for all women. Many women are stressed to exhaustion by their multiple roles, and have no time for exercise, rest, and attention to their lifestyle needs. Approaches to prevention, cure, and rehabilitation are not designed specifically for the needs of women, and nonmedical personal support services are inadequate or lacking.

These health care deficiencies are the outgrowth of a fundamental problem—the pervasiveness of discrimination against women at every level. In order to investigate the health needs of women, evaluate the care that they currently receive, and work to improve access and quality, one must first understand the normative standards established for women in society, and the ways that women's experiences have been perceived, catalogued, and analyzed.

References

Aaron, H. (1991). *Serious and unstable condition: Financing America's health care.* Washington, DC: The Brookings Institute.

Abromovitz, M. (1992). *Regulating the lives of women: Social welfare policy from colonial times to the present.* Boston: South End Books.

Agan, R. D. (1987). Intuitive knowing as a dimension of nursing. *Advances in Nursing Science, 10,* 63–70.

Amaro, H. (1993). Testimony on women's health research. In *Senate committee: Labor and human research.* Unpublished manuscript.

American Medical Association. (1992). Physicians and domestic violence. *Journal of the American Medical Association (JAMA), 267,* 3190–3193.

Amott, T., & Matthaei, J. (1991). *Race, gender and work: A multicultural economic history of women in the United States.* Boston: South End Press.

Anati, E. (1963). *Palestine Before the Hebrews.* London: Jonathan Cape.

Angell, M. (1993). Caring for women's health—what is the problem? *New England Journal of Medicine, 329,* 271–272.

Ashley, J. (1976). *Hospitals, paternalism and the role of the nurse.* New York: Teachers' College Press.

Barker-Benfield, J. (1976). *The horrors of the half-known life: Male attitudes toward women and sexuality in nineteenth century America.* New York: Harper & Row.

Bassuk, E. (1992). Women and children without shelter: The characteristics of homeless families. In M. Robertson & M. Greenblatt, (Eds.). *Homelessness: A national perspective.* New York: Plenum Press.

Bem, S. L. (1993). *The lenses of gender.* New Haven: Yale University Press.

Bernstein, B., & Kane R. (1981). Physicians' attitudes toward female patients. *Medical Care, 19,* 600–608.

Binder, L. (1992). Entitlement and ethical developments in emergency medicine. *Academic Emergency Medicine, 4,* 8–10.

Blackwell, R. E., Carr, B. R., Chang, R. J., DeCherney, A. H., Haney, A. F., Keye, W. R., Rebar, R. W., Rock, J. A., Rosenwaks, Z., Seibel, M. M., & Soules, M. R. (1987). Are we exploiting the infertile couple? *Fertility and Sterility, 48,* 735–739.

Boston Women's Health Collective. (1992). Our bodies, ourselves. New York: Simon and Schuster.

Brown, L., & Gilligan, C. (1992). *Meeting at the crossroads: Women's psychology and girls' development.* Cambridge, MA: Harvard University Press.

Brown, M. (1992). Economic considerations in breast cancer screening for older women. *Journal of Gerontology, 47,* 51–58.

Centers for Disease Control and Prevention. (1990a). Black and white difference in cervical cancer mortality, U.S. 1980–87. *Morbidity and Mortality Weekly Report, 39,* 245–248.

Centers for Disease Control and Prevention. (1990b). Ectopic pregnancy surveillance. *Morbidity and Mortality Weekly Report, 39,* 9–17.

Chesler, P. (1989). *Women and madness.* San Diego: Harcourt Brace Jovanovich.

Cohen, S., Schwartz, J. E., Bromet, E. J., & Parkinson, B. M. (1991). Mental health stress and poor health behaviors in two community samples. *Preventive Medicine, 20,* 306–315.

Colliere, M. F. (1986). Invisible care and invisible women as health care providers. *International Journal of Nursing Studies, 23,* 95–112.

Corea, G. (1992). *The invisible epidemic: The story of women and AIDS.* New York: HarperCollins.

Daly, M. (1978). *Gyn/Ecology: The Metaethics of Radical Feminism.* Boston: Beacon Press.

Ehrenreich, B., & English, D. (1973). *Witches, midwives and nurses: A history of women healers.* Old Westbury, NY: Feminist Press.

Eisler, R. (1988). *The chalice and the blade.* San Francisco: Harper.

Ethics Committee, Society for Academic Emergency Medicine. (1992). An ethical foundation for health care: An emergency medicine perspective. *Annals of Emergency Medicine, 21*, 1381–1387.

French, M. (1992). *The war against women.* New York: Summit Books.

Freund, P. E. S., & McGuire, M. B. (1991). *Health, illness and the social body: A critical sociology.* Englewood Cliffs, NJ: Prentice Hall.

Frymer-Kensky, T. (1992). *In the wake of the goddesses: Women, culture and the biblical transformation of pagan myth.* New York: Fawcett Columbine.

General Accounting Office. (1993). *Screening mammography: Higher medicare payments could increase costs without increasing use* (GAO/HRD-93-50). Washington, DC: Author.

Gilligan, C. (1982). *In a different voice.* Cambridge, MA: Harvard University Press.

Gilligan, C., Lyons, N., & Hanmer, T. (1990). *Making connections: The relational worlds of adolescent girls at the Emma Willard School.* Cambridge, MA: Harvard University Press.

Goldenberg, N. (1979). *Changing of the gods.* Boston: Beacon Press.

Gomes, C., Given, B., & Given C. (1992). Caregivers of elderly relatives: Spouses and adult children. *Health & Social Work, 17*, 282–289.

Googins, B., & Burden, D. (1987). Vulnerability of working parents: Balancing work and home roles. *Social Work, 20*, 295–300.

Grahn, J. (1993). *Blood, bread and roses: How menstruation created the world.* Boston: Beacon Press.

Greer, G. (1971). *The female eunuch.* New York: McGraw-Hill.

Hale, C. B. (1992). A demographic profile of African Americans. In R. L. Braithwaite & E. Taylor (Eds.), *Health issues in the black community.* San Francisco: Jossey Bass.

Hansen, K., & Philipson, I. (Eds.). (1990). *Women, class and the feminist imagination: A socialist-feminist reader.* Philadelphia: Temple University Press.

Lack, D. Z. (1982). Women and pain: Another feminist issue. *Women & Therapy, 1*, 55–64.

LaRosa, J. H., & Pinn, V. W. (1993). Gender bias in biomedical research. *Journal of the American Medical Women's Association, 48*, 145–151.

Levy, K. (1992). *The politics of women's health care.* Las Colinas, TX: Ide House.

Lorber, J. (1994). *Paradoxes of gender.* New Haven: Yale University Press.

Love, S., & Linsey, K. (1990). *The breast book.* New York: Addison-Wesley.

Martin, E. (1987). *The woman in the body: A cultural analysis of repro duction.* Boston: Beacon Press.

Matteo, S. (1993). *American women in the '90's: Today's critical issues* Boston: Northeastern University Press.

McBarnette, L. (1988). *Women and poverty: The effects on reproduc tive status.* London: Haworth Press.

McBride, A. B. (1987). Developing a women's mental health agenda *Image, 19,* 4–8.

McBride, A. B. (1988). Mental health effects of women's multiple roles. *Image, 20,* 41–48.

McCray, E. (1986). The cooperative needlestick surveillance group Occupational risk of the acquired immunodeficiency syndrome among health care workers. *New England Journal of Medicine 314,* 1127–32.

McDowell, K. (Ed.). (1991). *Adverse effects: Women and the pharma ceutical industry.* Toronto: Women's Press.

Miller, J. B. (1986). *Toward a new psychology of women.* Boston: Beacon Press.

Mushlin, A., & Fintor, L. (1992). Is screening for breast cancer cos effective? *Cancer, 69,* 1957–1962.

National Leadership Commission on Health Care, U.S. (1989). *For the health of the nation: A shared responsibility.* Ann Arbor: Health Administration Press.

Ovrebo, B., Ryan, M., Jackson, K., & Hutchinson, K. (1994). The homeless prenatal program: A model for empowering pregnan women. *Health Education Quarterly, 21,* 187–198.

Reverby, S. (1987). *Ordered to care: The dilemma of American nurs ing 1850–1945.* New York: Cambridge University Press.

Rich, A. (1976). *Of woman born: Motherhood as experience and insti tution.* New York: Norton.

Rodrique, J. M. (1990). Black women and the birth-control move ment. In E. C. Dubois and V. L. Ruiz (Eds.), *Unequal sisters.* New York: Routledge.

Rosenberg, R. (1992). *Divided lives: American women in the 20th cen tury.* New York: Hill & Wang.

Schieber, G. J., Poullier, J. P., & Greenwald, L. M. (1991). Health care systems in twenty-four countries. *Health Affairs, 10,* 22–28.

Scutt, J. A. (1990). *The baby machine: Reproductive technology and the commercialization of motherhood.* London: Merlin Press.

Stone, M. (1976). *When god was a woman.* New York: Harcourt Brace Jovanovich.

Volberding, P., & Jacobsen, N. (1992). *AIDS clinical review.* New York: Marcel Decker.

Wenger, N. K. (1990). Gender, coronary artery disease and coronary surgery. *Annals of Internal Medicine, 112,* 557–558.

World Health Organization. (1946). Preamble to the constitution of WHO. New York: Office of Records, WHO.

Young, R. F., & Kahana, E. (1989). Specifying caregiver outcomes: Gender and relationship aspects of caregiving strain. *The Gerontologist, 29,* 660–666.

2

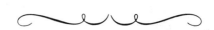

The Traditional Model of Women's Growth and Development

A Deficiency Theory

Judith Bernstein
Judith A. Lewis

A woman is not a pear tree
thrusting her fruit in mindless fecundity
into the world. . . .
    Marge Piercy, "Right to Life"

Judeo-Christian and Islamic societies are founded on a woman's creation myth that has had profound implications for the status of women in society, the conceptualization of normative standards for women, and modern approaches to their health care. Eve was born of Adam's rib, a part, not the whole, and a nonvital organ at that, unconnected to heart or brain. She was not only a part—partial, incomplete, tangential, and dependent. She was also dangerous, because her moral inadequacies led her to fall under the sway of the serpent, causing humankind to be expelled from the Garden of Eden and to be denied access to the tree of knowledge. These two aspects of the female persona, incompleteness and threat, are the basis of the psychology of women as it has been defined by traditional psychosocial and psychoanalytic theory.

Freud, the father of psychoanalysis and the progenitor of the deficiency theory of women's development, lived in a time of intense debate about the future of women in society. His lifetime spanned two eras in the women's rights struggle: the period of "domesticating the state"—winning suffrage, limiting the work day, and establishing the minimum wage and restricting child labor—and the era of "claiming the rights of men"—contraception, work after marriage, and access to higher education (Rosenberg, 1992).

Freud was certainly revolutionary in delineating the power of libido, describing the process of male identity development, and introducing the concept of a struggle between ego, the logical self and the controlling force for civilization, and id, the primitive core impulses. His theories about women, however, were unfortunately not based on science. Even knowledge of female anatomy was woefully inadequate in Freud's time. Prior to 1800 women were depicted anatomically as internalized males (Martin, 1987), and as late as 1890 it was asserted that higher education would mysteriously deprive women of reproductive capacity (French, 1992).

Freud was also handicapped by the lack of modern research methods—the use of controls and systematic sampling. Without these tools, he was left to make sense of his experience as a therapist for women in a very personal way, through interpretation of the tiny handful of clinical cases available to him: women of the nineteenth century Viennese upper class who presented for treatment of psychiatric symptoms. Although his observations were interesting and perhaps valid for those particular patients, they were tightly bound to his time, culture, and world outlook, and were not an accurate description of the process of development of female identity. Instead, the new discipline of psychoanalysis and the psychotherapy that followed became a powerful social force for conservatism and maintenance of the status quo, for intellectual justification of the oppression of women, and for the continuation of inequality in society. Three theories, in particular, proved especially inaccurate and damaging when applied to women, and because of their profound effect deserve exploration—the concepts of sex as destiny, autonomy as adulthood, and woman as threat.

Sex as Destiny

According to the tenets of psychoanalysis, young girls make an early, shocking discovery that they lack male genital organs and are therefore incomplete, inadequate, damaged, scarred (Freud, 1905a). This is the concept of penis envy, which is thought to be central to identity formation for young women. According to Freud, the main task of puberty is assimilating and accepting genital mutilation. In order to make a correct adaptation to an adult female persona, women must accept the passive role of being entered, i.e., must switch to vaginal orgasm as the major source of sexual stimulation, and give up their active source of sexual pleasure, clitoral stimulation, which is labelled infantile (Freud, 1905b; Hall, 1964; Chafetz, 1978). Men, because they had external sexual organs, were permitted to be the active principal, while women, with internal organs only, were required to act out the passive role in sexuality and in life.

Psychoanalysts who followed in this tradition insisted that women internalize the discrimination they faced in order to be normal. As late as the 1950s, Helene Deutsch, one of Freud's most articulate followers, diagnosed as mentally ill any woman who was unwilling to receive all of her fulfillment in life through others, who did not desire marriage or children, and who would not accept masochism as the dominant female principle and make peace with her subservient position in society (Deutsch, 1945). Anger expressed by women at their lot in life was further evidence of resistance to a feminine identity; if it persisted, they could be institutionalized, and were (Chesler, 1989). Because rational thought (masculine) was acceptable, and emotional distress (feminine) was not, women could also be committed for hysteria, or in more recent times subjected to shock therapy with no prior diagnosis or other form of treatment. Vapors, fainting spells, and hypochondria, however, have come down to us from Freud's time as suitably female (passive) and therefore acceptable, albeit untreatable.

Such theories of sex as destiny have now been exposed as having no basis in either female physiology or the experiences of women. The reality such ideas were actually based on was nothing other than the necessity for women in the late 19th and early 20th centuries to accommodate themselves to marriage relationships in which they had no power to control their decisions, their finances, or their lives, and little hope of meeting their sexual or other needs.

Autonomy as Adulthood

Another, equally important area of female inadequacy was women's lack of individuation, or drive for autonomy. The concept of the adult as an autonomous self, abstract, bounded, separate, self-sustaining, molecular and de-contextualized, may have been developed by Freud, but actually has its origins in concepts fundamental to Western philosophy: Newtonian physics; Calvinist principles of justice and the work ethic; the sanctity of the individual, his rights and entitlements as reflected in law; and the support for the competitive spirit and territorial acquisition provided by social Darwinism (Miller, 1986). Young boys, according to this perspective, are forced by Oedipal conflict to separate from their mothers, and this first early separation provides a model for autonomous action throughout life. Young girls, who do not undergo this process of separation, are inferior (Robbins & Siegel, 1985). Adler, one of the pioneers of modern psychiatry, recognized that there is a constant striving on the part of men to dominate women, and a resistance to domination on the part of women; such tension causes both sexes much emotional pain (Adler, 1957).

But the human condition "is to grow and live in groups" (Miller, Jordan, Kaplan, Stiver, & Surrey, 1991), and women have been assigned by society as carriers of enormous social responsibilities that require affiliation, not separation: emotional contact, empathy, maintaining marriage relationships, and childrearing. This creates a double bind; if a woman accepts her feminine designation and fulfills her accepted role, she often experiences poor self-esteem, because the work of women is devalued. She may appear in the psychologist's office for treatment of anxiety and depression. Yet the woman who opts for a male identified role may also experience distress as a result of distancing herself from emotions in order to become acceptable, and the experience of internal conflict between gender personae.

Freud assessed the world as a man of the upper class in a society that accorded him dominance. As Jean Jordan has described (1990), the message of a dominant group to an inferior group is "Your reality is inferior; it has no validity." And so the reality of women's lives and experiences was suppressed, and replaced by elaborate theories that had a basis in the experience and knowledge of men. Women have had great difficulty, until recently, speaking their truth.

Freud's successors have continued the tradition of judging women's lives and needs by the experience of men. Eric Erikson, author of an elaborate schema that portrays developmental tasks and goals for all ages of life, considered only his interviews with men in devising his categories. Chesler (1989) quotes a 1965 *Dedalus* essay in which Erikson states his beliefs about women's identities. "Young women," he says, "often ask if they can have an identity before they know whom they will marry and for whom they will make a home" (as quoted in Chesler, 1989, p. 76). The answer may not be so obvious to us, but to Erikson it was quite clear—women are somehow incomplete and unfinished until they marry, when it is the task of the mate to provide them with an adult identity. Chesler also exposes Bettleheim, another disciple of Freud, who shares this world view: "As much as women want to be good scientists and engineers, they want first and foremost to be womanly companions of men and mothers" (as quoted in Chesler, 1989, p. 79). This is woman's destiny as decided independently by male or male dominated theorists of psychology and psychiatry.

In the 1970s a survey was undertaken in California to ascertain the opinions of practicing clinical psychologists about what constituted a healthy adult woman (Broverman, Vogel, Broverman, Clarkson, & Rosenkrantz, 1972). A mature, healthy, socially competent male was judged from a list of possible traits to be aggressive, independent, objective, not easily influenced, active, logical, worldly, adventurous, self-confident and able to separate ideas from feelings. A healthy woman, on the other hand, was described by a list of traits similar to those ascribed to children: easily influenced, submissive, passive, illogical, sneaky, dependent, and unable to separate ideas from feelings (Braverman et al., 1972, p. 63).

Research psychologists have not fared better than their clinical colleagues. Kohlberg's (1981) widely used levels of moral development, for example, were based only on interviews with men. On this scale, which values abstract, logical justice over interpersonal responsibility and connection, women rarely develop to an "adult" level of moral reasoning (Miller, 1986). In models of intellectual development, human experience is similarly defined by men's experience. Perry (1968), in his landmark study of Harvard University students, discarded the few interviews with women and used only the data from men. It is not surprising, therefore, that these scales, too, ignore or invalidate women's ways of knowing, and leave women at a supposed lower level of development (Belenky, Clinchy, Goldberger, & Tarule, 1986). The negative effects of the pressure to conform to male norms on the self-esteem of young girls have been clearly chronicled in recent work by Gilligan and others (Brown & Gilligan, 1992; Gilligan, Lyons, & Hanmer, 1990).

Traits that are highly prized in women, such as intuitiveness, gentleness, tenderness, and the ability to be loving and caring, are devalued when they are applied to men (Gilligan, 1982). Even the object relations school of psychoanalysis, which has sought to reconcile with Freud's obvious inaccuracies, sees altruism, empathy, and the search for relationship as a diminution of the individual self (Jordan, Surrey, & Kaplan, 1983). But men, too, need affiliation and emotional congruity and integrity for a complete and satisfying life (Jordan, 1987; Jordan, 1990). The views of women on which the mental health disciplines are founded have done damage to the emotional health of both women and men. Because these discriminatory standards have provided the basis for defining development, health needs, and treatment methods, they have done enormous damage to the physical health of women as well.

If subjugation of those qualities assigned to women means that men suffer loss as a consequence, why has such a system of inequality persisted? Granted, those who have immediate power are often loath to let it go, but human history is full of examples of progress against the odds. What has given patriarchical social organization so much authority to repress, devalue, and silence women? Why have women's experiences and health needs been so dramatically ignored? The answer lies in a third precept inherited from early psychoanalysis, woman as threat (potential castrator).

Woman as Threat

There are five main ways that women have been perceived as elementally dangerous to men and to society, and they all have implications for the health of modern women.

First is the power of female sexuality. Patrilineal society is ruled by dualism, with reason, justice, and logic representing the forces of good. Arrayed against these forces of civilization is the pagan feminine power of sexual impulse and emotional drive, to be resisted at any cost (Eisler, 1988). Oedipus suffered at the hands of woman. Eve got involved with a snake, Freud's metaphor for phallus, and Adam lost his birthright of knowledge as a result. Witches were thought to derive their power from their sexuality (Ehrenreich & English, 1979). Women in Moslem cultures are so dangerous they must be swathed from head to toe. Mary, the only woman of significance in the Christian tradition, could be respected only as mother, not as woman, and even then only as a perennial virgin, nonsexual and therefore quasi-adult. In the modern state of Israel, Orthodox religious doctrine decrees that honorable women remain indoors, and disobedient wives may be divorced against their will and deprived of all rights, including property and child custody (French, 1992). Women must sit separately from men in temple lest the mere sight of them tempt men away from God. Yet in truth it is the sexuality of men that is dangerous to women, if there be danger. It is patrilineal society that has permitted rituals of defloration that involve taking and breaking, from the medieval *droit de seigneur*, the right of the first night, to today's gang rapes and ritual sexual scorecards. Among a college population, 22 percent of the males admitted to having had sex with unwilling partners, and more than a third of women today have been victims of incest or other sexual abuse (Jordan, 1987). If the victim is perceived as threatening, there is rationalization for victimization.

Second, women are dangerous because they have the power of mystery. In earliest prehistory, it was women who were attendants of the goddesses and privy to religious ritual. There was a place in the pantheon for female as well as male principles of godhood (Frymer-Kensky, 1992). And of course things happen in female bodies that are beyond the experience of men, the mysteries of natural cycling, of reproduction, of giving food of their own bodies to nourish children. In the Sumerian myth of Enki, the male god principle tries to form a creature on his own and fails, and has to admit his defeat to Nihmah, his female counterpart.

Women are also threatening because they are emotional, and less enculturated to maintain control at any cost. The Sumerian Erdu lament and the Greek chorus of mourners exemplify the power of an emotional woman. The word *hysterical* is actually derived from the Greek for wandering uterus. Women are "the other," and the unknown is always terrifying. To deal with this fear, man remade the other in his own image. Goddess attributes were subsumed, and male experience superimposed on women's lives.

Third, women are the vehicle of generational continuity in society, the empty vessels that store the future. Once inheritance became patrilineal, men needed to control the behaviors of women in order to assure their genetic patrimony. The chastity belts of the middle ages may have come off, but the reproductive choice currently available to women is perceived as a major threat, as we see from the involvement of the state in issues of abortion, contraception, reproductive treatment options, and research. Rigid control of women's behavior during pregnancy and even her body positions during labor and delivery reflect both the fear of these feminine functions and the value of women's bodies as property for progeneration (Martin, 1987). Even menopause, as Martin goes on to describe, has been clouded by this view of women as property. Menopause, which is not an illness but a normal evolution of the life cycle, is described as deficit (property losing worth): ovaries *wither*, become *unresponsive*, and *fail*, and the endocrine system is now *unbalanced*. Clearly a female body that is no longer able to produce heirs has lost a major part of its value.

Fourth, in the modern world women are an economic asset. If a woman works at home, she provides services in home management and child care that a man could not afford to replace. If she works outside the home, and her income is essential to family survival, she is still providing the vast majority of those unpaid services. Women represent an economic threat if they are not under male control, because they might leave and take their work power with them. If they are on their own, as head of household, and they threaten to withdraw the services of nurture, society could not begin to pick up the tab for child care or elder care.

Fifth, women are a threat because they are unclean. This is the aspect of threat that has most pervaded modern medicine. In patriarchal society, blood spilled in war and violence is somehow acceptable, but blood spilled by women in the natural processes of menstruation and childbirth is taboo. From the earliest of physicians to modern psychology, women's natural body functions have been redefined as illness and injury. Galen, for example, described menstruation as a bloodletting, a plethora (Crawford, 1981), and the psychoanalyst Havelock Ellis saw it as women being "periodically wounded . . . in even the healthiest of women, a worm gnaws periodically at the root of life" (Ellis, 1904, p. 284). This is of course the rationale behind ritual immersion bath required monthly after menses for women in Orthodox Judaism (the *mikvah*). The phrase most commonly used even today to describe menstruation, the curse, reflects the strength of the stigma associated with bleeding. Only in the last decade has it become possible to advertise feminine hygiene products explicitly in magazines or on television. Young girls still go through agonies to obtain a gym excuse or be excused from class to go to the bathroom when bleeding. Women have been entrusted with cleaning up all of society, from cleaning babies' bottoms to nursing to domestic labor outside the home; the taboo against uncleanliness extends from women's bodies to their functions in society. Gloria Steinem has written a very amusing essay entitled, "If Men Could Menstruate" (Steinem, 1992) in which she asserts that if men could menstruate, then menstruation would become an enviable, boastworthy masculine event to be celebrated with ritual, and "Congress would immediately fund a National Institute of Dysmenorrhea to help stamp out monthly discomforts (p. 308)." Medicalization of natural function is the way modern society gets around the taboo. This may have made the problem manageable for the male half of mankind, but it has created a system of medical care that does not meet women's needs, and acts most often to silence women's thinking and violate women's feelings and self-respect. Washburn (1977) suggests an interesting hypothesis, that myths and rites arise at moments of psychological danger. If this is so, society has codified some very destructive solutions to the crises represented by those feared aspects of women: denial of female sexuality, denial of female identity, forced persistence of childhood, and somatization of conflict into reproductive illnesses.

The second half of the 20th century has seen both a revolution against male dominance and a backlash against women for refusing to be docile. In *The War Against Women*, Marilyn French (1992) describes an institutional war against women, fought on medical, economic, and legal grounds, and a cultural war against women, fought in the realms of art and literature, advertising media, and the entertainment world. Susan Falludi (1991) in *Backlash: the Undeclared War against American Women* offers extensive corroboration. But it is a poem by Marge Piercy (1982) that shows us best what must be kept in mind in any journey through the landscape of women's health care:

> A woman is not a basket you place
> your buns in to keep them warm. Not a brood
> hen you can slip duck eggs under.
> Not a purse holding the coins of your
> descendants until you spend them in wars.
> Not a bank where your genes gather interest
> and interesting mutations in the tainted
> rain, any more than you are . . .
>
> We are all born of woman, in the rose
> of the womb we suckled our mother's blood
> and every baby born has a right to love
> like a seedling to sun. Every baby born

unloved, unwanted is a bill that will come
due in twenty years with interest, an anger
that must find a target, a pain that will
beget pain . . .

You may not use me as your factory.
Priests and legislators do not hold
shares in my womb or my mind.
This is my body. If I give it to you
I want it back. My life
is a non-negotiable demand.

Right to life,
Circles on the Water,
pp. 263–265
Used with permission.

References

Adler, A. (1957). *Understanding human nature.* New York: Fawcett Publications.

Belenky, M. F., Clinchy, B. M., Goldberger, N. R., & Tarule, J. M. (1986). *Women's ways of knowing.* New York: HarperCollins.

Broverman, I., Broverman, D., Clarkson, F. (1970). Sex role stereotypes: A current appraisal. *Journal of Social Issues, 28,* 59–78.

Brown, L., & Gilligan, C. (1992). *Meeting at the crossroads: Women's psychology and girls' development.* Cambridge, MA: Harvard University Press.

Chafetz, J. (1978). *Masculine, feminine or human?* New York: Peacock Books.

Chesler, P. (1989). *Women and madness.* San Diego: Harcourt Brace Jovanovich.

Crawford, P. (1981). Attitudes to menstruation in 17th century England. *Past and Present, 91,* 47–73.

Deutsch, H. (1945). *The psychology of women.* New York: Grune & Stratton.

Ehrenreich, B., & English, D. (1979). *For her own good.* New York: Doubleday Anchor.

Eisler, R. (1988). *The chalice and the blade.* San Francisco: Harper.

Ellis, H. (1904). *Man and woman.* London: Walter Scott.

Faludi, S. (1991). *Backlash: The undeclared war against American women.* New York: Dial/Doubleday.

French, M. (1992). *The war against women.* New York: Summit Books.

Freud, S. (1905a). Three essays on the theory of sexuality. In J. Strachey (Ed. and Trans.) *The standard edition of the complete psychological works of Sigmund Freud.* London: Hogarth Press.

Freud, S. (1905b). *Three contributions to the theory of sex* (A. A. Brill, Trans.). New York: Dutton.

Frymer-Kensky, T. (1992). *In the wake of the goddesses: Women, culture and the biblical transformation of pagan myth.* New York: Fawcett Columbine.

Gilligan, C. (1982). *In a different voice.* Cambridge, MA: Harvard University Press.

Gilligan, C., Lyons, N., & Hanmer, T. (1990). *Making connections: The relational worlds of adolescent girls at Emma Willard School.* Cambridge, MA: Harvard University Press.

Hall, C. (1964). *A primer of Freudian psychology.* New York: Mentor Books.

Jordan, J. V., Surrey, J. L., & Kaplan, A. G. (1983). Women and empathy. *Work in Progress: The Stone Center, 2,* 1–16.

Jordan, J. V. (1987). Clarity in connection: Empathetic knowing, desire and sexuality. *Work in Progress: The Stone Center, 20,* 1–13.

Jordan, J. V. (1990). Courage in connection: Conflict, compassion, creativity. *Work in Progress: The Stone Center, 45,* 1–12.

Kohlberg, L. (1981). *The philosophy of moral development.* San Francisco: Harper & Row.

Martin, E. (1987). *The woman in the body: A cultural analysis of reproduction.* Boston: Beacon Press.

Miller, J. B. (1986). *Toward a new psychology of women* (2nd ed.). Boston: Beacon Press.

Miller, J. B., Jordan, J. V., Kaplan, A. G., Stiver P., & Surrey, J. L. (1991). Some misconceptions and reconceptions of a relational approach. *Work in Progress: The Stone Center, 49,* 3–16.

Perry, W. (1968). *Forms of intellectual and ethical development in the college years.* New York: Holt, Rinehart and Winston.

Piercy, M. (1985). Right to life, pp. 263–265. *Circles on the water.* New York: Alfred Knopf.

Robbins, J. H., & Siegel, R. J. (Eds.). (1985). *Women changing therapy: New assessments, values and strategies in feminist therapy.* New York: Harrington Park Press.

Rosenberg, R. (1992). *Divided lives: American women in the 20th century.* New York: Hill & Wang.

Steinem, G. (1992). If men could menstruate—. In M. L. Anderson & P. H. Collins (Eds.), *Race, class and gender* (pp. 308–310). Belmont, CA: Wadsworth.

Washburn, P. (1977). *Becoming woman: The quest for wholeness.* New York: Harper.

3

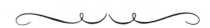

Relational Psychology

A Reframing of the Strengths of Women

Judith Bernstein
Judith A. Lewis

Some women wait for themselves
around the next corner
and call the empty spot peace
but the opposite of living
is only not living
and the stars do not care.

Some women wait for something
to change and nothing
does change
so they change
themselves.

Audre Lorde, *"Stations"*
(1986)
Our Dead Behind Us, *pp. 14–15*
Used with permission.

The original thinkers who founded the mental health disciplines changed the world fundamentally. They showed us that human behavior is motivated by natural laws that can be analyzed and understood; once these laws are grasped, techniques can be developed to change human motivation and action. But as we have seen, women have waited and waited for their experience to be examined, and their ways of relating, knowing, communicating to be understood. They have waited a very long time, hoping that what gives meaning to their lives will be valued. But as Audre Lorde says, waiting is not living, and women have generally had to change themselves to adapt to the expectations of a male-dominated society. They have watched, discouraged and angry, as psychiatrists and psychologists kept snipping away at traditional precepts, trying to make a fit, and failing.

Now the waiting is over. New paradigms have been developed, fueled by the feminist upsurgence of the 1970s and the resulting body of scholarship in women's studies. New approaches in physics contributed background support in suggesting that the natural world is less static and logical than previously understood, and in imparting new value to concepts women use to describe events and feelings: flow, waves, connection, relativity, and multiplicity. Psychologists, sociologists, and educators, some working in collective groups and others independently, have used in-depth interviews, a phenomenologic approach, to study women's lives, identities, relationships, knowledge, morality, and communication. From this research has emerged a fledgling theory of relational or self-in-relation psychology.

In *Toward a New Psychology of Women*, Jean Miller (1986) set the stage, describing the adaptations women have made to subordinate status. She outlined a new direction for healthy conflict, the reclaiming of women's characteristics as strengths. Skills in making and maintaining relationships, nurturing, peacemaking, and honesty about vulnerability and weakness were reframed as characteristics beneficial to both individuals and society. "Humanity's highest necessity," she said, "is intense, emotionally connected cooperation and creativity . . . for human life and growth" (p. 25). Objectives for health included physical, sexual, and emotional frankness; creativity and self-nurture as well as nurture for others; an end to objectification, the treatment of women as things; private and public equality; authenticity; and reclamation of conflict.

This agenda provided a basis for rethinking all aspects of women's functioning. The problem was not that women did not develop correctly to fit existing models of human growth, but that traditional models had failed to describe or permit gender differences. In *In A Different Voice*, Carol Gilligan (1982) examined the process of moral choice in women, and discovered that the standards women use are different from the principles of abstract, universal justice applied by males. The women Gilligan studied used a different set of constructs, a language of "selfishness" and "responsibility." High value was placed on an obligation to exercise care and avoid harm. Moral dilemmas were seen in terms of conflicting responsibilities. Progression toward solution appeared to begin with issues of concern for self-survival (conceptualized as "selfishness"), moved through a focus on goodness and avoiding harm, and finally arrived at decision through a process of reexamination and evaluation of relationships based on a reflective understanding of care. Resolution through negotiation was preferred, rather than confrontation, and conflict caused discomfort. The question was not what action is universally right, but who am I in the context of my own needs and the needs of others.

Female identity is thus formed, not by individuation, but within relationship contexts; identity and intimacy are not separate stages for women, as Erickson would have it, but interconnected. The highest level of masculine moral and intellectual reasoning, as traditionally defined, includes an ability to extend morality beyond considerations of fairness to concern with relationships. As men and women develop into full maturity, Gilligan asserts, their paths lead to greater convergence in judgment, but their developmental processes are very different.

A working group of psychologists and psychiatrists from the Stone Center at Wellesley College has put together a series of essays, *Women's Growth in Connection* (Jordan, Kaplan, Miller, Stivey, & Surrey, 1991), that provides a sharp contrast to traditional ideas based on self-development or individuation. Identity formation is described as an interactional process rooted in intimate attachment, from the earliest relationship with the primary caretaker to connections with peers, love relationships, and adult agency within community. Such interactions are made possible by empathy, which requires affective surrender and cognitive restructuring. Women's vulnerability, connectedness, emotionality, and ethic of nurture are the skills that permit empathy and the value system on which it is based. The differences described in play between young girls and boys (Lever, 1976; Lever, 1978), which have been used to describe boys' socialization for success and girls' for dependence, would be reinterpreted; the turn taking, informality, negotiation, and intimacy characteristic of girls' play are preparatory work for the affective attachments that will give meaning to their lives.

Women certainly achieve adult status, despite the infamous consensus of California psychologists (Broverman, Broverman, & Clarkson, 1970), but not as a fixed place in a logical hierarchy. Adulthood is rather a continued process of relationship differentiation, a mutual adaptation to the growth and development of each person in the relationship. The goal of such connections is mutual empowerment rather than dominance or power-over. Empathy in community translates to a group action model that utilizes negotiation. Recognizing and meeting one's own needs are conceptualized as self-empathy, a formulation which gives permission to women to care for themselves as well as others.

Psychologic dysfunction or psychiatric illness is seen as a failure of connection, with neurotic behaviors of narcissism, codependence, and masochism framed as failures in mutuality. Transference is seen as a relational phenomena, an empathetic environment conducive to the work of therapy. The goals of marriage counseling would be facilitation of mutuality, support for courage in connection, safety for expression and transformation of anger, and encouragement of "good" conflict characterized by authenticity, exploration of differences, and reintegration of interests based on expansive growth of both parties. Application of self-in-relation and other feminist theory to the dynamics of psychotherapy is described in Robbins and Siegel's (1985) anthology, *Women Changing Therapy*.

As this new discipline evolves, there will be many new discoveries and exciting spinoffs. Hancock (1989), for example, builds on Gilligan's studies of young women (Gilligan, Lyon, & Hanmer, 1990; Brown & Gilligan, 1992). In *The Girl Within* she discusses an elaboration of the nonlinear theory of female growth, the idea that most women remember a time of self-efficacy and power and centeredness in their lives, before the adaptations to a male-dominated society that occur during adolescence, and that this young girl can be returned to as a source of strength for the adult woman. Similarly, self-in-relation theories derived from examination of women's experience are currently being evaluated for their benefit to men for whom they might provide alternate explanations for boy-mother conflict, and the deficiencies common to most boy-father interactions. Relational theory has been used in marital counseling, to help men gain the intimate connections they desire but have been socialized to reject (Bergman, 1991). Research conducted at the Stone Center on issues specific to minority women, as seen through a relational approach, includes, for example, cultural diversity (Coll, 1992), Black single-parent families (Malson, 1986), psychological effects of discrimination (Turner, 1987), and Black women's career development (Turner, 1984).

Revaluing of female perspectives and a movement toward power-with rather than power-over have been suggested, on a larger scale, as essential to future peace, progress, and protection of the environment and the quality of human life (Eisler, 1988). The neolithic world described in Eisler's (1988) *The Chalice and the Blade* may have been kinder to women than our present form of social organization, but there is no ideal time to which we can return. We cannot simply go back to the future; new conditions and evolving human conscious-ness require new social forms. But we can and must take with us from the past the contributions of women that have proven valuable to society as a whole.

Such a perspective would not substitute the stereotyping of women by men with stereotyping of women and men by women. In *The Lenses of Gender*, Bem (1993) writes about androcentrism, or male centered-ness, and biological essentialism, or sex and destiny. But even more importantly, she writes about gender polarization as

> not just the historically crude perception that women and men are fundamentally different from one another but the more subtle and insidious use of that perceived difference as an organizing prin-ciple for the social life of the culture. . . . A cultural connection is thereby forged between sex and virtually every other aspect of human experience, including modes of dress and social roles and even ways of expressing emotion and experiencing sexual desire. (p. 2)

It will not do, she suggests, to simply flip the straightjacket of the sexual lens inside-out, and establish a new world where so-called women's perspective dominates. A comprehensive new paradigm for the health of women must recognize variety among men and women across all of society, and make room for the positive quality of diversity in gen-der attributes for any new norms that evolve.

A perspective of mutuality in relation would thus provide a frame-work for validating women's strengths as well as understanding men's struggles for growth and connection. In health it would provide sup-port for major social change: elimination of violence against women, addiction, hunger, homelessness, child abuse, and racial, ethnic, and gender discrimination. Women would make reproductive choices based on their own ethical constructs of responsibility and care, and be encouraged to use comfortable, woman-friendly coping mechanisms such as advocates to counter feelings of vulnerability and violation encountered in the health care system (Gilligan, 1982). The label of dependency that stigmatizes women and impairs quality of health and health care would thus be recast as a positive quality, interdependence. Passivity would be transformed into the positive quality of peacemak-ing, and emotionality would become empathy. Women would be assisted to learn self-empathy and meet their health and lifestyle needs.

Women would feel free to propose alternatives to traditional medical treatments that are more in keeping with their identities, their knowledge formats, and their ethical codes. They would be encouraged to grow, obtain education, and be supported to work as they wish without the stress that currently compromises many intimate affiliations. They would, in short, be healthy.

And society would understand that

A strong woman is a woman who craves love
like oxygen or she turns blue choking.
A strong woman is a woman who loves
strongly and weeps strongly and is strongly
terrified and has strong needs. A strong woman is strong
in words, in action, in connection, in feeling;
she is not strong as a stone but as a wolf
suckling her young. Strength is not in her, but she
enacts it as the wind fills a sail.

What comforts her is others loving
her equally for the strength and for the weakness
from which it issues, lightening from a cloud.
Lightening stuns. In rain, the clouds disperse.
Only water of connection remains,
flowing through us. Strong is what we make
each other. Until we are all strong together,
a strong woman is a woman strongly afraid.

Marge Piercy (1985), "For strong women"
Circles on the Water, pp. 257–258
Used with permission.

References

Bem, S. L. (1993). *The lenses of gender: Transforming the debate on sexual inequality*. New Haven: Yale University Press.

Bergman, S. J. (1991). Men's psychological development: A relational perspective. *Work in Progress: The Stone Center, 48*, 1–13.

Broverman, I. K., Broverman, D. M., Clarkson, F. E. (1970). Sex-role stereotypes and clinical judgements of mental health. *Journal of Consulting and Clinical Psychology, 34*, 1–7.

Brown, L., & Gilligan, C. (1992). *Meeting at the crossroads: Women's psychology and girls' development*. Cambridge, MA: Harvard University Press.

Coll, C. G. (1992). Cultural diversity: Implications for theory and practice. *Work in Progress: The Stone Center, 59*, 1–13.

Eisler, R. (1988). *The chalice and the blade*. San Francisco: Harper.

Gilligan, C. (1982). *In a different voice*. Cambridge, MA: Harvard University Press.

Gilligan, C., Lyons, N., & Hanmer, T. (1990). *Making connections: The relational worlds of adolescent girls at Emma Willard School*. Cambridge MA: Harvard University Press.

Hancock, E. (1989). *The girl within*. New York: Fawcett Columbine.

Jordan, J. V., Kaplan, A. G., Miller, J. B., Stiver, I. P., & Surrey, J. L. (1991). *Women's growth in connection*. New York: Guilford Press.

Lever, J. (1976). Sex differences in games children play. *Social Problems, 23*, 478–487.

Lever, J. (1978). Sex differences in the complexity of children's play and games. *American Social Review, 43*, 471–483.

Lorde, A. (1986). *Our dead behind us*. New York: Norton.

Malson, M. R. (1986). Understanding Black single parent families: Stresses and strengths. *Work in Progress: The Stone Center, 25*, 1–22.

Miller, J. B. (1986). *Toward a new psychology of women* (2nd ed.). Boston: Beacon Press.

Piercy, M. (1985). *Circles on the water*. New York: Alfred Knopf.

Robbins, J. H., & Siegel, R. J. (1985). *Women changing therapy*. New York: Harrington Park Press.

Turner, C. (1984). Psychosocial barriers to Black women's career development. *Work in Progress: The Stone Center, 15*, 1–13.

Turner, C. (1987). Clinical application of the Stone Center approach to minority women. *Work in Progress: The Stone Center, 28*, 1–17.

4

The Female Voice
Women's Ways of Knowing and Communicating

Judith Bernstein
Judith A. Lewis

> *Where language and naming are power*
> *silence is oppression, is violence.*
> *Adrienne Rich (1979)*

Belenky, Clinchy, Goldberger, and Tarule (1986) interviewed 135 women from college campuses and an "invisible college" consisting of parenting self-help programs. These interviews were rigorously analyzed and interpreted according to a very high standard of qualitative research methodology, and the results published in *Women's Ways of Knowing: The development of self, voice and mind.* Five categories of knowing were generated; not surprisingly, these are quite different from those that emerged from Perry's 1970 study of epistemological development among male Harvard University students.

The first of these categories of knowing is *silence,* the childlike condition of being seen but not heard. Women in general speak less than men, despite cultural stereotypes of talkative women (LaFrance & Mayo, 1979; Argyle, Salter, Nicholson, Williams, & Burgess, 1970), and only 1 in 12 writers today is female (Olsen, 1978). The silence described in this first category of knowing, however, is qualitatively different, a silence of repression and oppression and obliteration, as suggested by Rich (1979).

Men commonly rely on visual imagery to describe the process of knowing. They use metaphors like *enlightenment, blind justice,* and *veil of ignorance* that enable them to keep a distance from the object in perspective. In contrast, women talk about *speaking up, being silenced* or *not heard,* metaphors of voice for intellectual and ethical development, reflecting the need to get close to know. Language is a tool for representational thought, and women who accept silence accept obedience, passivity, and dependence along with it. They feel *deaf and dumb* and are unable to recognize their gifts of intelligence. They tend to be limited to present tense, concrete thinking, and specific situations, and find it very difficult to describe a self.

Women who fit the second category, *received knowledge,* do a lot of listening, and their language is studded with *should* and *ought.* They listen to friends and authorities, and their concept of self is based on external referents.

In the third category, *listening to the subjective inner voice,* women become their own authorities. Knowledge is based on intuition and personalized experience. This type of knowing is most consistent with stereotypes of feminine behavior, and occupies a low position in the male scale of epistemology. Women speaking a subjective or personal truth have little chance of being listened to in the public arena. Several routes for entry into subjectivism were described by informants: the failure of male authority, experience of violence against women, and loss of trust. Distrust extended for many to the world of science, which had rejected their way of looking at the world.

In the fourth category, *procedural knowledge,* women adopt the voice of reason. They speak in measured tones, and use conscious, deliberate, and systematic analysis. Form predominates over content, and all approaches based on logic are equally acceptable. Although the format of this perspective is similar to male rational thought, several elements are distinctively female: sharing small truths, refusing to judge, and willingness to collaborate in groups.

The last category, *constructed knowledge,* appears to combine the skills developed in procedural knowledge with truths devised from the inner voice. "We create the world at the same time as we talk about it," said one informant. Or, as the editors put it, "the knower is an intimate part of the knowing" (Belenky et al., 1986, p. 132). This is truth in context, with passion and no pretense of all things being equal. It is characterized by moral imperatives, commitment, and action to effect change. The commitment described is never to abstract ideas alone, but to ideas embedded in relationships and experiences acquired in them. The example these women set was a "refreshing blend of idealism and realism . . . an integration of care and feeling with work" (p. 152).

Each of these categories of knowing is established, validated, and maintained in adaptation to or reaction against cultural and political stereotypes about talk. In *Nonverbal Communication: The Unspoken Dialogue*, Burgoon, Buller, and Woodall (1989) have assembled extensive documentation of the extent to which gender assignment is specified and codified in communication. In *Language and Woman's Place*, Robin Lakoff (1989) reviews similar material in a very readable but less scholarly version. Gender differences clearly affect both delivery style (verbal and nonverbal expression) and speech content. These differences have been characterized as primary or genetic, secondary or physically related, and tertiary or learned (Birdwhistell, 1970), so they encompass both nature and nurture. The vast majority of gender distinctions, however, seems to be the result of acculturation; women are trained to be affiliative and reactive, and their speech reflects this training, while men are taught to be dominant and proactive, and demonstrate these characteristics in both verbal and nonverbal behavior (LaFrance & Mayo, 1976; Mulac, Studley, Weimann, & Bradac, 1987).

Men talk and women listen (Hilpert, Kramer, & Clark, 1975), and men interrupt more (Zimmerman & West, 1975; Kennedy, 1983). College men speak first in class, and do not require the permission to speak characteristic of women (Aries, 1987). Women begin sentences with disclaimers and hesitation words (*maybe, perhaps, well . . .*) and end them with tag questions (*isn't it?*) to soften their stance (Lakoff, 1973). There are gender-specific pitches and tones that indicate subordinate station, such as the high-low glide and the sentence with rising inflection that requests confirmation (Brend, 1975).

Gender differences appear in nonverbal communication as well, with women using more independent symbols (Ickes & Barnes, 1977) and illustrations (Baglan & Nelson, 1982), especially hands palm up, which denotes vulnerability and powerlessness (Friesen, Elkman, & Walbott, 1979). Both posture (Mehrabian, 1969) and facial expressions (Eakins & Eakins, 1978) express submissiveness, with women's frequent smiles denoting both embarrassment and inhibition of aggression (Mackey, 1976). The personal distance chosen by women expresses desire for affiliation, compared to the greater distance comfortable for males (Argyle et al., 1970).

Although these gender differences generally apply, individuals can override them; there are certainly submissive men and dominant

women whose signals are quite different from the patterns described
Similarly, both verbal and nonverbal behaviors may change according
to context, being more so in some settings and less so in others. In
addition, cultural signals vary considerably. Eye contact that might be
interpreted one way among Whites will mean something quite different among African Americans and something else entirely among African Blacks (Hall, 1981). Although gender differences in content vary
similarly according to individual, context, and culture, there are defi-
nite patterns that can be identified. Deborah Tannen (1990) summarizes these well in *You Just Don't Understand: Men and Women in
Conversation.*

Men see conversation, Tannen asserts, as a tool to achieve status,
exchange facts, solve problems, and bolster independence; their style
is asymmetrical, and prepared for contest and challenge. They wish to
be respected rather than liked. Women, in their desire for affiliation,
use conversation to achieve rapport and consensus. They share more
private information, and engage in "troubles talk," a sharing of daily
challenges that expects empathy, not solution. Their style is symmetri-
cal, and they prefer being liked to being respected. Men interrupt (competitive overlap), while women chime in and finish sentences
(cooperative overlap). A man may see the act of arguing as a form of
intimacy, while to a woman conflict might be an admission of failure.
These differences, in their extremes, are profound expressions of previously discussed differences in self-concept, identity formation, and
social expectations.

Feminist research methods have been devised in an effort to find,
value, and understand the silenced voice of women. Graham (1984)
cites semi-structured interviews as the principal means by which
researchers collaborate with respondents to create a shared sense of
the data (reality) of their lives. Interviewing appeals to feminists,
Shulamit Reinharz states in *Feminist Methods in Social Research*
(1992), because it permits access to people's thoughts, feelings, and
memories in their own words, an antidote to centuries of silencing
women or interpreting them through the words and works of men.
Ethnography permits documentation of the dailiest of activities,
analysis from the subjects' own perspective, and placement of individuals in familial, peer network, and social context. This relational
approach values the connectedness of women as well as their unique
personality. Oral histories are particularly important, because they
affirm the value of women's lives, and because they record the
person's own forms of expression, and can transcend differences of
class and race and culture between researcher and subject. Exhibits

that combine oral history with contextual photographs make history tangible (Reinharz, 1992).

In the medical domain, lack of response to all three components of women's voice—knowledge, verbal style, and verbal content—has a significant impact on the health of women and their access to care. The practice of medicine rarely elicits women's understanding of themselves and their own situation. Women in both patient and nurse roles are seldom given permission to speak or are seldom listened to if they speak in their own terms (Waitzkin, 1991). Nurses, who are primarily women, have had difficulty finding a voice in the medical environment (Fee, 1983; Ashley, 1976). Their own ways of knowing have been devalued, and they have been instructed, not just by the medical system but by nursing as well, to replace them with exclusively rational data gathering. Only recently have medical professionals begun to rely openly on intuition, sensing, and skilled pattern recognition, all examples of women's ways of knowing which have been used covertly since the inception of nursing (Agan, 1987; Correnti, 1990; Rew, 1988; Muff, 1990). Even gossip is being revalued as a legitimate form of women's communication, and its role in the development of professionalism among nurses is being investigated (Laing, 1993). Yet the doctor-nurse game, in which nurses offer recommendations while appearing passive and doctors accept recommendations if they can claim them as their own, still rules many hospitals, despite lip service given to team approaches (Stern, 1980). The importance of therapeutic touch and verbal stream to healing, commonly used nursing techniques, have yet to win acceptance among physicians despite supporting research (Freedman, 1972; Hall, Rotter, & Rand, 1981; Morrow, 1988).

The issues of verbal style and content, in the sense that they clearly reflect differences in who women are, what they want, how they connect, and how they survive in society, go to the heart of problems of discrimination in health care. A female patient expressing either submissive attitude or rage against oppression is on a collision course with a medical system that is patriarchal and intent on maintaining its power and control over patients and other health workers. Changes in the structure and content of the medical interview are mandatory before women can find their voice in health, either as patients or as health professionals.

Roter and Hall (1994) suggest seven communication transforming principles that would improve the quality of the health care encounter: (a) respect for the patient's story; (b) respect for the patient's expertise and insight; (c) respect for the emotional context of physical illness; (d) maximization of the usefulness of the physician's expertise; (e) acknowledgment of the emotional content of patient-physician communication; (f) mutual expectation of reciprocity and negotiation; and (g) facilitation of change by consciously avoiding stereotyped roles and expectations.

References

Agan, R. D. (1987). Intuitive knowing as a dimension of nursing. *Advances in Nursing Science*, *10*, 63–70.

Argyle, M., Salter, V., Nicholson, H., Williams, M., & Burgess, P. (1970). The communication of inferior and superior attitudes by verbal and non-verbal signals. *British Journal of Social and Clinical Psychology*, *9*, 221–231.

Aries, E. (1987). Gender and communication. In C. H. P. Shaver (Ed.), *Sex and gender*. Newbury Park, CA: Sage.

Ashley, J. (1976). *Hospitals, paternalism and the role of the nurse*. New York: Teachers' College Press.

Baglan, T., & Nelson, D. J. (1982). A comparison of the effects of sex and status on the perceived appropriateness of nonverbal behaviors. *Women's Studies in Communication*, *5*, 29–38.

Belenky, M. F., Clinchy, B. M., Goldberger, N. R., & Tarule, J. M. (1986). *Women's ways of knowing*. New York: HarperCollins.

Birdwhistell, R. (1970). *Kinesics and context: Essays in body motion communication*. Philadelphia: University of Philadelphia Press.

Brend, R. M. (1975). Male-female intonation patterns in American English. In B. Thorne & N. Henley (Eds.), *Language and sex: Difference and dominance*. Cambridge, MA: Newbury House.

Burgoon, J. K., Buller, D. B., & Woodall, W. G. (Eds.). (1989). *Nonverbal communication: The unspoken dialogue*. New York: Harper & Row.

Correnti, D. (1990). Intuition and nursing practice implications for nursing educators: A review of the literature. *Journal of Continuing Education in Nursing*, *23*, 91–94.

Eakins, B. W., & Eakins, R. G. (1978). *Sex differences in human communication*. Boston: Houghton Mifflin.

Fee, E. (Ed.). (1983). *Women and health: The politics of sex in medicine*. Farmingdale, New York: Baywood Publishing.

Freedman, N. (1972). The analysis of movement behavior during the clinical interview. In A. Siegman & B. Pope (Eds.), *Studies in dyadic communication*. New York: Pergammon.

Friesen, W. V., Elkman, P., & Walbott, H. (1979). Measuring hand movements. *Journal of Nonverbal Behavior*, *4*, 97–112.

Graham, H. (1984). Surveying through stories. In C. Bella & H. Roberts (Eds.). *Social researching: Politics, problems, practice*. London: Routledge & Kegan Paul.

Hall, J. A., Rotter, D. L., & Rand, C. S. (1981). Communication of affect between patient and physician. *Journal of Health and Social Behavior*, *22*, 18–30.

Hilpert, F. P., Kramer, C., & Clark, R. (1975). Participants' perceptions of self and partner in mixed sex dyads. *Central States Speech Journal*, *26*, 52–56.

Ickes, W., & Barnes, R. (1977). The role of sex in self-monitoring in unstructured dyadic interactions. *Journal of Personality and Social Psychology*, *35*, 315–330.

Kennedy, C. W., & Camden, C. (1983). Interruptions and nonverbal gender differences. *Journal of Nonverbal Behavior*, *8*, 91–108.

LaFrance, M., & Mayo, C. (1979). A review of non-verbal behaviors of women and men. *Western Journal of Speech Communication*, *43*, 96–107.

LaFrance, M., & Mayo, C. (1976). Social differences in gaze behavior during conversations: Two systematic observational studies. *Journal of Personality and Social Psychology*, *33*, 547–552.

Laing, M. (1993). Gossip: Does it play a role in the socialization of nurses. *Image*, *25*, 37–43.

Lakoff, R. (1973). Language and women's place. *Language in Society*, *2*, 45–79.

Lakoff, R. (1989). *Language and woman's place*. New York: Harper Torch.

Mackey, W. C. (1976). Parameters of the smile as a social signal. *Journal of Genetic Psychology*, *129*, 125–130.

Mehrabian, A. (1969). Significance of posture and position in the communication of attitude and status relationships. *Psychological Bulletin*, *71*, 359–372.

Morrow, H. (1988). Nurses, nursing and women. *International Nursing Review*, *35*, 22–26.

Muff, J. (1990). Myth and image of the female in nursing. *Imprint*, *37*, 96–98.

Mulac, A., Studly, L. B., Weimann, J. W., & Bradac, J. J. (1987). Male/female gaze in same sex and mixed sex dyads: Gender linked differences and mutual influence. *Human Communications Research*, *13*, 323–344.

Olsen, T. (1978). *Silences*. New York: Delacourte Press.

Perry, W. (1970). *Forms of intellectual and ethical development in the college years.* New York: Holt, Rinehart & Winston.

Reinharz, S. (1992). *Feminist methods in social research.* New York: Oxford University Press.

Rew, L. (1988). Nurses' intuition. *Applied Nursing Research, 1,* 27–38.

Rich, A. (1979). *On lies, secrets and silence: Selected prose 1966–78.* New York: Norton.

Roter, D. L., & Hall, J. A. (1994). *Doctors talking with patients, patients talking with doctors: Improving communication in medical visits.* Westport, CT: Auburn House.

Stern, L. I. (1980). Male and female: The doctor-nurse game. In J. P. Spradley and D. W. McCurdey (Eds.), *Conformity and conflict.* Boston: Little Brown.

Tannen, D. (1990). *You just don't understand.* New York: Ballantine.

Waitzkin, H. (1991). *The politics of medical encounters.* New Haven: Yale University Press.

Zimmerman, D. H., & West, C. (1975). Sex roles, interruptions and silences in conversation. In B. Thorne & N. Henley (Eds.), *Language and sex: Difference and dominance.* Cambridge, MA: Newbury House.

5

The Interaction
of Gender, Class,
and Race

Judith Bernstein
Judith A. Lewis

In this chapter we will examine some of the stereotyped roles and expectations that interfere with health and treatment of illness. The traditional normative standards that have labeled women as deviant or less than adult have been used throughout American history to stereotype even further those differences derived from culture, race, and class (Turner, 1987). When the freed slave Sojourner Truth, speaking at a Women's Emancipation meeting, cried out from the heart, "And ain't I a woman?" she was speaking out for those who have not even been eligible for the dubious benefits of female status in our society.

Social Norms, Gender, and Emotional and Physical Health

Norms are not just descriptions or expressions of societal expectations; they are *enforcers* of social rules. For those women who do not belong to the normative middle class or white majority in the United States, the enforcement of majority-based social norms can be a burden and a barrier to health and health care.

Regulation by teaching of norms begins within a child's primary nurturing relationship (Levine, 1977), and is enforced by the extended family, school systems, and, as a last resort, administrative and legal institutions (Coll, 1990). Growing up with racial or cultural identity and values distinct from those of the dominant majority is usually associated, in the United States, with restricted access to social and economic resources, and a daily life experience of prejudice, racism, or classism. Age, religion, sexual orientation, physical ability, religion, race, and ethnicity also shape definitions of health and illness, reactions of health care providers, and socioeconomic and cultural barriers to health care (Department of Health and Human Services [DHHS], 1990; Andersen & Collins, 1992).

Race, class, and gender can be additive factors. Often the experience of being a woman of color in the United States is described as double jeopardy, or triple jeopardy if poverty is also involved, as though being different is itself the problem. This kind of focus solely on pejorative aspects of gender and racial/ethnic status shows just how deeply discrimination roots itself in thinking, writing, and language. Barriers to health care are not the result of race, gender, and age (negatively perceived individual characteristics); they are the product of codified rac*ism*, sex*ism*, and age*ism* (characteristics of the socioeconomic structures and institutions developed and maintained by powerful interest groups).

Partly because of these barriers, many minority women base their health practices on alternative health care cultures that often combine beliefs and knowledge from their countries of origin with Native American healing traditions. Some of the mistrust of institutionalized medicine is the result, as Snow (1993) describes in *Walkin' Over Medicine*, of "experiences that all of these individuals have encountered as low income African Americans [or Latinas or Asian women] in a society where people are *not* created equal" (p. 31). But more importantly, these health cultures developed because they provide an explanatory system that is consistent with the world view of the group and provide acceptable methods of maintaining wellness and coping with illness (Weidman, 1979; Kleinman, Eisenberg, & Good, 1978).

Traditional remedies are usually short term, affordable, and assign causation. Compare orthodox medical prescriptions for hypertension, for example, with traditional therapies for "high blood," the African American way of understanding the problem. The medical model is static (once you have the disease, you always have it); addresses only the physical level of causation; requires expensive, fixed-dose, lifelong treatment, even when symptom free; designates the physician as expert; and places the patient in the role of passive recipient. In contrast, the African American construct integrates mind, body, and community; relates intensity of therapy to intensity of symptom perception; relies on inexpensive, short term treatment; designates the individual with her self-knowledge as expert; aims for a goal of achieving balance; and avoids the blame attached to the word "hypertension" which most people interpret as being nervous or hyperactive (Satcher & Ashley, 1974). It is no surprise that doctors' medicine is not necessarily seen as superior (Satcher & Creary, 1984).

Social Norms, Gender, and Emotional Health

Growing up Black or Hispanic or Appalachian is a rich and valuable cultural inheritance, a source of strength, energy, and meaning (Malson, Mudimbe-Boyi, O'Barr, & Wyer, 1990; DuBois & Ruiz, 1990). It also, however, implies inheriting the experience of being devalued in American society. When Black teens talk vividly of being "dissed" or disrespected, or made "less than," they speak for many groups in American society.

A positive sense of self, validated by the external world, is the basis for both mental and physical health. We have seen how women across race and class have had to struggle to take back who they are from the dominant society, and reclaim as strengths those characteristics of female behavior, such as the priority of relationship over individual competition, that patriarchal society has labeled as weaknesses. In order to achieve a definition of health that is appropriate, women of color, or diverse culture, and those who are not middle or upper class must reframe their diversity, validating with pride those characteristics that have served them well.

The extended family is an excellent example of a nonnormative form devalued by American society, often interpreted as a failure of individuals to become autonomous. A self-in-relation orientation would instead see this organizational form as a triumph of the human spirit and will to survive, and a major positive factor in outcomes for health and illness. In an extended family, often composed of both intergenerational relatives and nonrelated but equally important individuals, there are multiple care givers to whom a child can turn for nurturance and validation, as expressed, for example, in the Spanish phrase "*mija*" ("*mi hija*," or "my daughter"), which can be used from any loving adult to a child. Such a collectivity may form an integral part of an adult woman's social life and support system, both emotionally and economically. Elderly women in an extended family system have a valued and essential place. They are not burdens to be disposed of in nursing homes, as is often the case in the dominant culture, but serve important and necessary functions in their children's household (Andersen & Collins, 1992). Roles in Black dual-earner families may be more flexible, often combined or exchanged, with men assuming more household chores (Hill, 1972). And the single-parent family, which deviates from the American ideal of mom, pop, and two children, may actually be a subunit of an extended family that has considerable coping resources. Several groups of researchers have categorized the strengths of the Black single-parent family, and have rejected the label of deviance that has been common in sociology literature (Billingsley, 1968; Brandwein, Brown, & Fox, 1974; Malson 1986). Lesbian couples often create extended families through friendship networks that provide similar strength and support. Health care delivery and definitions of health and illness must be relevant to these adaptive, nonnormative family formats.

But adapting to a hostile world cannot be done without suffering. In addition to gender discrimination, women of color and immigrant populations are the survivors of histories that include systematic rape, conquer and plunder, slavery and lynching, police brutality, forced sterilization, and unwarranted institutionalization in mental hospitals and prisons. When not actively oppressed, they have been shamed, humiliated, ignored, unheard. The stress of multiple roles and the dual persona required to maintain authenticity within one's own group yet still survive among the dominant group can do damage to emotional (Vega & Miranda, 1985) and physical health (Krieger, 1990). Lillian Rubin (1976), who interviewed hundreds of working class families to discover their realities and perspectives, summarizes her research with the powerful statement: "For, in the working class, the process of building a family, of making a living for it, of nurturing and maintaining the individuals in it costs "worlds of pain" (p. 215). This is even more true for women of color, who experience both gender and racial discrimination, and may also have to cope with the restrictions of poverty. Even women in the Black professional middle class, as Terry McMillan (1992) describes in the novel *Waiting to Exhale*, share many issues in common with their working class counterparts. The assessment of emotional health for women, and treatment for emotional illness, must take into account the struggle to survive in a discriminatory society.

Social Norms, Gender, and Physical Health

Discrimination in American society is mirrored in the health care system and in health outcomes. The Society for the Advancement of Women's Health Research cites seven topics of concern for all medical specialties, listed in abridged form by Harrington and Estes (1994): (a) lack of information on a variety of diseases that primarily affect women; (b) failure to include women in research study populations; and when women are included in research, the lack of analysis by gender, age, race, and socioeconomic factors; (c) failure to consider modulating factors such as endogenous or exogenous sex hormones, different life stages, lifestyles or psychosocial issues when designing treatment regimens; (d) dearth of knowledge about the pharmacokinetics of drugs in women and the impact of age and hormonal status on drug metabolism; (e) underrepresentation of women professionals in both senior research and policy-making positions across the medical specialties; (f) importance of longitudinal studies to understand changes that occur with different life stages; and (g) acknowledgment that the low self-esteem of many women, occurring as a result of the socialization process that begins during childhood and adolescence and continues into maturity, profoundly affects choices throughout a woman's life.

The *Report of the National Institutes of Health: Opportunities for Research in Women's Health* (1991) summarizes current trends in women's health and identifies four issues related to susceptibility, status, prevalence, and differences. These issues are discussed below.

1. Women constitute the larger population and will be the most susceptible to disease in the future

Women live longer than men, 78.6 years versus 71.8 years according to 1989 life expectancies (National Center for Health Statistics [NCHS], 1992), but experience more disability associated with chronic disease (Manton, 1988; Verbrugge, 1985). Women now constitute 72 percent of the group over age 85 (United States Bureau of the Census, 1990), and face the problems that accompany old age, osteoporosis and Alzheimer's disease, for example, in increasing numbers.

2. Women overall have worse health than men

In 1990, of the 7 million women over age 75, 2 million were unable or limited in their ability to carry on major activities of daily living (National Center for Health Statistics, 1992). The National Institutes of Health [NIH] report also indicates that quality of life for women lags behind that of men, with women reporting 25 percent more sick days and 35 percent more bedridden days because of infections, respiratory disease, injury, and other acute conditions, even when reproductive conditions are eliminated from calculation.

Emily Friedman (1994), in *An Unfinished Revolution: Women and Health Care in America*, describes the situation succinctly:

> Women are the primary users of the health care system. They average one third more visits, one fourth more hospital discharges, and 5% more hospital days than men. Of all nursing home residents, 75% are women, as are 81% of those over the age of 85. Women represent 60% of Medicare beneficiaries and the vast majority of adults who receive Medicaid benefits. (p. 13)

Yet in life expectancy for women, the United States ranks quite low on the list of industrialized nations (see Table 5-1).

3. Certain health problems are more prevalent in women than men
The NIH report also lists many conditions that are more common in women: (a) more women than men die of stroke at all stages of life (90,000 each year), and half of all women (but only 31 percent of men) die within the first year of a heart attack; (b) the pattern of heart attacks is different, with later onset and 90 percent of all heart disease deaths in women occurring after menopause; (c) depression is twice as common in women, and osteoporosis affects one third to one half of all postmenopausal women, causing 50,000 deaths a year; (d) 6 million women each year acquire a sexually transmitted disease, and 15–20 million are chronically infected with either herpes virus or human papillomavirus (HPV); (e) women are the fastest growing population with AIDS; (f) they are 15 times as susceptible to thyroid disease, and have a much higher prevalence of rheumatoid arthritis and other autoimmune diseases; (g) diabetes, anemia, gall bladder disease, spastic colon, osteoarthritis, and chronic bronchitis also occur more frequently in women; (h) domestic violence is a major health hazard for women, with one woman being attacked somewhere in the United States every 15 seconds. Between 2 and 4 million women are physically battered each year (DHHS, 1992). Women may live longer than men, but they have more chronic disease and less quality of life (Verbrugge, 1985).

Genetic differences account for some of these discrepancies. Women produce more autoantibodies, monoclonal immunoglobulins, and specific antibodies after immunization, and have increased T-cell proliferation compared to men, all of which contribute to superior immune

TABLE 5-1   Life Expectancy at Birth, According to Sex:

Selected Countries, 1989 (In years)

Country	Women
Japan	82.5
France	81.5
Switzerland	81.3
Netherlands	81.1
Canada	80.6
Spain	80.3
Sweden	80.1
Hong Kong	80.1
Norway	80.0
Italy	79.9
Australia	79.6
Greece	79.4
Germany	79.2
Finland	79.0
Austria	78.9
UNITED STATES	78.6
England	78.4
Portugal	78.2
Belgium	78.2
Denmark	77.9

Data from: National Center for Health Statistics. (1993a).

protection (Webster, 1990). But these protective effects on mortality may be far offset by increased morbidity related to women's social environment and the type and level of stressors they experience (Nathanson, 1975), although some researchers suggest that the increased incidence in chronic disease experienced by women is just as much a function of differential socialization in the recognition and reporting of symptoms and in the use of formal health care (Verbrugge, 1976; Mechanic, 1976).

4. Certain health problems are unique to women

Cancer is the leading cause of premature death in women (American Cancer Society, 1991), with breast cancer the most prevalent cancer, but lung cancer the leading cause of cancer death (51,000 deaths in 1991). The initial presentation of HIV disease and its course are different in women, who often have menstrual irregularities or abnormal Pap smears as their first AIDS-linked event (Anastos & Marte, 1989), and die sooner after diagnosis (Harrington & Estes, 1994). Today more young women become smokers than young men (American Cancer Society, 1991). One million women each year are treated for pelvic inflammatory disease, and rates of ectopic pregnancy and involuntary infertility have quadrupled. Infant mortality is often considered to be one of the most sensitive markers for judging the quality of a health care delivery system (DHHS, 1992), and the United States ranks low among developed nations for healthy pregnancy outcome.

Detection bias based on assumptions about gender results in underdiagnosis and misdiagnosis of serious illnesses that are prevalent in women; for diagnosis of lung cancer, for example, sputum Pap smears are ordered much more frequently in men than in women with the same symptomatology (Wells & Feinstein, 1988). Differences have also been identified in access to treatment for women compared to men, with therapeutic procedures for coronary heart disease the most commonly cited example (Ayanian & Epstein, 1991). Provider behavior in medical encounters has been demonstrated to be profoundly influenced by gender (Hall, Rotter, & Katz, 1988; Bernstein & Kane, 1981).

Minority Status and Gender

The effects of gender discrimination on health are compounded by racial and ethnic discrimination and resulting poverty. The percent of minority populations with private health insurance remained the same from 1977 to 1987 for Whites, but decreased from 57 percent to 49 percent for African Americans and from 57 percent to 46 percent for Hispanics (Scupholme, DeJoseph, Strobino, & Paine, 1992). Woolhandler and Himmelstein (1988) conclude that lack of adequate insurance leads to reverse targeting of preventive measures. Non-English speakers also receive fewer screening tests (Marks et al., 1987). Barriers to screening for cervical cancer result in later stage diagnosis and excess mortality for minority women (Peters, Bear, & Thomas, 1989;

Holland, Foster, & Louria, 1993; Becker et al., 1994). African Americans receive fewer therapeutic procedures for treatment of breast cancer, and are less likely to have the benefit of reconstructive surgery (Diehr et al., 1989; Sartoriano, Swanson, & Moll, 1992). Race differences add to gender differences in access to treatment for myocardial infarction (Peterson, Wright, Daley, & Thibault, 1994) and identification of candidates for renal allograft (Soucie, Neylan, & McClellan, 1992). Cancer incidence rates show an increase over the last several decades of 27 percent among Blacks and only 12 percent among Whites, while mortality rates have increased by 34 percent for Blacks compared to 9 percent for Whites (DeVita, 1985).

Three central health problems common to United States minority women have been identified (Public Health Service Task Force on Women's Health, 1995; DHHS, 1992):

1. Higher maternal and infant mortality rates, higher neonatal death rates, and higher postneonatal death rates. Maternal mortality in 1991 was 7.2/100,000 for the United States as a whole, but 18.1/100,000 for African American women (NCHS, 1993). Black babies are twice as likely as White ones to die before the first birthday. Low birth weight, which accounts for 60 percent of infant deaths, is almost 3 times higher among racial/ethnic minorities, especially African-American women (12.4 percent) and mainland Puerto Rican women (9.1 percent).

2. A greater prevalence of chronic diseases among racial/ethnic minority women, such as diabetes, hypertension, cardiovascular disease, and certain types of cancers such as cervical cancer.

3. A life expectancy lower by 5–7 years, attributable to higher chronic disease rates and restricted access to medical care systems, particularly for early detection and prevention of disease.

Excess mortality is exemplified by calculation of years of life lost for five of the six leading causes of death before the age of 65 (in years lost per 100,000 women): *cancer* (947 for Blacks, 822 for Whites); *heart disease* (834 for Blacks, 341 for Whites); *accidents* (683 for Blacks, 537 for Whites); *homicide* (494 for Blacks, 99 for Whites); cerebrovascular diseases (238 for Blacks, 87 for Whites); and *HIV* (215 for Blacks, 24 for Whites). Only for suicide was the Black/White ratio reversed (Department of Health and Human Services, 1991). The mortality rate among African American women for cardiac and cerebrovascular disease has not improved at all in the last 40 years, despite immense technological advances.

Opportunity Structure and Health

Health services researchers have worked hard in the last decade to develop this profile of the health consequences of gender and racial discrimination. Many questions and gaps in knowledge remain to be explored, but the most significant issue is the use to which these facts are put. The highly political process of *naming*, or social policy debate, involves struggle over the conceptual framework to be constructed from data generated by these studies of discriminatory health practices (Stone, 1988).

The social problem of teen pregnancy is a case in point, a struggle between two political poles that place responsibility in two different locations. One point of view targets the breakdown of the Black family, the abdication of parental responsibility, and the culture of drugs and criminality, and proposes reduction in welfare benefits as a policy of deterrence. The opposing point of view takes cognizance of the experience of teen pregnancy in Puerto Rico, where the pregnant teen is following an accepted cultural norm, and receives support from an extended family. Under these circumstances, adolescent pregnancy does not create serious health problems for mother or child. On the United States mainland, however, where pregnancy among Puerto Rican teens is associated with negative psychological, social, educational, and economic impacts (Furstenburg, 1976; Guttenmacher, 1981; Bercerra, & deAnda, 1984), negative health outcomes for mother and child are described. The minority perspective identifies the recent increase in pregnancy rates for minority teens under the age of 18 as an adaptive response by young women of color to existing dysfunctional social structures that narrow their possibilities, and suggests that adolescent pregnancy will not decrease without widespread redistribution of social services and opportunities for education, jobs, and adequate housing (Williams, 1991). Maxine Baca Zinn (1990) expresses this perspective on causation:

> Instead of blaming minorities ... we must examine those macrostructural conditions that shape intimate relationships. The racial underclass is not destroying itself by a culturally deficient family structure, but millions of human lives are being destroyed by economic forces. Socio-economic circumstances limit the range of choices people can make about their everyday living arrangements. As poor urban residents struggle with the problems of everyday life, they may appear to be engaging in maladaptive coping tactics. Yet what may seem like poor coping strategies are often the result of severely limited options. (p. 375)

The first position blames the minority teen for her uncontrolled sexuality, and devises educational and punitive policies to control it; the second position assigns responsibility to those in the larger society who make the political decisions that shut off meaningful alternatives to youthful childbearing, and suggests changes in the opportunity structure as a remedy (Nathanson, 1991).

Lack of opportunity is illustrated by the fact that 36.4 percent of Mexican American women and 13.2 percent of African American women have completed eight years of education or less, compared to only 8 percent of White women (United States Census Bureau, 1992). In medical care, access to an opportunity structure translates into access to services. In 1991, 79.5 percent of White women received first trimester prenatal care, compared to 61.9 percent of African Americans, 65 percent of Puerto Rican women, 59.7 percent of Native Americans, and 58.7 percent of Mexican Americans. In 1992, 34 percent of Hispanics and 22.3 percent of African Americans were uninsured, compared to 16.1 percent of Whites (NCHS, 1993). And when health care is provided, it is often substandard. For example, surgery is delayed or denied for many Black women with hip fractures, and a significantly higher number of these women are likely to be nonambulatory on discharge, compared to White women (Furstenberg & Mezley, 1987).

Without expanded opportunity, attempts to enforce majority norms will not curb either teen pregnancy or welfare dependency. Political and social struggle over both the assignment of responsibility for deviance from social norms, and the accuracy of the underlying paradigm is key to eliminating barriers to quality health care for women of color.

Minority women, who are the health caretakers and responsible agents for themselves and their families, are likely to be in poor health themselves, experience a high rate of emotional symptoms or psychologically induced illnesses, and be at increased medical risk, especially during pregnancy and childbirth (Zambrana, 1988). Language, belief systems, poverty, and lack of insurance, educational exposure, and transportation have all been cited as barriers to care (Friedman, 1994), but the greatest barrier of all is the lack of respect for minority women's value systems and ways of expressing themselves. Universal access to health care, although it would be a great step forward, would not in itself be sufficient without changes that would also make the health care delivery system respectful of woman and responsive to the specific needs of minority women (Lee & Estes, 1990). In order to accomplish change, the women who need health services most must be involved in defining their requirements and suggesting innovative new ways of approaching problem solving A team must be created from within the communities themselves, and combined with the energies of minority women within the health professions, to lead those interested in health care improvement in culturally relevant research, program development, prevention campaigns, and curative efforts.

Audre Lorde (1984) sets us our tasks for the next decades:

> Our future survival is predicated on our ability to relate with equality. As women we must root out internalized patterns of oppression within ourselves if we are to move beyond the most superficial aspects of social change. . . . The future of our earth may depend on the ability of all women to identify and develop new definitions of power and new patterns of relating across differences. The old definitions have not served us, nor the earth that supports us. . . . We have built into all of us old . . . structures of oppression, and these must be altered at the same time as we alter the living conditions that are a part of those structures. . . . Change means growth, and growth can be painful. But we sharpen self-definition by exposing the self in work and struggle together with those we define as different from ourselves, although sharing the same goals. For Black and White, young and old, lesbian and heterosexual women alike, this can mean new paths to our survival. (p. 502)

References

American Cancer Society. (1991). *American Cancer Society facts and figures, 1991.* Atlanta: Author.

Anastos, K., & Marte, C. (1989). Women: The missing persons in the AIDS epidemic. *Health/PAC Bulletin, 19,* 6–13.

Anderson, M. L., & Collins, P. H. (Eds.). (1992). *Race, class and gender.* Belmont, CA: Wadsworth.

Ayanian, J., & Epstein, A. (1991). Differences in the use of procedures between men and women hospitalized for coronary heart disease. *New England Journal of Medicine, 325,* 221–225.

Becker, T., Wheeler, C., McGough, N., Parmenter, C., Jordan, S., Stidley, C., McPherson, S., & Dorin, M. (1994). Sexually transmitted diseases and other risk factors for cervical dysplasia among southwestern Hispanic and non-Hispanic women. *Journal of the American Medical Association (JAMA), 271,* 1181–1188.

Bercerra, R. M., & deAnda, D. (1984). Pregnancy and motherhood among Mexican-American adolescents. *Health and Social Work, 9,* 106–123.

Bernstein, B., & Kane, R. (1981). Physicians' attitudes toward female patients. *Medical Care, 19,* 600–608.

Billingsley, A. (1968). *Black families in white America.* Englewood Cliffs, NJ: Prentice Hall.

Brandwein, R., Brown, C., & Fox, E. (1974). Women and children last: The situation of divorced mothers and their children. *Journal of Marriage and Family, 36,* 498–514.

Bureau of the Census. (1992). Current population reports, Series P-20, No. 462. Educational attainment in the United States: March 1991 and 1990. Washington, DC: US Government Printing Office.

Coll, C. G. (1990). Developmental outcome of minority infants: A process oriented look into our beginnings. *Child Development, 61,* 270–289.

Department of Health and Human Services. (1990). *Minority aging.* DHHS Publication HRS-P-DV-90-4. Washington, DC: Author.

Department of Health and Human Services. (1992). *Healthy people 2000: National health promotion and disease prevention objectives.* Boston: Jones & Bartlett.

DeVita, V. (1985). Cancer prevention awareness program: Targeting Black Americans. *Public Health Reports, 100,* 253–254.

Diehr, P., Yergan, J., Chu, J., Fiegl, P., Glaefke, G., Moe, R., Bergner, M., & Rodenbaugh, J. (1989). Treatment modality and quality differences for black and white breast cancer patients treated in community hospitals. *Medical Care, 27,* 942–958.

Dubois, E., & V. L. Ruiz (Eds.). (1990). *Unequal sisters: A multi-cultural reader in U.S. women's history.* New York: Routledge, Chapman & Hall.

Friedman, E. (1994). An unfinished revolution: Women and health in America. New York: United Hospital Fund.

Furstenburg, F. F. (1976). *Unplanned parenthood: The social consequences of childbearing.* New York: Free Press.

Furstenberg, A. L., & Mezey, M. D. (1987). Differences in outcome between black and white elderly hip fracture patients. *Journal of Chronic Disability, 40,* 931–938.

Guttenmacher Institute. (1981). *Teenage pregnancy: The problem hasn't gone away.* New York: Author.

Hall, J., Roter, D., & Katz, N. (1988). Meta-analysis of correlates of provider behavior in medical encounters. *Medical Care, 26* 657–675.

Harrington, C., & Estes, C. (Eds.). (1994). *Health policy and nursing: Crisis and health reform in the U. S. Health Care Delivery System.* Boston: Jones and Bartlett.

Hill, R. (1972). *The strengths of Black families.* New York: Emerson Hall.

Holland, B., Foster, J., & Louria, D. (1993). Cervical cancer and healthcare resources in Newark, New Jersey, 1970–1988. *American Journal of Public Health, 83,* 45–48.

Kleinman, J. C., Eisenberg, L., & Good, B. (1978). Culture, illness and care: Clinical lessons from anthropologic and cross-cultural research. *Annals of Internal Medicine, 88,* 251–258.

Krieger, N. (1990). Racial and gender discrimination: Risk factors for high blood pressure? *Social Science Medicine, 30,* 1273–1281.

Lee, P., & Estes, C. (Eds.). (1990). *The nation's health.* Boston: Jones & Bartlett.

Lemer, G. (Ed.). (1992). *Black women in white America.* New York: Vintage Books.

Levine, L. M. (1977). Child rearing as a cultural adaptation. In P. H. Lederman, S. R. Tulkin, & A. Rosenfeld (Eds.), *Culture and infancy: Variations in human experience.* New York: Academic Press.

Lorde, A. (1982). Age, race, class, and sex: Women redefining difference. In *Sister outsider.* Freedom, CA: Crossing Press.

Malson, M. R., Mudimbe-Boyi, E., O'Barr, J., & Wyer, M. (Eds.). (1990). *Black women in America: Social Science perspectives.* Chicago: University of Chicago Press.

Malson, M. R. (1986). Understanding Black single parent families: Stresses and strengths. *Work in Progress: The Stone Center, 25,* 1–22.

Manton, K. G. (1988). A longitudinal study of functional change and mortality in the United States. *Journal of Gerontology, 43,* S153–S160.

Marks, G., Solis, J., Richardson, J., Collins, L., Birba, L., & Hisserich, J. (1987). Health behavior of elderly Hispanic women: Does cultural assimilation make a difference? *American Journal of Public Health, 77,* 1315–1319.

McMillan, T. (1992). *Waiting to exhale.* New York: Pocket Star Books.

Mechanic, D. (1976). Sex, illness behavior and the use of health services. *Journal of Human Stress, 2,* 29–40.

Nathanson, C. (1975). Illness and the feminine role: A theoretical review of data, theory and method. *Social Science and Medicine, 2,* 13–25.

Nathanson, C. (1991). *Dangerous passage.* Philadelphia: Temple University Press.

National Center for Health Statistics. (1991). *Health United States, 1990.* DHHS Publication No. 91-1232. Washington, DC: US Government Printing Office.

National Center for Health Statistics. (1992). *Health United States, 1991.* Hyattsville, MD: Public Health Service.

National Center for Health Statistics. (1993). *Health United States, 1992.* Hyattsville, MD: Public Health Service.

National Center for Health Statistics. (1992). National Health Interview Survey Cancer Control Public Use Record. Hyattsville, MD: National Center for Health Statistics.

National Institutes of Health, Office of Research on Women's Health (1992). *Opportunities for research on women's health.* Washington, DC: NIH.

Peters, R., Bear, M., & Thomas, D. (1989). Barriers to screening for cancer of the cervix. *Preventive Medicine, 18,* 133–146.

Peterson, E. D., Wright, S. M., Daley, J., Thibault, G. E. (1994). Racial variation in cardiac procedure use and survival following acute myocardial infarction in the Department of Veterans Affairs. *Journal of the American Medical Association, 271,* 1175–1180.

Public Health Service Task Force on Women's Health Issues. (1985). Women's health: Report of the Public Health Service task force on women's issues. *Public Health Reports, 100,* 74–106.

Rubin, L. B. (1976). *Worlds of pain.* New York: Basic Books.

Sartoriano, J., Swanson, M., & Moll, P. (1992). Nonclinical factors associated with surgery received for treatment of early-stage breast cancer. *American Journal of Public Health, 82,* 195–198.

Satcher, D., & Ashley, M. (1974). Barriers to hypertension control in urban areas. *Urban Health, 3,* 12–13.

Satcher, D., & Creary, L. B. (1984). Family practice in the inner city. In R. E. Rakel (Ed.), *Textbook of family practice* (3rd ed., pp. 226–237). Philadelphia: Saunders.

Scupolme, A., DeJoseph, J., Strobino, D., & Paine, L. (1992). Nurse midwifery care to vulnerable populations: Phase I: Demographic characteristics of the National CNM Sample. *Journal of Nurse Midwifery, 37,* 341–348.

Snow, L. F. (1993). *Walkin' over medicine.* San Francisco: Westview Press.

Soucie, J., Neylan, J., & McClellan, W. (1992). Race and sex differences in the identification of candidates for renal transplantation *American Journal of Kidney Diseases, 19,* 414–419.

Stone, D. (1988). *Policy paradox and political reason.* New York: HarperCollins.

Turner, C. (1987). Clinical application of the Stone Center approach to minority women. *Work in Progress: The Stone Center, 28,* 1–17.

Vega, W. M., & Miranda, M. R. (1985). *Stress and Hispanic mental health.* Washington, DC: U.S. HSSD/NIH.

Verbrugge, L. (1976). Females and illness: Recent trends in sex differences in the United States. *Journal of Health and Social Behavior, 17,* 387–403.

Verbrugge, L. M. (1985). Gender and health: An update on hypotheses and evidence. *Journal of Health and Social Behavior, 26,* 156–182.

Weidman, H. (1979). The transcultural perspective in health and illness. *Social Science and Medicine, 13B,* 85–87.

Weksler, M. (1990). A possible role for the immune system in the gender-longevity differential. In M. Ory & H. Warner (Eds.), *Gender, health and longevity: Multidisciplinary perspectives.* New York: Springer.

Wells, C. K., & Feinstein, A. (1988). Detection bias in the diagnostic pursuit of lung cancer. *American Journal of Epidemiology, 128,* 1016–1026.

Williams, C. (1991). *Black teenage mothers: Pregnancy and childbearing from their perspective.* Lexington, MA: Lexington Books.

Woolhandler, S., & Himmelstein, D. (1988). Reverse targeting of preventive care due to lack of health insurance. *Journal of the American Medical Association (JAMA), 259,* 2872–2873.

Zambrana, R. E. (1988). *A research agenda on issues affecting poor and minority women: A model for understanding their health needs.* London: Haworth Press.

Zinn, M. B. (1990). Minority families in crisis: The public discussion. In K. Hansen & I. Philipson (Eds.), *Women, class, and the feminist imagination: A socialist-feminist reader* (pp. 363–379). Philadelphia: Temple University Press.

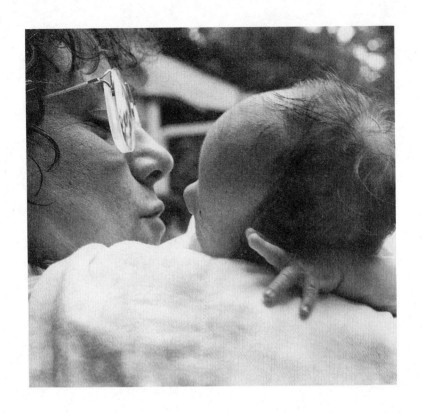

Part Two

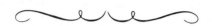

Women Across the Life Cycle: The Maturational Process

6

Adolescence

Sarah S. Strauss
Bernardine A. Clarke

I am fourteen
and my skin has betrayed me
the boy I cannot live without
still sucks his thumb
in secret
how come my knees are
always so ashy
what if I die
before morning
and momma's in the bedroom
with the door closed.

I have to learn how to dance
in time for the next party
my room is too small for me
suppose I die before graduation
they will sing sad melodies
but finally
tell the truth about me
There is nothing I want to do
and too much

that has to be done
and momma's in the bedroom
with the door closed

Nobody even stops to think
about my side of it
I should have been on Math Team
my marks were better than his
why do I have to be
the one
wearing braces
I have nothing to wear tomorrow
will I live long enough
to grow up
and momma's in the bedroom
with the door closed

Audre Lorde (1978)
"Hanging Fire" pp. 96–97
The Black Unicorn
New York: W. W. Norton

Adolescence, the period between childhood and adulthood, represents an important developmental transition. G. Stanley Hall characterized adolescence as a time of storm and stress (Muuss, 1975). Although this notion remains popular, for the majority of adolescents, including adolescent women, who are the focus of this chapter, the movement from girlhood to womanhood is relatively smooth, despite dramatic physical, cognitive, emotional, and social changes.

These changes offer challenges and opportunities to parents, caregivers, and adolescents. Because adolescence is a time when physical changes and health needs unique to this period may reestablish consistent contact between caregivers, there are many opportunities for health promotion. Understanding the nature of changes within transition periods (e.g., adolescence) and the special risks and concerns in regard to gender suggests a framework for care providers of adolescent women that focuses on health promotion, at the individual and community level.

Schumacher and Meleis (1994) identify types of individual transitions that are applicable to individuals: developmental, situational, and health-illness. These authors note that categories are not mutually exclusive. In this vein, situational and health-illness transitions occur concurrently and can potentially impede the developmental transition. For example, the pregnant and parenting adolescent encounters elements of both developmental and situational transitions. Schumacher and Meleis provide examples of a number of situational transitions, including family changes. Situational transitions encountered by adolescents may include divorce of parents and/or other losses, such as the death of friends. Examples of health-illness transitions that primarily affect adolescent women include eating disorders. Clearly, both situational and health-illness transitions in adolescence interact with ongoing developmental transitions; therefore, it is important to evaluate all health related concerns in the context of development, both physical and psychosocial.

Physical Development

For the adolescent woman, the years between ages 12 and 20 encompass a physical maturation process that culminates in reproductive maturity. The neuroendocrine system controls these physical changes. One important factor affecting hormonal regulation of changes is critical body weight. This process for girls proceeds on a different trajectory than for boys. Several differences can be highlighted (Slap, 1986). For example, young women have more subcutaneous fat than young men with lean body mass decreasing from 80 percent to 75 percent. In boys it increases from 80 to 90 percent The mean age of menarche in the United States is 12.8 years (age range 10 to 16.5 years) with the duration of puberty lasting about 4 years. Puberty follows peak height velocity by 1 year. Its onset is earlier than for boys and lasts longer. (For a more detailed discussion of differences between female and male growth patterns, suggested references can be found at the end of the chapter.)

Sexual maturation (see Figure 6-1) is typically graded using stages developed by Tanner (1962). These stages reflect progressive development of secondary sexual characteristics that in turn reflect increased levels of estrogens and androgens. For females this scoring system assesses breast and pubic hair development. Table 6-1 summarizes this information, and notes the percentage of females having onset of menarche at the various stages. Eighty percent of young women experience menarche at Stages 3 and 4.

Cognitive, Emotional, and Social Development

Many clinicians and theorists view adolescence as divided into phases: early (12–13 years), middle (14–16 years), and late (about 17–19 years) (Erikson, 1968; Strauss & Clarke, 1992; Mercer, 1983; Nelms, 1981). Strauss and Clarke's (1992) framework using three developmental patterns (immature, transitional, and mature) and nine areas (domains) within each pattern (coping, self, family, partner, infant, thinking, risk taking, goals, and interpersonal style) can serve as a guide for clinicians in assessing, diagnosing, and managing health concerns and needs of the adolescent woman (see Table 6-2). For the nonpregnant adolescent, the infant would be omitted; if the adolescent woman is not sexually active and has no partner, assessment in this domain can focus on needs and concerns in regard to establishing relationships with the opposite sex. Although this framework was developed and validated with pregnant and parenting adolescent women, it provides a pragmatic perspective for better understanding issues in psychosocial development and their implications for health care for all adolescent women.

Cognitive Changes

Pivotal to understanding the health needs of the adolescent woman is understanding how thinking is altered during the transition from childhood to adulthood. Reasoning changes from syllogistic thinking in childhood to propositional thinking in adolescence. Syllogistic thinking

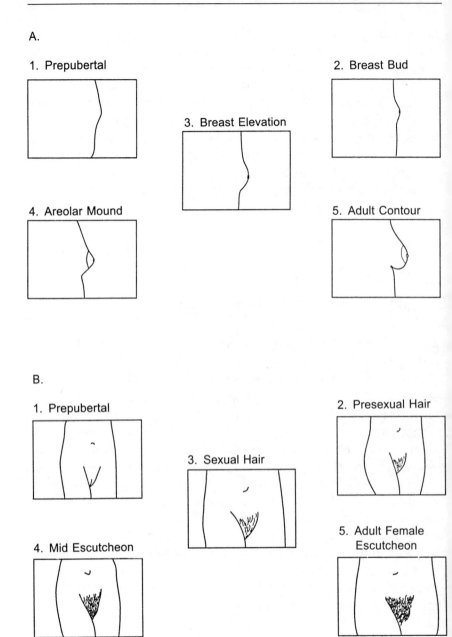

FIGURE 6-1. Tanner Staging: A. Breast, B. Pubic Hair

TABLE 6-1   Sexual Maturation in Females

Stage	Onset of Menarche	Breast Development	Pubic Hair
1		no breast tissue	no pubic hair
2	10%	breast buds	sparse downy hair medial aspect, labia majora
3	20%	enlargement of breast and areola	darkening, coarsening, curling of hair; pattern extends up and lateral
4	60%	areola and nipple form a mound on top of under-lying breast tissue	hair adult consistency, confined to mons
5	100%	adult; areola and breast smoothly contoured	hair on medial thighs

Data from: Litt, I. F. (1990). *Evaluation of the adolescent patient.* Philadelphia: Hanley & Belfus, pp. 42–43; and Tanner, J. M. (1962). *Growth at adolescence* (2nd Ed.). Blackwell, England: Oxford.

involves understanding a general rule governing the immediate and concrete (e.g., saying "thank you," when given something). Propositional thinking involves using symbols for symbols or moving from the here and now to a nonimmediate world of possibilities, including the future, the past, and distant places (Elkind, 1984). Adolescents can think about thinking; children think, but not about thinking. While this new ability offers great opportunity, it also possesses inherent traps. Elkind (1984, 1985) labels these as personal fable and imaginary audience. He sees these thinking patterns as explaining and influencing many risk-taking and help-seeking behaviors and health beliefs in adolescence. Further, these thinking patterns predominate during the transitional phase (Strauss & Clarke, 1992). The immature adolescent thinks more like the older child; thinking is more concrete and behavior is more impulsive. Events such as intercourse and pregnancy are often not logically sequenced in terms of cause and effect in emotionally charged situations. In fact, situations involving health and illness are likely to be perceived as quite threatening, and reversion to more immature forms of thinking may be apparent.

Elkind (1984) identifies cognitive conceit and assumptive realities as the major pitfalls in the thinking of older children. When using assumptive realities, the adolescent girl may possess fallacious hypotheses; errors are explained in terms of the fallacious thinking (e.g., intercourse needing to last 2 hours in order to become pregnant). Because

TABLE 6-2   Adolescent Decision-Making Patterns

Concepts	*Patterns*		
	Immature	*Transitional*	*Mature*
Coping	unable to describe ways to deal with problems; others initiate problem solving	uses emotional strategies (i.e., walking out, crying); identifies appropriate help	seeks information on self-care; discusses problem, identifies alternatives
Self (personal boundaries)	unable to own and identify uniqueness of likes and dislikes about self	description of self is inconsistent; sees superficial changes in relations	sees self as unique; defines self as unique individual
Family (personal boundaries)	decisions controlled by family	takes responsibility for decisions with family support	makes independent decisions; seeks family advice
Partner	shows only superficial concern	may glorify, idealize; does not project future	shows reciprocal interactions; projects future
Infant (if parent)	child playmate; named by others	ambivalent and inconsistent; can comfort but may be overwhelmed	able to comfort; describes child as unique
Egocentrism	others not affected by behavior; school important because mother says so	school important; concrete, self-focused	school important for future job
Risk-Taking	unable to identify self-protection information	erratic pattern of self-protection	consistent self-protective behavior
Goals	is unable to identify goals	has only superficial, general goals and no alternative plans	is able to describe 3 goals; recognizes problems; has alternatives
Interpersonal style	makes limited eye contact; is unable to answer	giggles; is dramatic	expands on answers; initiates questions

thinking during times of stress tends to be more egocentric at every phase, the girl may argue and refuse to relinquish her viewpoint or belief. This behavior is particularly frustrating for parents, and it is the basis for many parent-child conflicts in the young adolescent. Cognitive conceit also fuels conflicts between parents and young adolescents. The young adolescent girl believes in her own perfection, hence she has difficulty acknowledging mistakes. Parents and other adults, however, have many noticeable flaws, and the young adolescent is quick to point these out. These glitches in thinking set the stage for parent-child power struggles that can be perpetuated well beyond childhood unless parents have assistance in defusing argumentative behavior arising out of these cognitive processes. These cognitive constructions can also be major impediments to health promotion efforts in this age group.

The more mature adolescent will report a fairly accurate realistic description of events and admit to fallacious reasoning in certain situations. She is also better able to understand others' viewpoints, and therefore she is more likely to seek and listen to advice.

Chronologic age cannot be used alone to predict where the adolescent woman will be in the maturity of her thinking patterns. In addition, life experiences, emotional stability, family support, parental discipline and maturity, and health status are important factors to be considered. Therefore, it is important for health care providers to fully understand how audience and fable permeate thinking during this period, and how other life situations interact with adolescent developmental processes.

Because adolescents can think about thinking, they become preoccupied about what others are thinking, about their thoughts and their actions. This is manifested in self-consciousness. The adolescent woman may be reluctant to come to the health care provider to ask for contraception because of an imaginary audience and what the provider might be thinking. Personal fable or a pervasive sense of invulnerability ("it can't happen to me") may further influence health seeking in regard to contraception. Imagining two young people engaging in sexual intercourse whose thinking around an emotionally charged activity is dominated by preoccupation with the partner's thinking, and thinking the partner knows what they are thinking, combined with a sense of being invulnerable, provides some insight into increasing unplanned pregnancies and sexually transmitted diseases in this population. Breaking through some of the cognitive constructions of adolescence requires an understanding of maturation processes and repeated, nonthreatening discussions of concerns and behaviors that may result in serious consequences. It also helps us better understand why some of our traditional educational intervention strategies are not as effective as we would like them to be.

Identity, independence, and development of significant love relationships outside the family are the major tasks of adolescence. Emotional (and cognitive) development in childhood and adolescence occurs within the context of social units—family, neighborhood, friendships, school, church, and the larger community. By the time the adolescent girl reaches puberty she has experienced over a decade of foundational life experiences and relationships that she brings with her to the health care setting. Development of an identity, the major task of adolescence (Erikson, 1968), requires separation from significant persons (e.g., the mother) and development of boundaries for the self.

Self

Much of the development of self-awareness occurs through interaction with others. These interactions around the issues of identity occur in the family, with peers, at school, and in adolescence, with members of the opposite sex. Factors such as family relationships, parenting styles, child temperament, birth order, skill acquisition during childhood, success in school, and friendships all interact and contribute to social and emotional development and definition of a unique and positive sense of self.

Descriptions of self yield clues to maturity of thinking and how the adolescent girl views herself. Clinicians have used self-description (e.g., three likes and dislikes) as part of assessment (Strauss & Clarke, 1992). Immature adolescents usually cannot identify three likes and dislikes, and the likes and dislikes identified typify concrete thinking, such as dress, hair, dichotomous personal attributes (nice/nasty), and other superficial characteristics. Transitional adolescents begin to describe inner qualities (e.g., fun to be with) but they continue to define self based upon external factors such as possessions and relationships with others. Some focus more on negative characteristics (e.g., bad attitude that is reflective of self-absorption). The more mature adolescent girl describes a more complete view of herself that includes several positive as well as some negative characteristics.

Family

The immature adolescent is still dependent on her family for most needs. Although conflicts with family members may be reported, these will generally not be of the same intensity as those described by transitional adolescents and/or their parents. Because of the need to separate from family in developing an identity, family conflict is at its peak for the transitional adolescent girl. Arguments and refusal to accept parental advice are frequently reported by both adolescents and parents. Simultaneously, relationships with peers and boys become increasingly important. The more mature adolescent girl may seek parental input on decisions and acknowledge the value of her parents' perspective, even though she disagrees with them.

Exposure to parental depression, alcoholism, substance abuse, and other mental disorders (e.g., schizophrenia); existence of chronic conditions (e.g., learning problems and attentional deficits); and all forms of abuse, including unremitting exposure to violence in family, neighborhood, and communities may present significant obstacles to developing a positive sense of self during adolescence. Adolescent girls experiencing these problems, especially in the context of dysfunctional families, often do not receive support to develop coping skills. This is especially true for the immature and transitional adolescent. Day-to-day problems encountered by adolescent girls include conflicts with parents, teachers, and peers (especially boyfriends); disappointments in regard to school activities and competition; and mood swings in regard to hormonal changes.

Anger is frequently expressed in outbursts followed by withdrawing from the conflict and a self-imposed period of isolation (Strauss & Clarke, 1992). This behavior suggests some beginning ability to cognitively appraise threat, but responses to threat continue to be primarily defensive and emotionally based. Younger adolescents tend to use more impulsive, emotion-based strategies (e.g., hitting). Older adolescents are better able to use problem-focused coping strategies (e.g., talking the problem over). Parents and other significant adults, however, must usually initiate the "talk," consistently model information-seeking behavior and problem resolution, and insist on the adolescent practicing these strategies. In our study of pregnant and parenting adolescent women, the majority of the adolescents reported that problems that initiated angry outbursts were never brought back up and resolved (Clarke, 1993). Therefore, the environment is important in supporting the development and use of problem-solving coping strategies.

Moral Development

Kohlberg's theory of moral development, frequently cited in child development literature, was based upon his early research with male subjects and hence does not adequately address moral reasoning strategies used by women (Muuss, 1988). Gilligan's (1982) work focuses on sex differences in moral reasoning and introduces a feminist perspective into moral developmental theory (Muuss, 1988). When Kohlberg administered the moral dilemmas to women, sex differences were found. According to his theory, adolescent women usually attain a rating at Stage 3, good girl/nice boy; adolescent males typically score at Stage 4, law and order (whether judgment maintains or violates the existing social order). The moral dilemma usually cited is Heinz's problem (only an expensive drug that Heinz cannot afford can save his wife). In responding to this dilemma, women typically approve of Heinz's theft of the drug to save his wife while men tend to believe that Heinz's stealing must be dealt with fairly, using principles of law and justice. Since the latter is scored as a higher level of moral reasoning using Kohlberg's system, women are penalized for responding with increased sensitivity and caring (Muuss, 1988).

Gilligan (1982), a student of Kohlberg, attempted to address gender differences in moral decision making. Her work supports the notion that women approach moral and other issues, such as violence, from a fundamentally different perspective than do men; hence women are not "lower" than men in their moral reasoning. She postulates two moral voices: (a) the justice orientation preferred by most males that reflects equality, reciprocity, autonomy, and individuation; and (b) the interpersonal network orientation, preferred by women (Muuss, 1988). Developmentally, Gilligan (1982) suggests a two-level theory of moral reasoning for women: orientation to self-interest and identification of goodness and responsibility to others, with a transition period between them.

These reasoning differences have implications in understanding reasoning processes in regard to peer pressure and a variety of health issues that may present moral and ethical concerns, such as self-care during pregnancy (smoking cessation) or elective abortion. Adolescents, especially younger adolescent women, are likely to focus more on self and express limited or no concern verbally or behaviorally for the fetus, an orientation quite distressing to health care providers.

Common Health Problems

Developmental/Lifestyle Concerns

Adolescence is generally considered to be a healthy time of life. Vital statistics report that most deaths (over 80 percent) of persons 15 to 24 years of age are due to violent causes, specifically, accidents, suicide, and homicides. However, four out of five injury victims are male, with an adolescent being killed in an accident every 20 minutes (Neinstein, 1991). Morbidities more likely to involve the female adolescent include pregnancy, sexually transmitted diseases (STDs), running away, and suicide. One in eight teens will run away from home at least once.

Risk-taking behavior arises out of discrepancies between physical, cognitive, and emotional development. Environment must mediate these discrepancies. Poverty areas also have higher rates of fires, homicides, unintentional shootings, drownings, and motor vehicle accidents (Neinstein, 1991). Availability of cars, alcohol, and drugs also increases risk significantly for injury and other morbidities.

Behaviors that typify risk taking in young women, such as substance abuse and early sexual experimentation with multiple partners frequently resulting in pregnancy and contraction of STDs, are also those identified as symptomatic of depression arising from poor self-esteem, coping with chronic illness, family and school/learning problems, and abuse. Therefore, clinicians must sort out whether risk-taking behaviors arise from normative transitions, and transitional thinking and problem solving, or involve other significant risk factors. This clinical decision-making guides the management plan for the adolescent woman and determines the plan of care.

Sexual and Reproductive Problems

Responses to Menarche
Among ancient peoples, menstruating women were envied for their mythological powers, and their intimate connection to creation and the rhythms of the earth and moon, and feared for the harm they could do (from turning milk sour if they violated the taboo against handling food, to throwing the world into essential chaos if they violated the taboo against mixing blood with water). Until recent times, women menstruated rarely in their lives because of later onset and repeated pregnancy followed by long periods of lactation.

It is no wonder, with this history, that the advent of menstruation is still met in our society with a mixture of eagerness, unease, confusion, and denial of its significance. In contemporary society menstrual blood is not taboo; it is hidden, not magical. Menarche represents a milestone in maturation toward adulthood, but it also represents maturation into the secondary status of the female role. The adolescent's behavior may be more closely monitored and regulated after first menstruation because of the potential for pregnancy, and there are major changes in closeness and conflict within the mother-daughter dyad (Danza, 1983). Adolescent girls describe menstruation as "more bothersome, debilitating and unsanitary than do their mothers" (Fogel & Woods, 1995, p. 63). Changes in body image may be greeted with acceptance or denial, with significant effect on self-esteem and lifestyle patterns (Doan & Morse, 1985).

The majority of teens are prepared for menarche, if at all, with hygienic or pregnancy-related information. Adolescent health care providers can intervene, in many situations, to change the focus of preparation to include recognition of the emotional milestone that menarche represents (Logan, Calder, & Cohen, 1980).

Dysmenorrhea

Because the early postpuberty annovulatory cycles are rarely associated with menstrual cramping, the incidence of painful menstruation rises as young women move through the teen years (Klein & Litt, 1983). Endometriosis, the growth of endometrial tissue outside the uterine cavity, has been found to be a significant cause of persistent dysmenorrhea in adolescents. Because this is a progressive, chronic disease, it requires attention early in the process to reduce pain and preserve options for future fertility (Redwine, 1987). Cervical polyps can also cause painful menses by blocking outflow. Once pathology has been ruled out as a cause of dysmenorrhea, symptoms may be treated with antiprostaglandins, beginning a day or two prior to expected menstruation.

Abnormal puberty

Many young women and their mothers express ambivalent feelings about the advent of menses. Because menses may normally begin as early as age 10, health visits and visits in later school years provide opportunity to evaluate breast development and provide anticipatory guidance. Family history of onset of menses as well as expectations for onset based on development of secondary sexual characteristics assists parents in identifying appropriate books, materials, and opportunities for discussion. Many mothers express some anxiety about preparation and request age-appropriate literature and suggestions from care providers.

The preadolescent girl's onset of menarche is correlated with maternal and even more so, older sister's age of menarche (Litt, 1990). Litt suggests that if a young woman is more than one year older than when her mother or older sister began menses, she should be considered to have primary amenorrhea (never menstruated). The relationship between pubertal development and menarche is so consistent that young female who has not reached Sexual Maturation Rate (SMR) 2 by age 13 may be considered to have primary amenorrhea, as does the young woman who has begun to have pubertal changes that cease for more than 2 years (Litt, 1990, p. 104). Secondary amenorrhea is absence of monthly menses of more than 3 months' duration in a previously menstruating female.

Menarche operates on a social as well as biological clock (Rierdan & Koff, 1990), and girls who think of themselves as "on time" in their development report fewer adverse menstrual symptoms. Girls who mature either early or late have long been thought to be at a social disadvantage (Faust, 1960, 1983).

Litt (1990) indicates that the etiologies of primary and secondary amenorrhea in the adolescent may be considered simultaneously. Congenital structural anomalies (e.g., imperforate hymen, and vaginal and uterine agenesis) and chromosomal disorders (e.g., Turner Syndrome and testicular feminization) are responsible for 20–40 percent of the cases of primary amenorrhea. Other causes include (a) *pregnancy*, which should always be ruled out; (b) *chronic illness*, (e.g., pituitary and hypothalmic tumors, thyroid disease, poorly controlled diabetes mellitus, sickle cell anemia, thalassemia major, adrenal insufficiency or hypersecretion, compromised tissue oxygenation [e.g., heart disease and cystic fibrosis], and compromised nutrition [e.g., anorexia nervosa and inflammatory bowel disease]); (c) *drugs*, including illicit drugs (e.g., heroin, methadone, and marijuana), prescribed drugs (e.g., hormones, methyldopa [an antihypertensive], phenothiazines [antidepressants], vitamin A, radioisotopes [e.g., I 131]), and some chemotherapeutic agents; (d) *gynecologic problems* (e.g., ovarian tumors and cysts, and endometrial hyperplasia); and (e) *emotional stress*. Management depends on etiology.

Primary amenorrhea

Turner syndrome, the most common chromosomal anomaly to cause primary amenorrhea, is also characterized by short stature and sometimes a webbed neck and widely spaced nipples. The amenorrhea is the result of dysgenetic, undifferentiated gonads. Early diagnosis permits more effective treatment with exogenous estrogens and progestins to allow breast development and monthly withdrawal bleeding from a usually normal uterus. Estrogen therapy will also prevent osteoporosis.

Secondary amenorrhea

Many of the causes of amenorrhea, such as chronic illness, tumors, and drugs, could cause primary or secondary amenorrhea. A careful history focusing on family sexual and drug histories, as well as weight loss/gain, exercise, physical growth patterns, abnormal hair development, acne, galactorrhea, abdominal pain, and headache or visual disturbances, must be obtained (Litt, 1990). Pregnancy must also be considered in adolescent as well as post pill amenorrhea which may continue for up to 18 months in adolescents. References by Litt (1983; 1990) at the end of the chapter provide greater detail.

Other Factors Affecting Sexuality

Adolescent women have many concerns and needs around sexual and reproductive functions, and numerous factors influence how they define and express their sexual identity. Because defining an identity is the primary developmental task of the adolescent, integrating one's sexual identity assumes major importance. Adolescents must cope with dramatically changing bodies and new feelings that these bodies produce. These changes necessitate exploration, testing, and validation of themselves as men and women. While there are many ways that sexuality can be explored and feelings expressed, for many adolescents, exploration involves engaging in sexual intercourse at an early age. Environmental factors (e.g., family values and behavior, peer pressure, and sexually explicit advertising) and internal factors (e.g., maturity of thinking) influence adolescents' sexual decisions.

By age 15, 26 percent of females have experienced sexual intercourse, and by age 20, 75 percent. Antecedents of early sexual behavior include early maturation, poor communication with parents, lack of parental supervision, perceptions of what one's peer group is doing and poor academic performance (Brooks-Gunn & Furstenberg, 1989). For example, early maturing girls are likely to have older friends, and this is associated with intercourse, smoking, and drinking (Brooks-Gunn, 1988). Also, while physically mature, they are likely to be quite immature in their thinking and decision making, and likely to be easily led by older friends.

Of even greater concern is the continuing pattern of failure to initiate effective contraception and adequate protection against STDs given the decision to have sexual intercourse. Brooks-Gunn and Furstenburg (1989) indicate that the percentage of teens who use birth control only occasionally or not at all is substantial. An earlier study by Zabin and Clark (1981) indicated that one third of teens attending a family planning clinic came because of possible pregnancy, and only 14 percent came prior to initiating intercourse. Embarrassment, ambivalence about the decision to be sexually active, concerns about confidentiality, and misinformation about parental consent and notification were all factors in contributing to procrastination (Brooks-Gunn & Furstenburg, 1989).

Finally, maturity of thinking and personal fable are important factors contributing to the impulsivity often underlying sexual decision making for young adolescent women. The decision of the immature adolescent to engage in intercourse is not clearly thought through. Casual contact with young males in close proximity, poor judgment, desire to please and be accepted, inability to connect act (sex) with consequence (pregnancy and STDs), and inadequate monitoring by responsible adults often set the stage for early sexual experiences. For the transitional adolescent woman, personal fable and imaginary audience are at their height, making pregnancy and STDs problems that happen to other people. Both the immature and transitional thinker are unlikely to insist that the male partner wear a condom. This would not occur to the immature adolescent, and the imaginary audience would inhibit the transitional woman. Finally, the role of alcohol and drugs must be considered. Sexual activity in adolescents is often initiated while under the influence of mind-altering substances. Therefore, the dynamics of development, thinking, and problem solving; the increasing number of environments which may not be supportive of developmental issues affecting adolescents; and mixed messages about contraception and initiation of sexual activity offer significant challenges to parents, teens, and health care providers.

Sexually transmitted diseases

The incidence of sexually transmitted disease is rising in all populations. The rapidity of the rise in adolescent populations is of considerable concern because of significant threats, both to development of the self and to physical health. Although real numbers are low and constantly changing, reported heterosexual acquired immunodeficiency syndrome cases in the 13- to 24-year-old group indicates that this is the most rapidly increasing subpopulation contracting this lethal sexually transmitted disease (Centers for Disease Control and Prevention [CDC], 1991). Further, the incidence of AIDS in adolescent women increased by 67 percent in 1990, more than twice the incidence for males (Hersch, 1991). Infection with the human immunovirus (HIV) and subsequent development of AIDS is frightening, but prevalence and morbidity of other STDs, such as gonnorhea, syphilis, herpes, human papilloma virus (HPV), chlamydia, and hepatitis B, in the adolescent population is even a greater cause for concern. Fuerst (1991) provides the following data on these diseases. HPV, a viral STD, is a culprit in venereal warts and increased risk of cervical cancer at a young age. There is only palliative treatment for genital warts. Chlamydia, caused by a bacterial organism, is currently the most prevalent STD and is responsible for 20–40 percent of pelvic inflammatory disease (PID) cases and subsequent female infertility; its devastating consequences are partially due to silent symptoms, hence it often remains untreated. One in six adults carries genital herpes caused by herpes simplex type 2; it is usually a silent infection that lasts a lifetime. During its periodic outbreaks, the open lesions, as those with other STDs, increase the risk for infection with HIV.

Women are particularly vulnerable to gynecological and reproductive sequelae from these infections during adolescence and young adulthood. They are often ignorant of symptoms of STDs or too embarrassed to seek treatment and exposure until serious problems occur. Undetected and/or untreated infections can result in infertility. In the presence of conception and pregnancy, there may be significant threat to embryonic and fetal development, including premature labor and delivery. For the infant, postnatal complications of untreated STDs such as syphilis, gonorrhea, and herpes include potentially serious mental handicaps.

Pregnancy

Every 31 seconds a teen becomes pregnant, with 40 percent of today's teens becoming pregnant at least once during adolescence, and every 2 minutes a teen gives birth (Neinstein, 1991). One fourth of teenage girls become pregnant before age 18, and 85 percent of these pregnancies are unintended (CDC, 1990). Adolescent pregnancy has been cited as a major health problem having significant psychological and social morbidity in addition to physical health risks for both the adolescent mother and her child, prenatally and postnatally. Teen mothers are likely to drop out of school and become single heads of households, and they are 50 percent more likely than nonparents to receive welfare (Hofreth & Hayes, 1987).

While numerous studies have reported many factors relating to the occurrence of teen pregnancy, a recent report by Holden, Nelson, Velasquez, and Ritchie (1993) assessed differences between pregnant and nonpregnant adolescents in three areas: cognitive, psychosocial, and reported sexual behavior. They found that the pregnant teens were more likely to be doing poorly in school, and less likely to use contraceptives. Compared to nonpregnant adolescents, they were also more likely to have a relative or friend who was an adolescent mother, and have expectations that childrearing would be easy. Although she did not have a nonpregnant comparison group, Clarke's (1993) finding in her predominantly African American inner city sample of pregnant adolescents parallel this report. Fifty-nine percent had failed at least one grade; one third of the sample became pregnant in middle school; and 80 percent thought they knew enough to raise a child. Findings such as these have significant implications for health care providers, both in terms of managing individual care and in developing programs to prevent early sexual activity and first pregnancies, as well as in working with parenting adolescent mothers and preventing unplanned subsequent pregnancies.

Decision making in regard to the pregnancy is one of the first major concerns facing the adolescent and her family. The caregiver usually becomes involved with the adolescent in the process of confirming the pregnancy. The girl and her family, and often the father of the child, are in a situational crisis at this point. How the girl and/or the family respond to a positive confirmation of pregnancy depends on a number of factors. Maturity of the adolescent and family support, resources, and values guide these decisions about the pregnancy. Parents, particularly mothers, often respond initially with anger and acute disappointment. In Clarke, Strauss, Munton, Fleming, and Kish's (1994) study, a significant number of mothers of the pregnant adolescents were young mothers. Expressions of wanting things to be different for their daughters were common.

Approaches to management will vary. Caregivers must present all options and be familiar with laws governing parental notification. Resnick, Beringer, Stark, and Blum (1994) reported that in their sample of 184 adolescents, all consulted at least one individual before obtaining an abortion, but that one fourth who were mostly older did not consult an adult prior to pregnancy counseling. The adolescents in this study perceived their mothers and male partners as the most important and helpful people in decision making. Family communication needs to be supported, and short-term crisis counseling may be helpful for adolescent women, parents, and partners.

Further, many pregnant adolescents may have other obstacles to caring for themselves. Results from Holden et al.'s (1993) and Clarke et al.'s (1994) studies suggest a high incidence of special needs learners who may not learn best from traditional teaching strategies involving oral communication and printed material combined with rushed caregivers in crowded health care settings. Fragmentation of care, receiving health care in different settings from different providers who may or may not understand the special needs of this developmental period, is also problematic.

Parenting

Of the one million adolescent women who become pregnant each year in the United States, half carry their pregnancies to term and only 12,000 choose adoption (Hofferth & Hayes, 1987). The overwhelming majority of adolescents who carry their pregnancies to term elect to keep the infant. Because of their egocentrism and immaturity, appropriate decision making that addresses the needs of the infant may be a problem. For example, adolescent mothers have been shown to be more physical in handling their infants and less affectionate, as well as less verbal than older mothers (Osofsky & Osofsky, 1970; Greene, Sandler, Altemeier & O'Connor et al., 1981). Clarke et al. (1994) found, however, that a parenting, decision-making intervention coinciding with well-child visit over the first 2 years of life improved parent-child interaction and home environment, and reduced parenting stress.

Assistance and support in the parent role must consider the adolescent parent's thinking and decision-making competence. Comprehensive rather than categorical services to adolescent families and use of a consistent professional provider appear to offer a more efficacious approach in achieving consistent and appropriate patterns of health seeking behavior (O'Sullivan & Jacobsen, 1992). Family support is also a key factor in assuring positive outcomes. Smith (1983) identified three patterns used by families to incorporate the adolescent mother and her infant into the family: role sharing, role binding, and role blocking. In the role sharing pattern, the family, particularly the grandmother, are involved in assisting the adolescent in caring for the infant and meeting her own developmental needs. This pattern is likely to be evident in families in which the adolescent may be immature or transitional. Two dimensions of role sharing have been identified: collaborative and turn taking. In collaborative role sharing the grandmother and adolescent mother work together to provide care for the infant. For example the grandmother might support her daughter by caring for the infant in the evening during final exam week. In turn taking, the grandmother might care for the infant during school hours but expect the adolescent mother to assume all care responsibilities when she returns home.

Role binding is a pattern in which the adolescent mother assumes most or all of the parenting responsibilities. A more mature adolescent mother who has completed or is nearing completion of school is likely to exhibit voluntary role binding; forced role binding occurs when the grandmother is unavailable or unwilling to assist the adolescent mother. Parental illness or family dysfunction may result in forced role binding pattern. Outcomes for the immature and transitional

dolescent mother and her infant caught in forced role binding may
ot be optimal. This is the adolescent mother who may be the most
n need of parenting programs such as surrogate mothers and a con-
istent professional provider who is knowledgeable about the special
eeds of adolescent families.

Finally, role blocking is reflected in families in which a significant
dult or adults, usually one or both grandparents, take over all parenting
esponsibilities. They are likely to assume guardianship of the infant,
nd the adolescent mother assumes the role of sibling with few if any
arental responsibilities. This pattern is evidenced in a variety of situ-
tions; it is most likely to be seen with very immature adolescents, but
nay occur if the adolescent and her family have ambitions for career
ducation or when the adolescent has significant physical or mental
ealth problems.

Smith (1983) identified role sharing as the normative pattern, and
nost care providers are at least partially correct in their belief that sup-
ortive families make a difference in developmental outcomes for ado-
escent mothers and their infants. We need to be aware, however, that
ome investigators have found that role binding adolescent mothers
ave higher teaching interaction scores than role sharing adolescent
nothers (Clarke, 1993). The issue becomes one of who is consistently
nd contingently involved with the infant. These studies did not
xamine grandmother interaction with the infant. Further, caregivers
eed to be aware of the potential for power struggles between the
randmother and the adolescent. This is particularly true when the
dolescent is a transitional thinker and not always able to put the needs
f the infant first. Statements such as "He's my child, but I need to
isten to the rest of this song before I change him," place many
randmothers in a quandary. Caregivers need to be able to discuss and
ssist in mediating these conflicts.

Abuse

Self abuse

Smoking. Smoking, because of the addictive potential of nicotine and
ecause of sequelae to the health of the smoker and others who have
hronic exposure to detrimental effects of smoke, should be considered
n abusive behavior. A recent study by Waldron, Lye, and Brandon
1991) found significant differences in smoking patterns in a national
ample of Caucasian adolescent males and females. More females than

males were smokers, because they adopted the habit earlier. More girls were likely to have tried smoking at least once and to have smoked more than once or twice. The investigators attributed this to the fact that the males were more involved in sports during adolescence, which may have inhibited early adoption. Rural adolescent girls were less likely to smoke excessively soon after adopting the habit than later possibly because of traditional values, and very religious adolescent women were less likely to adopt smoking than men. Although these findings cannot be generalized to other ethnic groups, they have implications for targeting prevention programs and encouraging participation in sports activities and exercise programs for young girls.

Alcohol and drug abuse. While recent adolescent use of illicit drugs has decreased, levels are still quite high when compared to use prior to 1965 (Werner, 1991). Werner also indicated that the prevalence of drug use is underestimated in recent large epidemiologic surveys because drug use among adolescents who are school dropouts, and hence at increased risk for drug use, is unaccounted for. Further, abuse of alcohol and tobacco have not declined among adolescents. A recent study of adolescents and young adults indicated that while males drink more and more often than females, the majority of both females and males consume alcohol, with a significant number consuming five or more drinks in a row during a 2-week period (National Institute on Drug Abuse, 1990). Reasons for consumption are somewhat distressing and reflect considerable risk: drinking to become intoxicated and to cope with problems (including anger and frustration). Medium to heavy drinkers expected to be more aggressive after drinking. In an earlier survey, 11 percent of 8th graders reported frequent alcohol consumption (an average of 5.6 oz. per week) (Maryland Department of Health & Mental Hygiene, 1982).

Risk factors have been identified in predicting drug and alcohol use (Newcomb, et al., 1986). These include poor academics, low religiosity, early alcohol use, decreased self-esteem, and psychopathology (e.g. depression). It is important to note that these factors are not influenced by gender or increased age, but may be increased for Native American and other ethnic groups when compared to Caucasians (Werner, 1991).

Given these statistics and risk factors, prevention of alcohol consumption, smoking, and drug use must occur before adolescence. Like prevention of early sexual activity, prevention rests on early intervention for young children and their families in the area of communication, parenting, development of positive feelings about self, and sound decision-making skills. Decision making is not learned quickly; many experiences and

"safe" failures may be required. These experiences are best provided
t younger ages when parents, teachers, and other significant adults
vho have more influence over the child's environment can better pro-
ect against adverse consequences. Primary prevention strategies in-
lude role playing refusal skills in response to peer pressure. In certain
ituations, parent and child/adolescent can reverse roles, with the
oung person advising the parent (or adult) about dangers of high-
isk behaviors. Teen theatre and peer counseling are also possibilities.

Persistent review of these behaviors during health-related visits by
are providers is useful, and some of the advice may be followed at
ome point. Adolescents who engage in high-risk behaviors are often
ransitional thinkers and tend to discount authority figures' advice,
ncluding that of the health care provider. As with other activities,
ersonal fable and imaginary audience may inhibit immediate accep-
ance of adult assessments of danger. Some clinicians cite research:
"What I am telling you is not just something I believe, but in a study
vith many young people around your age. . . ." Getting the adoles-
ent to think about the problem in another way is sometimes helpful.
\ colleague who is an expert in working with adolescents in a college
etting routinely asks for estimates of drinking, knowing that this group
vill underestimate drinking when asked to give numbers of beers,
lrinks, etc.; she then asks for amount of money spent each week on
lrinking. The adolescent must then consider the monetary cost. For
nany adolescents, this has never been addressed. For a group that also
ikes clothing, musical recordings, cars, and other material things, this
)ecomes an additional reason to consider reducing consumption.

Eating disorders. Females comprise 95 percent of the eating disorder
)opulation (Plehn, 1990). The incidence of anorexia nervosa and
)ulimia is increasing, with the incidence of anorexia nervosa being
bout 1 percent and bulimia about 4 percent (Zuckerman, Colby,
Vave, & Lazerson, 1986) in the college age population studied. Both
onditions are potentially life threatening illnesses that have common-
lities as well as differences. While both conditions arise out of dis-
orted body image and share the likelihood for coexisting disorders
e.g., depression, personality disorder, and substance abuse), anorexia
nervosa is most likely to affect younger adolescent girls (ages 13–17)
vhile bulimia affects the older adolescent female (ages 17 to early 20s).
'resentation of illness also differs, with anorexia being less difficult to
liagnose, particularly if serial height/weight records are available. The
norexic is at least 15 percent below ideal body weight, and usually
ndicates that she is dissatisfied with her weight and desires to be

thinner despite being within normal limits or below expected weight (Plehn, 1990; American Psychiatric Association, 1987). She may report fasting for days or eating low calorie foods and exercising anywhere from 3 to 5 hours, daily. Amenorrhea is often an early sign before weight loss. Bulimic behavior may also be exhibited by up to 50 percent of anorexics. Prolonged starvation results in manifestations of malnutrition, including osteoporosis from prolonged deficient calcium intake.

Bulimia is more difficult to identify, particularly in an initial contact. Vague gastrointestinal symptoms due to vomiting and laxative abuse may be the chief complaint. Weight is usually within normal limits and may fluctuate slightly, but not dramatically (Beresford & Hall, 1989). This condition is characterized by binging and purging (Plehn 1990). A single binge can include 1000 to 25,000 calories; foods selected are usually high carbohydrate junk food and can cost from $8 to $50 per binge (Plehn, 1990). Binges are usually secretive, although family members may report suspicions because of volume of food consumption and frequent trips to bathroom for vomiting and diarrhea. Laxatives are used to purge. Therefore, food becomes the narcotic, and the bulimic needs more and more frequent fixes of greater and greater amounts. Because of the money needed to purchase food and laxatives, the bulimic may steal.

Signs and symptoms that should alert care providers to suspect bulimia are hoarseness, reports of blood in emesis (which may frighten the adolescent into help-seeking behavior), swollen, but nontender parotid glands, and calluses and/or abrasions on the fingers, especially the index and second fingers (Plehn, 1990). Frequent vomiting can also cause conjunctival hemorrhages and broken capillaries on the cheeks. Abdominal bloating from laxative use may also be evident Laboratory studies are likely to indicate electrolyte imbalance, especially low potassium caused by vomiting.

These conditions require careful management. Yates and Sielin (1987) note that pharmacologic treatment is more helpful for bulimia than for anorexia, especially the use of antidepressants (e.g., tricyclates and monoamine oxidase inhibitors). These drugs appear to decrease carbohydrate craving and hence reduce binging. Evaluation for use of antidepressants should also be done for anorexic adolescents because 50 percent of adolescents with both bulimia and anorexia are also depressed (Palmer, 1990).

Inpatient treatment may be necessary under the following circumstances: (a) physical symptoms (e.g., weight loss below 15 percent persistent bradycardia of 50 or more beats per minute, core body temperature of 97°F or lower, or hypotension with a systolic reading less than 90), (b) medical complication, (c) suicide ideation, (d) persistant noncompliance with outpatient treatment, or (e) complete denial of need for help (Palmer, 1990).

Many adolescent women with these conditions can be managed on an outpatient basis, especially with adequate family and social network support. Palmer (1990) recommends use of food contracts in regard to food intake and weight gain for the anorexic. Flexibility in regard to what is eaten depends on the individual. If the adolescent is resistant, Palmer indicates she must be told exactly what to eat. Privileges are given if food intake and weight gain agreements within the contract are met. Regular meetings with a nutritionist are recommended as well as group and individual psychotherapy and support groups. Family therapy may also be necessary.

Abuse Inflicted by Others

Maltreatment of adolescents occurs at rates equal to or exceeding those of younger children (Council on Scientific Affairs, American Medical Association, 1993). Adolescent girls are more frequently reported as victims, especially of sexual abuse, possibly because of consequences (e.g., pregnancy and gynecological problems, and STDs) requiring help seeking. The Council on Scientific Affairs of the American Medical Association also reports that abusive parents of adolescents have a higher than average income and educational level and are less likely to have a parental history of abuse than parents abusing younger children. Further, many homeless, incarcerated, and runaway youth, and those who victimize parents and siblings have had prior maltreatment.

Adolescent girls living in homes with maternal male companions, stepfathers, and stepbrothers are at increased risk for sexual abuse (Clarke, 1986). In the presence of suspicious findings (e.g., pregnancy, STD, or report of sexual activity in adolescent girls), further questioning in regard to family relationships, and supervision by parents of after school activities, dating patterns, and relationships is necessary. If two or more of the following factors are present, sexual abuse may be suspected: reversal of family roles (e.g., adolescent acting as mother), running away, serious rebellion against the parent of the same sex (mother), low self-esteem, frequent psychomatic complaints unrelated to any apparent stressors, parental alcoholism and/or dysfunction, evidence of physical abuse, and STDs and/or pregnancy in very young or mentally/physically impaired teens (Brookman, 1983).

Abuse of all kinds has significant and grim long-term consequences for adolescent women, requiring careful case management and a multidisciplinary approach to care for a prolonged period. The primary care provider is strategically positioned to assess for evidence of abuse and provide initial counseling and referral, and monitor ongoing needs/concerns of the adolescent woman. Physical abuse may be evident from facial bruising and oral injuries or injuries sustained from pushing and falling, marks from beating with belts or other objects, or old scars. Although the adolescent may initially deny abuse, careful questioning in a nonthreatening manner throughout the history and physical examination may yield inconsistencies in the "story." The transitional adolescent is usually the "storyteller," and she has an internal model of what social norms are acceptable. Further, they may feel they deserved the beating, or the perpetrator may have threatened to harm the adolescent if the truth is revealed. Stories are not lies, but attempts to doctor the truth to make it more socially acceptable. Questions such as "What happened here [old scar on knee]?" "How did you get this [bruise on buttocks]?" "Can you tell me about this?" during the physical examination will yield considerable data from any adolescent. Eventually the adolescent may be able to verbalize the type and extent of the abuse as well as revealing the perpetrator and expressing a need for protection. The parent should be informed and assistance should be offered. If the provider feels reporting is necessary, this information should be shared with the adolescent and parent.

Information in regard to abuse is most likely to emerge in the context of caring and trust extended to both the adolescent and the parent or significant other. Establishing this relationship often requires time and more than one contact. Knowledge of community resources and services as well as reporting procedures is essential. In the case of severe physical and/or sexual abuse by a family member, the adolescent may need to be placed immediately outside the home. If the adolescent feels she is in danger as a result of abuse being revealed, this needs to be assessed; at this point, a social worker will need to be involved. Care providers also need to be aware of emergency services such as shelters. Depending on severity of the abuse, inpatient treatment may be necessary.

Sexual assault. In increasingly violent environments, sexual assault is a serious problem that health care providers encounter in caring for adolescent women. Physical injury, risk for acquiring STDs (possibly HIV), and long-term emotional sequelae requiring psychotherapy are probable consequences. Again, prevention is the preferred health promotion strategy. Some clues arise out of recent reports of adolescent sexual assault and acquaintance rape. In examining adolescent sexual assault victims' records at a large metropolitan hospital in Seattle,

Washington, to determine behavioral risk factors preceding the assault, one researcher found that 26 percent of the group were impaired by alcohol or other drugs, and 46 percent of the assaults occurred after social interactions with strangers in unprotected surroundings (Jenny, 1988). The time at which most of the assaults occurred was between 10 p.m. and 4 a.m. Given these statistics, anticipatory guidance would seem to focus on not becoming intoxicated, not talking to strangers, not staying out late, and avoiding isolated locations. However, many of the victims exhibited other risk-taking behaviors so that lifestyle issues and decision making around these issues must be addressed. The immature and transitional thinkers are most at risk in terms of impulsive decision making, and the care provider must use clear, concrete, and compelling examples, and be able to address all questions and oppositional responses with objectivity and appropriate humor.

Prevention of acquaintance rape, another widespread problem among adolescents, particularly the college age group, also necessitates preventive counseling. While this group of adolescent women may be older, chronologically, transitional thinking is frequently used in social and emotional situations involving sexual matters; needs for intimacy, love, and belonging often overwhelm the cognitive capacity the older adolescent possesses to make more logical decisions in matters of personal health. Further, alcohol consumption interferes with appropriate decision making. Questions about partying and drinking patterns are an essential part of the health history for adolescent women, and anticipatory guidance about ensuring safety in the social activities enjoyed by many adolescents should be a standard for all practitioners providing routine health care services to this age group.

Mental Health

Depression/Suicide
The rate of adolescent suicide has dramatically increased, with suicide being the third leading cause of death during adolescence. Incidence of self-reported depressive symptoms for 14–15-year-old girls runs as high as 47.7 percent (Hodgman & McAnarney, 1992). Suicide incidence for females is about one fourth the incidence for males, and females will have more attempts primarily because they tend to use less effective methods (e.g., drug overdose), while males use more violent, self-destructive means (e.g., guns).

The relationship between suicide and depression is not as direct as it might seem; most depressed adolescents are not suicidal, and many suicidal individuals are not depressed, as indicated by Hodgman and McAnarney (1992). Their paper notes that impulsivity is responsible for almost as many suicides as depression, with half of adolescent suicidal behavior occurring after less than 30 minutes of deliberation and one fourth with less than 15 minutes. While the latter is frightening to contemplate, diagnosis and treatment of depression, however, are essential in preventing many adolescent suicides.

Hodgman and McAnarney also indicate that adolescent depression and suicidal behavior, like that in adulthood, are now viewed as lifelong affective disorders on a continuum. Recent findings in regard to brain chemistry have found low levels of biogenic amines (norepinephrine and serotonin) in many forms of depression. These neurochemicals are viewed as essential for transmitting positive affective stimuli. While much remains to be learned, the biochemical basis of depression and suicide may be the same. In addition to biologic factors, situational and health factors triggering depression in adolescent women include loss, pregnancy, physical illness, seasonal and hormonal changes, and chemicals. Further, depression may be accompanied by other disorders covered in this chapter, including eating disorders, substance abuse, attention deficits and learning problems, and conduct disorders. Alcohol may also be a compounding problem in depression because it functions as a self-medication by temporarily increasing serotonin levels in the brain (Hodgman & McAnarney, 1992).

Assessment for depression during routine wellness visits and visits for health problems, both minor and major, is an essential part of the history for the female adolescent. Adolescents are usually in robust health, and when they seek help for any problem, a brief review of how their lives are going (school, relationships with family and friends, dating, partying, changes in sexual activity, etc.) takes only a few minutes, especially if the caregiver has already established a relationship. If a parent is available, verification that there have been no significant mood changes and psychological or physiological stressors can be accomplished.

Symptoms of depression in adolescents often typify normative behaviors expected in this age group: boredom and restlessness that is unabated (normative boredom is transient), persistent somatic symptoms that are often vague but not debilitating, acting out, flight to and from people (alternate between attention seeking and withdrawal), extreme attachment to a pet in the context of withdrawal, insomnia, weight loss/gain, fatigue, school failure, and preoccupation with death (Hodgman & McAnarney, 1992; American Psychiatric Association,

1987). Hodgman and McAnarney (1992) note that acting out behavior in girls is more likely to be self-destructive, that is, running away, becoming pregnant, and doing drugs.

Risk factors (e.g., concurrent problems identified above) and family history become important in weighing the symptoms. Pattern changes are also important. Young adolescents are concrete and may not be able to verbalize their unhappiness, fears, anger, and sadness. Further, stressed adolescents will regress in abilities to verbalize. The presenting symptoms and complaints may seem relatively minor; however, frequent minor complaints over time must be considered a proxy for more serious problems. Fragmentation of care and seeing multiple providers increases the likelihood that behavior patterns may not be identified or treated early.

Several assessment tools that are useful in clinical settings can provide serial objective data. This may be particularly important in that Hodgman and McAnarney (1992) believe that depressive illness and suicidal thoughts in adolescent patients are often overlooked by primary physicians. For at-risk adolescents, this type of data gathering should be a primary care standard. Hodgman and McAnarney (1992, p. 81) suggest an 8-item mood survey. The Beck Depression Inventory–Revised is a 21-item scale that covers a wide range of depressive symptoms including an item reflecting thoughts of suicide (Steer, Scholl, & Beck, 1990). Normative data have been gathered on diverse adolescent populations. A score of greater than 20 is suggested to screen for depression in nonclinical populations. The Center for Epidemiologic Studies of Depression Scale (CES-D; Radloff, 1977) is another scale that is frequently used; a cutoff score of 16 is indicative of depression.

Because of the neurochemical basis of depression, pharmacologic management has become a standard and should be accompanied by mental health counseling and psychotherapy. The primary care provider is responsible for monitoring the efficacy of ongoing treatment with both medication and therapy, therefore knowledge of common side effects of antidepressants and therapy modalities and identification of therapists who work effectively with adolescents and their families so that appropriate referrals can be made is essential. Adolescents who show signs of serious suicidal intent must be hospitalized. Although referral to a psychiatrist in these situations is likely, the availability of this type of care in emergency situations is an important factor; therefore, the primary care provider may be responsible for initiating treatment.

Assessment for suicide potential is much more difficult. Rotheram (1987) discussed problems with current evaluation strategies of suicide risk that have been developed primarily with adult suicide attempters: matching sociodemographics, psychometric assessments, psychological profiles, and identification of specific high-risk groups. Clinicians rely heavily on psychological profiles, particularly in the context of high-risk groups. Intense emotional reactions (e.g., anger), low frustration tolerance, suggestibility, depression, sudden mood elevation, feelings of hopelessness and worthlessness, preoccupation with death, perceiving the concept of death as pleasant or temporary are indicators of increased suicide risk (Rotheram, 1987). Other clues may include giving away possessions; remarks such as, "this will be the last time you see me"; interest in art, music, or literature with death themes; inquiring about the hereafter; accident proneness, carelessness, and death wishes; and chain smoking to relieve tension. At-risk groups include runaways, substance abusers, those with borderline and psychotic conditions, and adolescents with family stressors (e.g., marital strife, severe maternal depression, and family disorganization). In fact, Rotheram indicates that researchers have found up to 78 percent of suicide attempts are precipitated by family fights.

A major problem with these strategies is overestimate of risk. Rotheram (1987) suggests a model similar to that used to predict violence, one of imminent danger. That is, evaluation can be made only in close temporal proximity to the event. This model presents some difficulty for community-based primary care clinicians, however, who may not see their adolescent clients frequently. The psychological profiles and risk groups must continue to guide assessment and intervention. School nurses, teachers, parents (including foster parents), social workers, and school counselors may be better positioned to use the imminent danger model. This model certainly lends credence to the continuing movement to place health professionals delivering primary health care services in school settings.

Conduct disorders

In a survey on Isle of Wight of 10–11-year-old children, boys were reported to have conduct disorders three to four times more frequently than girls. However, prevention and early diagnosis and intervention with young children are the most successful strategies in amelioriating this disorder; therefore, caregivers who work with adolescent women, especially during pregnancy and early parenthood, are in strategic positions to make a difference. In addition, caregivers are likely to provide direct care and/or consultation in a variety of settings where they will come in contact with conduct disordered adolescent females and possibly their children, including detention centers, child psychiatric/mental health facilities, child development centers, day care facilities, and schools.

Gottlieb and Friedman (1991) note that both biological and environmental factors contribute to conduct disorders. The fact that depression, attention deficit disorder, and school/learning problems (specifically dyslexia) occur more frequently in this population suggests a genetic factor.

Assessment includes gathering a comprehensive picture of social, emotional, and cognitive function, in addition to physical appraisal from school, community, and family members, and the adolescent. Past and present history of diagnostic behavior, family function (including early attachment problems), abuse, and criminality should be ascertained. Direct interview of the adolescent is likely to yield an underestimate of the behavioral problems. The Conner's Parent and Teacher Rating Scales (Gayette, Conners, & Ulrich, 1978) and the Child Behavior Checklist (Achenbach & Edelman, 1979) are useful in providing objective data from family and teachers. Mental health referral is often essential as well as intervention to address the dysfunctional parent-child relationship. Other coexisting problems (e.g., depression and learning problems) may require stimulant and antidepressive medication. The long-term prognosis is not good. About half of conduct disordered adolescents continue to have significant social problems in adulthood.

Attention deficits and learning disabilities

Attention deficit hyperactivity disorder (ADHD) is not ameliorated by increasing chronological age. Murphy and Hagerman (1992) indicate that symptoms change with developmental stage. Adolescents tend to be less hyperactive than younger children, but inattentiveness continues and impulsivity increases. These symptoms in turn may diminish school performance, leading to a host of other difficulties often related to impulsivity (e.g., lying, cheating, stealing, social failure [no friends], and delinquency). Evidence that at least some learning disorders affect males to a much greater extent than females has been questioned by more recent studies. In a carefully controlled longitudinal study, Shaywitz, Shaywitz, Fletcher, and Escobar (1990) found that girls were equally affected by reading disabilities, but underidentified and underreferred for special help by schools. Based upon these findings, further research is needed for related disabilities in regard to gender prevalence. Because our society may consider a certain degree of flightiness and scatterbrained behavior as a behavioral norm for females, bias in referral for attentional and related organizational problems may also exist.

Up until a few years ago, use of medications such as methylphenidate (Ritalin) was stopped after childhood because of concerns in regard to growth and addiction to stimulants. It was believed that adolescents "outgrew" their attentional problems to some extent, and no longer needed medication. In addition, medication to increase concentration was prescribed only during school hours. Most pediatricians, child psychiatrists, and other specialists recognize now that these are lifelong disorders, and that ability to concentrate is also important for the learning that occurs during play and social interactions (Hazra, 1989; Kinsbourne, 1992; Mandelkorn, 1993). Adolescents and adults with these problems may need medication for school, work, and leisure activities.

Adolescents with ADHD are at increased risk for accidents, depression, suicide, and other impulsive behaviors that can have catastrophic consequences. These adolescents also need to meet their developmental tasks in regard to independence and vocational selection. Medication may be the difference between a successful, esteem-building work experience and being fired for incompetence and laziness.

Parents and care providers are often concerned about the potential for adolescents with ADHD to abuse their prescribed medications. Education of the adolescent about her medications and necessary precautions (e.g., carrying only needed amounts on trips, and never carrying them to school) are important. Careful parental and provider monitoring of the drugs are also necessary. The ADHD adolescent may over- or underdose his or her medication because of the primary disability, inattentiveness. Parents must be alert to friends who may take advantage of the adolescent. Keeping the medications under lock and key with a small accessible supply is advisable. Ongoing anticipatory guidance by the health care provider in regard to medications can further reinforce the necessity for careful precautions.

Chronic Conditions

Based on evaluation of data from several studies, Gortmaker and Sappenfield (1984) report 10–20 percent of the child population may have chronic health problems. A number of chronic conditions that in the past carried a poor prognosis now have survival rates into young adulthood and beyond. With gene therapy on the horizon, a number of diseases (e.g., cystic fibrosis) may be eventually curable. New and aggressive treatments for several cancers (e.g., some forms of leukemia and Hodgkins lymphoma) provide many youngsters with disease remissions lasting years. Young women with phenylketonuria (PKU) and cystic fibrosis are having children. Added to this group are survivors of birth defects and genetic syndromes who died at young ages a few years ago. Health care providers are faced with assisting these young people and their families to navigate the adolescent period and achieve their developmental tasks at their potential.

To better understand how adolescents with chronic conditions navigate adolescence, once again we need to consider the health problem in a developmental context. First, the nature of the health problem may cause some variation in ability to accomplish important developmental tasks, namely, consolidation of identity, independence from parents, establishment of love objects outside the family, and finding a vocation. For the chronically disabled adolescent woman, the experience of childbearing may be of great importance. The physically disabled adolescent with mental impairments also faces different issues with some tasks than the adolescent with cancer or insulin dependent diabetes.

Elkind (1985) extends his model of cognitive and affective development, specifically the concepts of the imaginary audience and personal fable, in analyzing how disabilities may influence the normative development of thinking processes in adolescence. Further, this model allows for greater generalization across disabilities. Therefore, this section will not focus on information in regard to specific health problems, but on how developmental phenomena unique to adolescence present themselves in the context of chronic problems.

Disabled adolescents and adolescents with chronic illness without cognitive impairments can be expected to achieve the Piagetian stage of formal operations that enables the adolescent to use propositional logic discussed earlier in the chapter. These new abilities can create new problems and disabilities for adolescents (Elkind, 1985). Formal operational thinking allows adolescents to reconstruct their childhood and view it more broadly from a different vantage point. They can consider alternatives to the childhood and parenting they experienced. For example, adolescents who have lost a parent in childhood do not mourn in the adult sense at the time because they do not understand death in the same way as in adolescence. When the adolescent can imagine how childhood may have been different and fully understands the permanence of the loss, true mourning occurs. This line of reasoning can also apply to disabilities. Adolescents with chronic conditions will also reconstruct their childhoods. They can understand what a childhood without a disability would be like and may mourn this loss. Cognitive constructions based upon the imaginary audience and personal fable can further contribute to this withdrawal and depression.

Adolescents are normally preoccupied with changes they are undergoing, and physical and personality shortcomings are magnified. Adolescents with chronic health problems are no exception. They are able to see the extent of their problems as others do for the first time and feel that others, including parents and care providers, have been dishonest with them. The adolescent with a chronic problem can imagine other scenarios and others' thoughts (e.g., assistance and support were available because people pitied her, or that people like her can be a "burden"). At this point withdrawal may occur. These assessments further fuel resentment and anger.

With personal fable factored into the equation ("Well, yes, I have this disease and it can be very serious, but those complications happen to other people, not to me"), denial of the condition and/or complications may occur. Further, a previously cooperative, cheerful girl may become a resentful, sullen adolescent who challenges caregivers, parents, and other significant adults over the management regimen.

As mentioned earlier, these cognitive constructions are at their height during the transitional period. This is also the time during which the adolescent girl is redefining her relationships with her family. For the more immature adolescent, the parent may still maintain some control over health decision making (e.g., appointments and medication administration). The transitional adolescent will demand greater control even when responsibility in consistently adhering to a prescribed regimen is erratic. Helping families avoid power stuggles over management and adherence issues is a major goal for the health care provider. Consulting with other specialists, second opinions, and individual and family psychotherapy are all strategies that may assist the adolescent in facing the limitations of the illness or problem. For example, young women with genetic defects (e.g., cystic fibrosis or PKU) should visit the genetic counselor if childbearing is desired. Open discussions in the presence of parents of what the adolescent can and cannot control in terms of decisions, both legally and ethically, should begin early, preferrably in middle and late childhood. As with sexuality, allowing the child to make decisions when developmentally appropriate, and practicing the decisional process, strengthens communication, which is critical in making the adolescent transition.

The adolescent woman needs to be aware that drinking, smoking, and sexual activity may also increase exposure to infectious diseases and pregnancy, events that may seriously exacerbate the chronic condition. Further issues in regard to childbearing and childrearing may come to the forefront. Depression over inability to master or sustain mastery of developmental tasks (e.g., independence from family and attending college away from home), feeling unattractive and undesirable to the opposite sex because of altered physical appearance, and having limited energy to work at a job are all issues that must be addressed. Family and individual counseling may be helpful in promoting communication and problem solving.

Health Promotion

In health matters, care providers often stress what patients must do to attain an optimal level of health that is generally defined as preventing the preventable (e.g., injuries in auto accidents from failure to wear seat belts) and promoting health (e.g., participating in aerobic exercise three to four times a week and eating a proper diet). Our approach to adolescents frequently is no exception—this is what you the patient must do to avoid STDs, unwanted pregnancy, and catastrophic injuries resulting from poor judgment, etc.

Focus groups were conducted with 160 youth, 10–18 years of age, and 70 parents and grandparents of youth of similar ages in order to identify potential strategies for influencing health-risk behaviors prevalent in adolescence (Public Health Reports, 1993). With the exception of safe sex practices and HIV infection, the young participants were well informed about risky behaviors and their health consequences, but engaged in these behaviors as part of a lifestyle accepted in the high-risk environments in which they lived. Knowledge is not enough to prevent engaging in these behaviors. Needs for love, home, family, and safety were cited as very important. These adolescents said they wanted to talk to someone they could trust, who knew what they were going through.

Therefore, this final commentary will not focus on specific strategies to teach adolescents about smoking, drinking, eating junk food, or having unsafe sex. As Louis Sullivan (1991) indicates, we already have many answers to these concerns. He said it best in a speech at Harvard University. We can no longer continue to blame risking prevalence of STDs, homicides, unintended pregnancies, and drug addiction on lack of research or lack of insights into possible solutions (p. 157). We have met ourselves going in circles on these pages reviewing conditions that possess the same risk factors that Sullivan reiterates: school failure, lack of family support and guidance, early initiation of deviant behavior, and inability to resist peer influences. He further stresses that about one in four youth "do it all," and therefore may not ever become mature, functional adults (p. 157). This includes adolescent women and their children for whom we care. The following are a few suggestions to guide care for adolescent women.

Providing Individual Care to the Adolescent Woman

Many health care providers are not comfortable providing individual services to adolescent women. Health care visits continue to be threatening for most adolescents, particularly if they anticipate a gynecological examination. In addition, interpersonal behavior of many immature and transitional adolescent women may not be particularly reinforcing for the care provider. The immature adolescent girl may refuse eye contact, squirm, and give the caregiver limited feedback in regard to responses to questions. "I don't know," and monosyllable answers are typical. The transitional adolescent woman may cover her anxiety by sullen responses, volunteering little information, especially in response to questions that she finds embarrassing (e.g., those dealing with sexuality). Another typical response of the transitional adolescent female is dramatic. This adolescent may project a very mature demeanor, but the behaviors described do not reflect mature judgment or actions. We have labeled this *pseudomaturity* (Strauss & Clarke, 1992). The caregiver who is not experienced in working with adolescents may initially assess a greater degree of maturity than actually present and develop a management plan that will be largely unsuccessful. The more mature adolescent woman is able to seek and act on information. Achieving this often requires persistent patience and consistency (repeating the facts), and support to the adolescent and parents through the immature and transitional phases.

Assessment and management of complex, multifaceted problems experienced by adolescent women require development and use of holistic models to guide practice. These models must incorporate integration of cultural, psychosocial, and biological theories. Skills in interviewing, listening, and counseling in sensitive areas are crucial for those working with adolescents. Complete histories may take more than one visit. All risk factors must be covered in the history. Sexual activity should be discussed toward the end of the interview in a nonthreatening manner.

The adolescent should be carefully prepared for the physical examination. The young adolescent may wish the mother to remain in the room. If major problems have not been identified in the history that require private discussion with the adolescent during the physical exam, the mother should stay. This is a good time to review stages of physical maturation and inquire further about friendships and parental limits, parental discussions of pubertal changes, dating, intercourse, and family habits (e.g., smoking and alcohol consumption). Breast self-examination can be demonstrated during the examination.

The transitional adolescent also needs to be carefully prepared for the physical examination. If the adolescent is sexually active and gynecological problems or pregnancy are suggested from the history, then a pelvic examination must be performed. Preparation should include both procedural as well as sensation information.

Time should be spent with the adolescent alone, the parent alone, and the adolescent and parent together. This requires more time than many caregivers spend in routine health visits.

Providing Community Care to the Adolescent Woman

Sullivan (1991) cited research that gives us important information about what works best:

1. One-to-one individual attention. A responsible, invested adult in every young person's life is essential. This can be a parent, teacher, counselor, or health care provider, or another adult who is able to care what happens.

2. Involvement of parents. Home visiting disadvantaged parents and assisting them with management of day-to-day problems with childrearing and monitoring family well being has proved efficacious.

3. Focus on schools. Young women need to acquire the basic skills. Pregnancy is cited as the main reason young women drop out of school. Setting up completion programs that offer job and social skill training and providing on-site child care may help many young women become employable. Comprehensive programs that include social and mental health services, after school child care, and primary health care should be developed.

4. Community involvement in developing comprehensive solutions to complex problems. Multiple agencies need to develop collaborative goals and plans, and pool resources where appropriate.

These recommendations require that health professionals not only provide individual services to adolescents and their families, but play an advocacy role in the community in development of comprehensive approaches to the new morbidities. They must talk about their experiences and expertise in caring. Participation in the development of integrated programs designed to address high-risk behaviors and practice decision making, specifically in regard to early sexual activity, drinking, smoking, drug use, and other potentially dangerous behaviors that arise out of impulsivity, is essential.

The best hope lies in individualizing programs at the community level. This permits programs to be appropriately adapted given health beliefs of the target group and the community. Cultural considerations and values of rural Iowa and urban areas of the Northeast, or the more homogeneous church group as opposed to a more diverse group in a school setting, could then be better accommodated. Such flexibility also allows high-risk behaviors that may be somewhat unique to the community to be addressed. Implementation in homes, school, church, youth groups, and other settings should begin at school age (at the latest). Workshops for parents and children together would be a first step to improving communication and providing settings where innovative approaches intrinsically appealing to young people could be implemented.

Puberty as Passage

The transition from girlhood to womanhood, like other life transitions, has the potential for both large gains and crippling losses. The young teen may, through trial and error in a safe setting, grow into an enriched sense of personhood that includes validation of female physical, emotional, and social self. Such a young woman would have the knowledge to recognize the limitations of gender-based societal expectations, the assurance to set her own goals, and the coping skills and energy to attack barriers.

At the other end of the spectrum is the young girl who lacks support for emotional growth and development, and experiences the transition to adulthood as a series of losses—of freedom and opportunity, self-esteem, and self-confidence. This is the young person at greatest risk for ill health.

The work of health care professionals, as defined within the medical model, has focused almost exclusively on adolescent reproductive issues—prevention of sexually transmitted disease and unwanted teen pregnancy—with both health care and social welfare policy aimed almost exclusively at control of adolescent behavior. This approach simply does not work, and is not in the best interests of either adolescents or society. If the goal of adolescent health care can be shifted from control to successful passage to a *full* womanhood, the individual, her family, and her community will be better served.

References

Achenbach, T. M., & Edelbrock, C. S. (1979). The child behavior profile: II, boys aged 12–16 and girls aged 6–11 and 12–16. *Journal of Consulting Clinical Psychology, 47,* 223–233.

American Psychiatric Association. (1987). *Diagnostic and statistical manual of mental disorders* (3rd ed., rev.). Washington, DC: Author.

Beresford, T. P., & Hall, R. C. W. (1989). Food and drug abuse: The contrasts and comparisons of eating disorders and alcoholism. *Psychiatric Medicine, 7*(3), 37–45.

Brookman, R. R. (1983). Adolescent sexuality and related health problems. In A. Hofmann (Ed.), *Adolescent medicine* (pp. 238–287). Menlo Park, CA: Addison-Wesley.

Brooks-Gunn, J. (1988). Antecedents and consequences of variations in girls' maturational timing. *Journal of Adolescent Health Care, 9,* 1–9.

Brooks-Gunn, J., & Furstenberg, F. F. (1989). Adolescent sexual behavior. *American Psychologist, 44,* 249–257.

Centers for Disease Control and Prevention. (1990). Premarital sexual experience among adolescent women, United States, 1970–1988. *MMWR, 39,* 929–932.

Centers for Disease Control and Prevention. (1991). Update: Acquired immunodeficiency syndrome—United States, 1981–1990. *MMWR, 40,* 358–363.

Clarke, B. A. (1986). Adolescent women. In J. W. Griffith-Kenney. *Contemporary women's health: A nursing advocacy approach* (pp. 208–277). Menlo Park, CA: Addison-Wesley.

Clarke, B. A. (1993). *Nursing role supplementation for adolescent mothers: Final report.* Bethesda, MD: National Institute for Nursing Research, National Institutes of Health.

Clarke, B. A., Strauss, S. S., Munton, M., Fleming, B., & Kish, C. (1994). Effects of nursing role supplementation on adolescent parent-child adaptation. Unpublished manuscript.

Council on Scientific Affairs, American Medical Association. (1993). Adolescents as victims of family violence. *Journal of the American Medical Association, 270,* 1850–56.

Danza, R. (1983). Menarche: Its effects on mother-daughter and father-daughter interactions. In S. Golub (Ed.), *Menarche.* New York: Lexington Books.

Doan, R., & Morse, J. (1985). The last taboo: Roadblocks to researching menarche. *Health Care for Women International. 6,* 277–283.

Elkind, D. (1984). Teenage thinking: Implications for health care. *Pediatric Nursing, 10,* 383–385.

Elkind, D. (1985). Cognitive development and adolescent disabilities. *Journal of Adolescent Health Care, 6,* 84–89.

Erikson, E. H. (1968). *Identity: Youth and crisis.* New York: W. W. Norton.

Faust, M. S. (1960). Developmental maturity as a determinant of the prestige of adolescent girls. *Child Development, 31,* 173–184.

Faust, M. S. (1983). Alternative construction of adolescent growth. In J. Brooks-Gunn & A. Petersen (Eds.), *Girls at puberty.* New York: Plenum Press.

Fogel, C. I., & Woods, N. F. (1995). *Women's health care: A comprehensive handbook.* Thousand Oaks, CA: Sage Publications.

Fuerst, M. L. (1991). An STD primer. *American Health, 10,* 45–46.

Gayette, H., Conners, C. K., & Ulrich, R. F. (1978). Normative data on the revised Conner's Parent and Teacher Rating Scales. *Journal of Abnormal Child Psychology, 6,* 221–236.

Gilligan, C. (1982). *In a different voice: Psychological theory and women's development.* Cambridge, MA: Harvard University Press.

Gortmaker, S. L., & Sappenfield, W. (1984). Chronic childhood disorder: Prevalence and impact. *Pediatric Clinica of North America, 31,* 3–17.

Gottlieb, S. E., & Friedman, S. B. (1991). Conduct disorders in children and adolescents. *Pediatrics in Review, 12,* 218–222.

Grahn, J. (1993). *Blood, bread and roses: How menstruation created the world.* Boston: Beacon Press.

Greene, J. W., Sandler, H. M., Altemeier, W. A., & O'Connor, S. M. (1981). Child-rearing attitudes, observed behavior, and perception of infant temperament in adolescent versus older mothers. *Pediatric Research, 15,* 442.

Hazra, M. (1989). Attention deficit disorder. *Bear in mind. Children's Hospital Newsletter, 6*(7), 1–2.

Hersch, P. (1991). Sexually transmitted diseases are ravaging our children: Teen epidemic. *American Health, 10,* May, 42–45.

Hodgman, C. H., & McAnarney, E. R. (1992). Adolescent depression and suicide: Rising problems. *Hospital Practice, 27,* 73–96.

Hofferth, S. L., & Hayes, C. D. (Eds.). (1987). *Risking the future: Adolescent sexuality, pregnancy and childbearing.* Washington, DC: National Academy Press.

Holden, G. W., Newson, P. B., Velasquez, J., & Ritchie, K. L. (1993). Cognitive, psychosocial, and reported sexual behavior differences between pregnant and nonpregnant adolescents. *Adolescence, 28,* 557–72.

Jenny, C. (1988). Adolescent risk-taking behavior and the occurrence of sexual assault. *American Journal of Diseases of Children, 142,* 770–772.

Kinsbourne, M. (1992). Quality of life in children with ADHD. *Challenge, 6,* 1–2.

Klein, J., & Litt, I. F. (1983). Menarche and dysmenorrhea. In J. Brooks-Gunn & A. Petersen (Eds.), *Girls at puberty.* New York: Plenum Press.

Litt, I. F. (1990). *Evaluation of the adolescent patient.* Philadelphia: Hanley & Belfus.

Logan, D., Calder, J., & Cohen, B. (1980). Toward a contemporary tradition for menarche. *Journal of Youth and Adolescence, 9,* 263–269.

Mandelkorn, T. D. (1993). Thoughts on the medical treatment of ADHD. *The CH.A.D.D.ER Box, 6*(3), 1, 7–9.

Maryland Department of Health & Mental Hygiene. (1982). *Drug Abuse Administration 1982 survey of drug abuse among Maryland adolescents: Report on alcohol use.* Annapolis, MD: Author.

Mercer, R. T. (1983). Assessing and counseling teenage mothers during the perinatal period. *Nursing Clinics of North America, 18,* 293–301.

Murphy, M. A., & Hagerman, R. J. (1992). Attention deficit hyperactivity disorder in children. *Journal of Pediatric Health Care, 6,* 2–11.

Muuss, R. E. (1975). *Theories of adolescence* (3rd ed.). New York: Random House.

Muuss, R. E. (1988). Carol Gilligan's theory of sex differences in the development of moral reasoning during adolescence. *Adolescence, 89,* 229–243.

National Institute on Drug Abuse. (1990, February). *1989 National high school senior drug abuse survey.* Press release. Washington, DC.

Neinstein, (1991). *Adolescent Health Care: A practical guide* (2nd ed.). Baltimore: Urban & Schwarzenberg, pp. 121–129.

Nelms, B. C. (1981). What is a normal adolescent? *American Journal of Maternal Child Nursing, 6,* 402–406.

Newcomb, M. D., Maddahian, E., & Bentler, P. M. (1986). Risk factors for drug use among adolescents: Concurrent and longitudinal analyses. *American Journal of Public Health, 76,* 525–531.

Osofsky, H. J., & Osofsky, J. D. (1970). Adolescents as mothers: Results of a program for low-income pregnant teenagers with some emphasis upon infants' development. *American Journal of Orthopsychiatry, 40,* 825–834.

O'Sullivan, A. L., & Jacobsen, B. S. (1992). A randomized trial of a health care program for first-time adolescent mothers and their infants. *Nursing Research, 41,* 210–215.

Palmer, T. A. (1990). Anorexia nervosa, bulimia nervosa: Causal theories and treatment. *Nurse Practitioner, 15,* 13–18, 21.

Plehn, K. W. (1990). Anorexia nervosa and bulimia: Incidence and diagnosis. *Nurse Practitioner, 15,* 24–25, 28, 31.

Public Health Reports. (1993). Designing health promotion approaches to high-risk adolescents through formative research with youth and parents. *Public Health Reports, 108 Suppl 1,* 68–77.

Radloff, L. (1977). The CES-D Scale: A self report depression scale for research in the general population. *Journal of Applied Psychological Measurement, 1,* 385–401.

Redwine, D. B. (1987). The distribution of endometriosis in the pelvis by age group and fertility. *Fertility and Sterility, 47,* 173.

Reirdan, J., & Koff, E. (1990). Premenarchal predictors of the experience of menarche: A prospective study. *Journal of Adolescent Health Care, 11,* 404–407.

Resnick, M. D., Beringer, L. H., Stark, P., & Blum, R. W. (1994). Patterns of consultation among adolescent minors obtaining an abortion. *American Journal of Orthopsychiatry, 64,* 310–316.

Rotheram, M. J. (1987). Evaluation of imminent danger for suicide among youth. *American Journal of Orthopsychiatry, 57,* 102–110.

Schumacher, K. L., & Meleis, A. (1994). Transitions: A central concept in nursing. *Image, 26,* 119–127.

Shaywitz, S. E., Shaywitz, B. A., Fletcher, J. M., & Escobar, M. D. (1990). Prevalence of reading disability in boys and girls: Results of the Connecticut Longitudinal Study. *Journal of the American Medical Association, 264,* 998–1002.

Slap, G. S. (1986). Normal physiological and psychosocial growth in the adolescent. *Journal of Adolescent Health Care, 7,* 13S–23S.

Smith, L. (1983). Incorporating the adolescent and her infant into the family. *Advances in Nursing Science, 6*(1), 45–60.

Steer, R. A., Scholl, T. O., & Beck, A. T. (1990). Revised Beck Depression Inventory scores of inner-city adolescents: Pre- and postpartum. *Psychological Reports, 66,* 315–320.

Strauss, S. S., & Clarke, B. A. (1992). Decision-making patterns in adolescent mothers. *Image, 24,* 69–74.

Tanner, J. M. (1962). *Growth at adolescence* (2nd ed.). Blackwell, England: Oxford.

Vaughn, V. C., & Litt, I. R. (1990). *Child and adolescent development: Clinical implications.* Philadelphia: W. B. Saunders.

Waldron, I., Lye, D., & Brandon, A. (1991). Gender differences in teenage smoking. *Women's Health, 17,* 65–90.

Werner, M. J. (1991). Adolescent substance abuse: Risk factors and prevention strategies. National Center of Education in Maternal and Child Health, Maternal and Child Health Bureau, Maternal Child Health Technical Bulletin. Washington, DC (1–11).

Yates, W. R., & Sieleni, B. (1987). Anorexia and bulimia. *Primary Care, 14,* 737–744.

Zabin, L. S., & Clarke, S. D., Jr. (1981). Why they delay: A study of teenage family planning clinical patients. *Family Planning Perspectives, 13,* 205–217.

Zuckerman, D. M., Colby, A., Wave, N. C., & Lazerson, J. S. (1986). The prevalence of bulimia among college students. *American Journal of Public Health, 76,* 1135–1137.

Recommended Resources for Further Information

Books

Litt, I. (1990). *Evaluation of the adolescent patient.* Philadelphia: Hanley and Belfus. [St. Louis: Mosby].

Litt, I. (1983). Menstrual problems during adolescence. *Pediatric Review, 4,* 203.

Audiovisual

Clarke, B. A. (1982). *Making growing groovy* [Series of 6 videotapes]. (Available from B. A. Clarke, Virginia Commonwealth University, PO Box 980567, Richmond, VA 23298-0567).

Munton, M., Clarke, B., Fleming, B., & Strauss, S. (1993). *How to know what to do* [Videotape]. (Available from B. A. Clarke, Virginia Commonwealth University, PO Box 980567, Richmond VA 23298-0567).

Strauss, S. S., & Clarke, B. A. (1993). *Adolescent decision-making inventory* [Videotape]. (Available from B. A. Clarke, Virginia Commonwealth University, PO Box 980567, Richmond, VA 23298-0567).

7

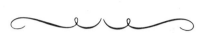

The Reproductive Years

Ellen Olshansky

Women's health is often discussed synonymously with reproductive health, and those years of a woman's life have historically been the focus of women's health, reflecting a societal value of women primarily for their (re)productive capacities. While this chapter focuses on the reproductive years of women's lives, it is with the belief and understanding that these years are only a piece of the *whole* of women's health and that, in fact, the reproductive years consist of more than the physiologic status of women's reproductive organs. Hence, this chapter examines the physical, psychosocial, and lifestyle dimensions that affect women systemically as well as those that result in reproductive conditions and disorders. In this chapter, the term *reproductive years* refers to the time span from the beginning of adolescence/puberty until the beginning of the perimenopausal years. Issues specific to adolescence and perimenopause are covered in other chapters.

The Physical Dimension: Meeting the Challenge for Health Maintenance

Physical health maintenance for women during the reproductive years consists of many factors. Specifically, nutrition, exercise, monitoring/ assessing physiological conditions, and treating problems early (preventive health care) highlight important issues in physical health maintenance. Many of these specific issues are addressed in a later section of this chapter. For now, the important points to emphasize are that women can best meet the challenge for health maintenance when the social context and sociopolitical factors are conducive to their doing so. That is, women can optimally maintain their health when they do not simultaneously have to confront racism, sexism, and classism, but instead have equal access to health care, to economic stability, and to other needed resources. The reality of most women's lives, however, occurs within a context of multiple physical demands and high energy emotional requirements related to work/career, pregnancy, parenting, and single parenting especially.

The Psychosocial Domain: Continuing Emotional Growth as an Adult

The psychosocial domain of women's health has recently received increased attention. Carol Gilligan (1982), Nancy Chodorow (1978), and Jean Baker Miller (1986), as well as Belenky, Clinchy, Goldberger, and Tarule (1986) are but a few of the scholars who are addressing women's psychosocial development in a new way. Prior to this work, the "accepted" developmental milestones for women were merely extrapolated from work on men and applied to women. Erik Erickson's (1950) eight developmental stages, based on a male model for maturation, were almost universally accepted as the norm against which to evaluate women's psychological development. "Normal" in this sense included autonomy and individuation with much less regard for developing relationships (other than a marital relationship). The newer work on women's development has revealed a new definition of *normal*, one in which the relational aspects of women's lives are emphasized. The presentation of the psychosocial developmental issues that follow are clearly informed by these newer works on women's development.

Accepting Responsibility

Women's traditional location of their responsibility has been in the home, nurturing children and husband, as well as parents. This remains a large part of women's responsibility, and the term "sandwich generation" is very apropos in describing women who simultaneously care for children and aging parents, often at very great emotional and economic cost (McBride, 1988). In addition, it is usually women who are the caretakers for aging spouses. While providing for family in terms of financial contribution has been less frequently emphasized as a significant part of women's roles, in truth many women have always had and met this responsibility. Single-parent families headed by women are not an invention of the late 20th century. Many women continued to work after marriage, but because their work was uncounted (take-home piece work), unrecorded for tax purposes (maids and nannies), or unacknowledged (work in the fields and stables on family farms), a myth was propagated of the stay-at-home wife and mother whose work was nonproductive in economic terms. Black women from antebellum days onward have been counted on to provide financially for their families (Hooks, 1982). And during wartime, while men were away at the front, women were encouraged by the "Rosie the Riveter" poster campaign to take over traditional male occupations, only to be dismissed from these positions when the war ended and the men returned. Thus, the concept of responsibility for women encompasses a great diversity that has not been reflected in traditional (patriarchal) views of women's roles.

A different way of conceptualizing the degree to which women accept responsibility, and thus the degree to which they have reached a particular level of psychosocial development, is to understand individual women's lives within their individual social context. For some women, life circumstances are so difficult that even food and shelter loom as impossible goals. A battered, homeless woman, by seeking assistance from a shelter for herself and her children, can be conceptualized to be accepting a high degree of responsibility. Thus, it is difficult, if not impossible, to generalize about what reflects acceptance of responsibility among mature women.

The following two vignettes represent very different situations and circumstances, but both represent a high level of responsibility:

A 30-year-old woman, living with her mother, her alcoholic husband, her two teenage children, and her 6-month-old grandchild, is receiving financial assistance from the federal government for the care of her children. She has had difficulty holding down a job as a house cleaner because she has had to stay home to care for her sick daughter (the mother of her grandchild) as well as for her ailing mother. Despite many obstacles, she has been able to provide balanced meals for the family as well as a clean, though crowded, home.

A 45-year-old woman, living with her husband, a successful lawyer, and her two children, ages 5 and 8, works part time at a local museum.

In her spare time, she volunteers for community activities and serves on the board of her children's private school.

Work and Career Identity

Similar to the concept of accepting responsibility, women have had varying experiences with careers and the extent to which they incorporate careers as part of their identity. Many women have developed very productive careers later in life, after they have met their traditional family responsibilities (Heilbrun, 1988). Other women have been precluded from developing careers as a result of the pressure of other responsibilities, or because of sexism and/or racism within the larger society. Class inequalities among women have given rise to semantic differences: unemployment versus work versus career are words that reflect a continuum of women's experiences around issues of "career identity." Some women are unemployed because of difficulty finding work, while others are unemployed by choice and may even be "independently wealthy." Some women refer to their jobs as "work," and others refer to their jobs as "careers" and as part of their professional identity. The meanings and perceptions of these various descriptors are important to understand in order to appreciate the range of women's experiences in this arena.

However women define themselves, there is no question that more women enter the formal work force now, and contrary to past patterns, stay there for most of their lives (see Figure 7-1), with no diminution of their traditional responsibilities (see Figure 7-2). More than 75 percent of all married female physicians, for example, perform all of their household work. In addition to providing the bulk of caretaking for their children, many working women also provide unpaid long-term care for their parents (at an average of 26 hours a week). The opportunity costs these women pay in loss of income and slowed career advancement have implications for their own old age in lost Social Security benefits and pensions. The loss in burnout and time for personal relationships and emotional growth is incalculable.

Recent media attention on the "superwoman" has contributed to a notion among women that this is the goal to which all women should aspire. Health care providers must be wary of the implications of such perceptions, for the superwoman image eludes most women in reality, as many women struggle to make ends meet and live at a very different end of the spectrum from the "You've come a long way, baby" media image of the highly successful, professionally dressed woman

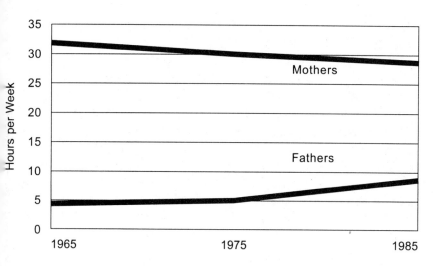

FIGURE 7-1   Trends in Housework Time by Parents of Preschoolers, 1965–1985
Data from: Moen (1992)

with two children, a husband, a dog, a cat, a large house, and a high-pressured corporate executive job.

For others, fertility issues confound career trajectories (Olshansky, 1987b) as infertility represents a confrontation with one's ability to achieve the "superwoman" image. Women may put careers on hold as they focus on trying to achieve pregnancy. When pregnancy does

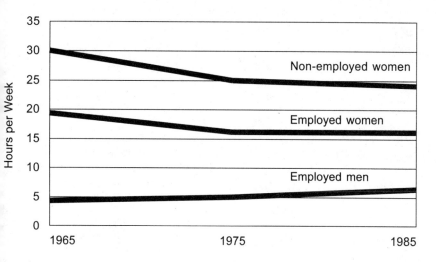

FIGURE 7-2   Housework Time by Gender, 1965–1985
Data from: Moen (1992)

not occur, they often see themselves as failures in motherhood as well as in their professional lives.

Another issue confronting women who work is systematic discrimination based on perceived dangers to their unconceived fetuses. Susan Falludi (1991) describes the incidence and prevalence of fetal protection policies which may serve to systematically limit women's access to those occupations which were traditionally male. While women have challenged these laws, the suits have been long and expensive, and the victories have not always included the restoration of actual and potential lost wages. The benchmark case was brought by the United Autoworkers' Union against Johnson Controls, Inc. It was not until the appeal in this case reached the level of the United States Supreme Court that the discriminatory nature of fetal protection policies was adjudicated.

Marriage and Enduring Relationships

Marriage has always been viewed as a normal developmental stage for women and men, though men who did not marry were not shunned as were the women who were deemed to be "old maids." The term *bachelor* for single men has not had the same negative connotation. From a feminist perspective, we can expand our definition of enduring relationships to include marriage as one kind of intimate relationship, but not inclusive of all forms of intimate relationships. Lesbian relationships strong friendships, nonmarital heterosexual relationships are all enduring relationships that include a certain degree of intimacy. In fact, the newer psychological literature on women's development (Belenky et al. 1986; Chodorow, 1978; Gilligan, 1982; Miller, 1986) emphasizes the strong need among women for connection with others in their lives. Connection refers to many and varied relationships.

The concept of "alternative families" must be incorporated into our understanding of women's lives. Society is currently in transition moving toward an acceptance of such families. With acceptance must come a change in nomenclature; it would be better to eliminate the term *alternative* because of its connotation of being compared to *normal*. Table 7-1 summarizes various family configurations.

Relationships with Parents: Negotiating Equality/Egality

As a woman matures throughout the years from puberty through menopause, her relationship with her parents undergoes change. O

TABLE 7-1 Various Family Configurations

Couple	two persons who live together; heterosexual or homosexual, or two persons who are not in a sexual relationship; married or unmarried; with child(ren) or without child(ren)
Single person	with child(ren) or without child(ren)
Extended family	group of related persons, often multigenerational, living together
Group living	group of related or nonrelated persons living together
Divorced couple	without child(ren); with joint custody of child(ren) or with only one parent with custody

course, not all women have parents who are living, or with whom they communicate, during these years of their lives. For those women who do, however, these changing relationships are significant to their psychosocial development.

These are the years when lesbian women often accept and validate their orientation, and must decide how best to negotiate acceptance of their identity and lifestyle by parents. Risks of rejection must be balanced against the benefits of enhanced self-esteem and freedom from the weight and discomfort of deception. The emotional upheaval often associated with "coming out" in that most vulnerable area of the parent-daughter relationship may manifest itself somatically. The health care provider who is culturally sensitive will probe gently for information about the connections between homophobia-induced life stress and current health status.

For all women, changing relationships with parents may occur along a trajectory of increasing and ongoing entanglement on the one hand, or enrichment on the other hand. These two ends of the continuum are very different from one another. Enmeshment includes lack of differentiation from family of origin, whereas enrichment includes encouragement of individual potential among members of a family while those members continue to have a strong family identity that does not threaten their individual identities. Adult women may mirror their family of origin or may break away from it to varying degrees. Their own identity development as mother or wife/partner may be similar to or distinct from that of their own mothers.

Significant changes that occur as women develop adult relationships with their own parents include several key factors. Many families experience a loss of connection as family members move away (mobility in our society has increased tremendously), as the nuclear family is less emphasized for some, and as there is more isolation for some family members. Many adult women begin to take on the role of parenting their own parents as their parents age, become disabled, and become more dependent. This shifting of roles is a significant developmental stage for women who take on this parenting role for both their own parents and their children (sandwich generation).

The Decision to Parent

The decision to parent is significant in women's psychosocial development, particularly as it is not always a decision. Women become pregnant despite their desire to prevent conception and often give birth despite their desire to abort. On the other end of the continuum, women are infertile and, despite seeking all means available to them to assist in conception, they remain infertile.

Even for those women who have no difficulty in becoming pregnant if they so choose, the decision to parent is fraught with much ambivalence. Some women describe how they have grown up with the idea that motherhood is what they "should" achieve. With changing societal mores, they now perceive that they have other choices that they had not previously considered, creating some ambivalence for them. Other women describe how they have grown up with the notion that they never wanted to become mothers, and now, as adults, feel criticized by many for what is considered to be a "selfish" decision.

For lesbian women, the choice to parent is complex, because of negative social attitudes and lack of legal and social recognition for lesbian families. The lesbian couple who approach a physician with a request for artificial insemination may be faced with homophobia or refusal to include the partner as an equal participant. Couples who shun the medical system and make their own arrangements for a donor may encounter legal risk, and may not have adequate protection against transmission of infection. In the HIV era, informal arrangements may be life threatening. Because lesbian marriage is not legally recognized in most states, attention must be paid up front to protecting the custody rights of the nongestating parent. In addition, cost of associated health care may be a problem, because insurance coverage may not be available under family benefits. Health care for women of reproductive age must be broadened to include the needs of the lesbian couple. Information should be provided about all available alternatives, from artificial insemination to adoption. Referral for counseling, if offered, should be to counselors who are informed about the specific issues to be weighed and who are also culturally competent.

From a feminist perspective, it is important to understand the social factors that contribute to women's perceptions of parenting and to assist individual women and their families to make those decisions that are best for them. The concept of *choice* as an underlying philosophy of feminism must be extended to the choice to parent or not. On one end of the continuum there is the lesbian woman who is pressed about birth control use or never offered information about alternatives for family building. On the other end there is the woman who chooses not to parent, and is made to feel abnormal or unnurturing. The health care practitioner who works with women needs to cultivate a professional self-presentation that goes beyond mere acceptance of difference to a mind set that permits celebration of diversity.

Common Health Problems

This section of the chapter addresses some of the common health problems encountered by women. The controversies around diagnosis and treatment of these common problems are discussed.

Systemic Illness

Cardiac Disease

Women have been thought to be practically immune from cardiac disease because estrogen is cardioprotective. While estrogen does have protective effects, it is far from accurate to state that premenopausal women are not at risk for cardiac disease, because they experience significant risk later in life (see Chapter 8). Preventive efforts in the middle years are particularly important because prevention of heart disease is accomplished through lifestyle changes. Patterns of good nutrition, regular exercise, and stress reduction can take many years to establish, and are best initiated as part of a lifetime orientation toward wellness, not a response to crisis. Specific risk factors include family history, smoking, obesity, sedentary lifestyle, elevated total cholesterol and low-density lipoprotein (LDL) to high-density lipoprotein (HDL) ratios, hypertension, and type A personality (Phipps, Long, Woods, & Cassmeyer, 1991).

Autoimmune Diseases

Two autoimmune diseases that affect a significant number of women are lupus erythematosus (LE) and multiple sclerosis (MS). Both of these conditions are chronic, having major lasting effects on the health of women. Lupus erythematosus is a disorder of the connective tissue that is believed to be caused by anti-DNA antibodies. Symptoms include swollen and tender joints, fever, malaise, and weight loss, as well as facial erythema and scalp hair loss. LE is more common in women and, in particular, in Black women (Dalton, 1990).

Multiple sclerosis is a chronic inflammatory condition, with consequent demyelination and scarring. It is believed to be caused by a virus that occurs in persons who are genetically susceptible (Hauser, 1994). Symptoms include weakness, tingling, numbness, and pain. These two diseases are examples of chronic conditions that have major and long-lasting effects on women's lives. As efforts continue to be made toward learning more about these diseases and their treatment, more effort must be directed toward assisting women to live with these diseases.

Arthritis

Arthritis heads the list of chronic diseases for women, and represents a major source of disability in later life. The reproductive years are often the time for emergence of the most crippling form of arthritis, rheumatoid disease. The pressures of raising children and assisting one's own older parents that characterize this period of life make it a very difficult time to learn to adjust to disability and the prospect of future limitations. Although symptoms of osteoarthritis do not usually begin before age 50, prevention must begin in the reproductive years, with avoidance of trauma, obesity, and joint stress, particularly joint problems related to occupational activity.

Occupational Injury and Illness

The World Health Organization (WHO) International Classification of Disease (ICD) codes were expanded in 1991 to include 64 diagnoses related to occupation (Mullan & Murthy, 1991). Clerical, sales, and service occupations, in which a majority of women are employed, all stress the musculoskeletal system, and may contribute to later-life arthritis. Other occupations such as cosmetology, nursing, textile and garment work, housekeeping, and laundry are associated with exposure to chemicals, irritants, and pathogens. Sexual harassment on the job, associated with stress-induced illnesses and depression, is experienced by 42–88 percent of working women (Levy & Wegman, 1988).

Working women who are, or desire to become, pregnant face many decisions. Our current knowledge about reproductive hazards in the workplace comes mainly from research performed on animals. Paul (1993) provides a comprehensive approach to occupational and environmental hazards to reproduction and suggests strategies for employers, health care providers, and policymakers.

Keleher (1991) suggests a three-factor evaluation focusing on the woman, the pregnancy, and the job. The results of this evaluation may suggest one of three courses of action. The first conclusion may be that all factors are normal, and the woman may continue in her current employment without modification. In a second scenario, the woman, the specific pregnancy, or the job has a characteristic that increases the risk, and this characteristic should be modified. The third scenario, which occurs in a minority of instances, is when the woman or the pregnancy precludes work, such as in the instance of preterm labor or uncontrolled diabetes mellitus.

Cancer

Cancer in women is a major health issue. In particular, breast cancer, lung cancer, cervical cancer, ovarian cancer, Hodgkin's and non-Hodgkin's lymphoma, skin cancer, and colon cancer present significant threats to the health of women. Table 7-2 includes the risks for women, according to age, of the major cancers. Only recently have the National Institutes of Health devoted money to the study of cancers of women, and required that women be included as subjects in clinical trials of new treatments. The recent Women's Health Initiative is a start in this area.

Breast cancer has received considerable attention within the last several years, particularly as the incidence has been rising, with the latest figure estimated at about one in nine women being diagnosed with breast cancer yearly. Yet until recently, scientific efforts have been haphazard at best. While research indicates that radical mastectomy is not always the best approach, many breast surgeons continue to recommend such procedures and do not offer the available alternatives (Love, 1990).

The example of breast cancer demonstrates the need for a higher level of research funding for diagnosis and treatment and health policy research for conditions that affect women. The controversies and ambiguities surrounding guidelines for and interpretation of mammograms, and political divisiveness regarding health insurance coverage for routine mammograms both highlight the need for more exploration. In particular, women would like to understand why the incidence of breast cancer is increasing, and begin to be able to pinpoint the contribution of environmental agents to this disease. Identification of a breast cancer

TABLE 7-2   Risk Factors for Major Cancers in Women

Lung cancer	cigarette smoking; environmental carcinogens; lung scarring and chronic interstitial fibrosis
Breast cancer	older age; menses beginning at or before 12 years old; menopause occurring at or after 55 years old; first full-term pregnancy at 30 years old or older; no pregnancies; family history of breast cancer
Cervical cancer	early incidence of first sexual intercourse; increased number of sexual partners; presence of human papillomavirus (certain types)
Ovarian cancer	nulliparous; history of infertility, endometriosis, and possible long-term use of ovulation-inducing drugs; more commonly occurs in age range of 40 to 65; family history of ovarian cancer
Colon cancer	family history of colon cancer; age 40 and over; low-fiber, high-fat diet
Skin cancer	fair skin pigmentation; history of sun exposure; history of genetic diseases that include low tolerance to sunlight; environmental exposures
Endometrial cancer	age 50 to 70; nulliparous; obese; presence of high blood pressure and/or diabetes; late onset of menopause; unopposed estrogen replacement therapy

risk gene has made possible the evolution of a clinical test for risk, but at best this development will affect only 5 percent of breast cancers, because the rest appear to be multifactorial. There are no primary prevention techniques available, only less than optimal secondary prevention techniques—clinical breast exam, coupled with mammography, which half the women at highest risk do not receive regularly, and self-exam, which is often practiced inconsistently and inaccurately (Hall, Adams & Stein, 1980).

Infections

Women are susceptible to many different kinds of infections. This section focuses on sexually transmitted diseases (STDs), human immunodeficiency virus (HIV) and acquired immuno deficiency syndrome (AIDS), and urinary tract infections (UTIs). STDs are summarized in Table 7-3. These infections are all preventable, but are prevalent within our society. The long-term consequences for women include sterility

TABLE 7-3 Summary of Sexually Transmitted Diseases

Type of STD	Treatment	Complications if Untreated
Gonorrhea	antibiotics; sexual abstinence until treated	cervicitis, salpingitis, urethritis
Chlamydia	antibiotics; sexual abstinence until treated	cervicitis, urethritis, bartholinitis
Pelvic inflammatory disease	antibiotics; remove IUD if present; bedrest; sexual abstinence until treated	infertility
Mucopurulent cervicitis	antibiotics; sexual abstinence until treated	endometritis, salpingitis
Bacterial vaginosis	metronidazole; antibiotics	PID postinstrumentation, postpartum, postsurgery
Trichomonal vaginitis	metronidazole	unknown
Candida vulvovaginitis	antifungal agents	not always transmitted sexually, but can be; complications unknown
Genital herpes	antiviral therapy (palliative); sexual abstinence during presence of active lesions	primary episodes may cause spontaneous abortion, neonatal herpes; premature birth; C-sections advised only if active lesions present in cervix or lower genital tract
Human papillomavirus	palliative treatment with liquid nitrogen, trichloroacetic acid, podophyllin, laser therapy	genital epithelial neoplasia; may cause anogenital or laryngeal papillomatosis in neonate
Syphilis	antibiotics	transmission to neonate; neurological disorders

infertility, chronic pain, and often self-esteem problems. STDs are discussed in detail in a later section of this chapter.

HIV and AIDS are receiving increasing attention as a critical risk to the health of women. Early in the developing knowledge of the AIDS epidemic, women were thought to be at no risk or minimal risk for what was considered to be the "gay disease." As we have learned more about this virus, we have begun to see it as an equal opportunity infection. In light of this knowledge, it is now apparent that we must target research toward women and HIV/AIDS. Women present with particular symptoms that are often different from those with which men present. For example, chronic vaginal yeast infections in women may be a symptom of HIV infection. With improved treatment of HIV infection with the drug AZT, many HIV-positive women are giving birth to HIV-negative babies, but the risk to infants of the virus crossing the placental barrier and the risk to the mother of exacerbating the progress of the HIV infection during pregnancy continue to be profound. More women must be included in drug trials as well as in general research about HIV/AIDS.

UTIs are the cause of about 6 million visits to health care providers in the United States each year, mostly among women of childbearing age. UTIs are rare in men under age 50. The most common cause of UTIs is gram negative bacilli, mostly *E. coli*. Overdistention of the bladder (commonly caused by infrequent voiding), mechanical introduction of bacteria during intercourse, and tampon and diaphragm use are predisposing factors. Pregnancy also increases susceptibility, as does clothing that fits tightly or is made of fabrics that permit moisture to accumulate, causing bacteria to proliferate.

Reproductive Disorders

In an ovulatory or egg-producing cycle, neurotransmitters produced by the arcuate nucleus at the base of the brain stimulate release of gonadotropin-releasing hormone (GnRH). The pituitary gland (the source of follicle-stimulating hormone [FSH] and luteinizing hormone [LH]) and the egg chamber in the ovary (the source of estradiol and progesterone) work together in elaborate synchrony with the uterine lining to orchestrate the events of the menstrual cycle, or adaptation to pregnancy if conception occurs. Figure 7-3 relates the events occurring within the ovary (on top) temporally with the endometrial lining of the uterus (in the middle) and the hormonal events (at the bottom) that result in both ovarian and uterine changes.

Ovarian Cycle

Folicular Phase   Ovulation   Luteal Phase

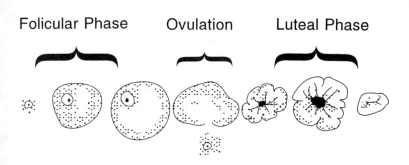

Endometrial Cycle

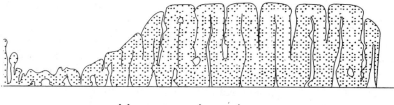

Hormone Levels

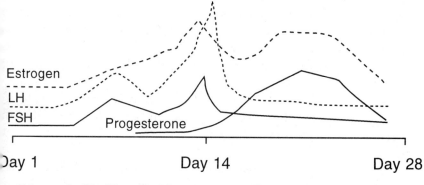

Estrogen

LH

FSH   Progesterone

Day 1   Day 14   Day 28

[Menses]   [Proliferative Phase]   [Secretory Phase   ]

FIGURE 7-3

Contraception

Because the large majority of contraceptive methods are used by women as opposed to men, it is crucial that health care providers understand the implications to women of the various methods available. Table 7-4 includes a summary of the various methods, side effects, costs, and contraindications of each method. From a feminist perspective, it is important to recognize that not all methods are available to all women, and that some methods, in fact, are encouraged for certain women (e.g., third world women are the ones on whom experimentation occurs). Table 7-5 illustrates use patterns among women of reproductive age, and Table 7-6 indicates the risk of failure for different methods. Oral contraceptives are most commonly used, and have the lowest failure rates at all ages, regardless of socioeconomic status.

Infertility

Infertility is medically defined as the lack of conception after at least 1 year of trying to conceive. From a nursing perspective, however, the medical definition is not necessarily the most meaningful to the women who are experiencing infertility. For some women, 3 months without conception is worrisome, particularly if the woman is 42 years old and has had several miscarriages. It is estimated that about 20 percent of couples in the United States experience infertility. This statistic does not reflect the infertility rates among unmarried women, nor is it clear how these statistics were obtained. Many women are not in heterosexual relationships, though they may want children. These women can be referred to as being "situationally infertile" by virtue of the situation of not having a male sexual partner (either by choice or by circumstance). Thus commonly presented statistics may minimize the true prevalence of infertility.

Most infertility can be diagnosed and treated with low-level technology (see Table 7-6). Success rates depend on age, the number of infertility disorders present, and the seriousness of the specific diagnosis (Garner, 1991).

Infertility is very distressing for many women, and often becomes their central identity as they become immersed in the work of trying to overcome infertility (Olshansky, 1987a). With the advent of assisted reproductive technology (ART), the work of fertility is prolonged as individuals and couples find it difficult to stop treatment when newer treatments are constantly being discovered (Olshansky, 1988). From a feminist perspective, however, these newer treatments can represent potential exploitation of women, and they highlight the inequities in

TABLE 7-4   Summary of Contraceptive Methods

Type	Benefits	Side Effects	Contraindications
Spermicides	no systemic side effects; nonoxynol 9 may have some protection against STDs; can buy over the counter	possible allergic reactions	allergic reactions; unreliable in using (low user effectiveness)
Condoms	possible prevention against STDs, particularly HIV; no systemic side effects; can buy over the counter	possible allergic reaction to latex	allergic reactions; unreliable in using (low user effectiveness)
Diaphragm and jelly/foam	no systemic side effects; nonoxynol 9 may have some protection against STDs	possible bladder irritation and UTIs; possible allergic reaction to jelly/foam	recurrent UTIs; allergic reaction to jelly/foam; unreliable in using (low user effectiveness)
Cervical cap	no systemic side effects; may be left in place for 48 hours without re-applying spermicide; may be able to fit a woman who cannot wear a diaphragm	possible allergic reaction to jelly/foam	cannot be worn during menses; may be difficult to insert; may be associated with cervical dysplasia; unreliable in using (low user effectiveness)
Contraceptive sponge	no systemic side effects; can buy over the counter	possible bladder irritation; possible allergic reaction	unreliable in using (low user effectiveness)
Oral contraceptives	very reliable/effective; sex can be spontaneous; may be protective against endometriosis and ovarian cancer	many potential systemic side effects	history of cardio-vascular problems; hypertension; smoking
Intrauterine device	very reliable/effective; sex can be spontaneous	some IUDs associated with pelvic inflammatory disease	PID
Norplant	reliable; sex can be spontaneous; contraceptive effects last for several years	various potential side effects to the hormone; changes in bleeding pattern; pain at insertion site	if desire pregnancy soon; long-acting
Depo provera	reliable; sex can be spontaneous	various potential side effects to the hormone; irregular bleeding; weight gain	if desire pregnancy soon; long-acting

TABLE 7-5   Use of Contraceptive Methods, Women Age 14–44 (in percentages)

Age	Female Sterilization	Male Sterilization	Pill	Diaphragm	Condom	IUD
15–19	2	0	59	1	33	0
20–24	5	2	68	4	15	0
25–29	17	6	45	6	16	1
30–34	33	14	22	9	12	3
35–39	45	20	5	8	12	3
40–44	51	22	3	4	11	4
Total	28	12	31	6	15	2

Data from: Mosher, W. D. (1990). Contraceptive practice in the United States, 1982–1988. *Family Planning Perspectives, 22*(5), 198–205.

access to care between upper- and upper-middle-class women versus lower-class women, for whom the expense of such treatment is prohibitive. However, denial of access to these treatments also poses the very important feminist issues of reproductive choice and allocation of resources. Table 7-7 includes a summary of the newest assisted treatments for infertility.

A feminist critique of the infertility literature includes an understanding of how infertility has traditionally been portrayed as a woman's problem, particularly as related to a woman's psychological ambivalence or failure of desire for pregnancy (Sandelowski, 1990). It is critical that health care providers appreciate the profound effect of the social views of infertility upon both women and men.

Unwanted Pregnancy

Over a million and a half pregnancies (30 percent of all pregnancies) end in abortion each year. Unwanted pregnancy is the other end of the continuum of infertility. From a feminist perspective, it is the concept of choice that unites both ends of this continuum. Women should have the right to make reproductive decisions, whether these decisions are reflected in access to infertility care or access to contraception and abortion. The social context has a major impact on this decision. Since the *Roe v. Wade* Supreme Court decision in 1973 that legalized abortion, controversy continues in the political arena. The recent wave of violence, witnessed by shooting deaths of physicians and staff who provided abortions to women, has heightened the controversy and has instilled fear in some health care providers who might consider offering abortion services to women. At present only 12 percent of residency

TABLE 7-6 Types of Contraceptive Failure (in percent): First Year by Age,
Marital, and Poverty Status, 1988

	Condom	Diaphragm	Abstinence	Spermicide	Pill
unmarried:					
(<200% poverty)					
age: <20	27.3	37.3	51.7	49.8	12.9
20–24	31.1	27	57.3	55.4	15
25–29	27	36.9	*	49.4	12.8
30+	20.8	*	*	39.6	9.6
(200% and over)					
<20	13.2	*	27.5	26.3	5.9
20–24	15.2	21.4	31.4	30	6.9
25–29	13	18.4	27.2	26	5.9
30+	2.8	14	*	*	4.4
married:					
(200% poverty)					
<20	51.3	*	*	*	26.8
20–24	29.3	39.8	54.7	52.8	14
25–29	19	26.6	38.3	36.7	8.8
30+	13.8	19.5	28.7	27.5	6.2
(200% and over)					
<20	*	*	*	*	12.9
20–24	14.2	20.1	29.5	28.2	64
25–29	8.9	12.8	19.2	18.3	4
30+	6.4	9.1	13.9	13.2	2.8

*insufficient data

Data from: Jones, E. F., & Forrest, J. D. (1992). Contraceptive failure rates based on the
1988 NFSG. *Family Planning Perspectives, 24*(1), 12–19.

programs provide training in abortion techniques, although the Residency Review Committee that oversees all training programs in obstetrics and gynecology has recently made abortion skills a mandatory part of the gynecology curriculum. Lack of services, problems of transportation to available services, and high out-of-pocket costs combine to reduce the availability of safe abortion.

TABLE 7-7   Newest Assisted Reproductive Technology Treatments

Abbreviation	Long Title	Description
IVF	in vitro fertilization	sperm retrieved by man through masturbation; eggs retrieved surgically; fertilization in petri dish; embryo(s) placed in uterus through cervix
GIFT	gamete intrafallopian transfer	sperm and eggs retrieved as in IVF, but then placed in fallopian tubes for fertilization to occur
ZIFT	zygote intrafallopian transfer	sperm and eggs retrieved as in IVF; fertilization in petri dish; zygote placed in fallopian tube
SUZI	subzonal insertion of sperm by micro-injection	sperm and eggs retrieved as in IVF; sperm injected directly into egg
ICZI	intracytoplasmic sperm injection	as SUZI, but only a single sperm is directly injected into egg

Premenstrual Syndrome: A Double-Edged Sword

Premenstrual Syndrome (PMS) is a somewhat vague diagnosis that has gained attention in recent years (Mitchell, 1991). The technical definition is that of a continuum of symptoms ranging from mild breast tenderness to severe uterine pain to suicidal ideation, with these symptoms reaching their peak of severity during the premenses (approximately the six days prior to actual beginning of menses) and reaching their nadir during the postmenses (approximately the 6 days after menstrual flow has ceased). The most accurate method of diagnosing this syndrome is in retrospect, after a woman has maintained a daily symptom log over at least a 2-month period. PMS is present if a pattern is detected that links symptoms with the timing of the menstrual cycle.

The recognition of PMS as an actual entity that women experience has created a "double-edged sword" for women. On the one hand, women's complaints have become recognized as "legitimate" rather than all in their head or due to hysterical reactions. This legitimation has resulted in serious attention paid to learning how best to relieve these complaints. On the other hand, however, this syndrome

TABLE 7-8   Symptoms of PMS

Symptoms may be very different for each individual woman, and the degree to which symptoms are experienced may vary as well. The key factor in diagnosing PMS is that the symptoms occur cyclically, with severity of symptoms high just before menses and falling with the onset of menses. The following are common symptoms experienced by different women.

irritability	bloating
tension	abdominal pain
anxiety	painful/tender breasts
mood changes	headache
sleep changes	backache
changes in sexual desire	swelling of hands and/or feet
increased cold sensitivity	difficulty concentrating
food cravings	hot flashes/sweats

has, at times, been used as a way of discriminating against women's effectiveness and ability. The diagnosis of "late luteal phase dysphoria" was recently debated as a possible addition to the recent edition of the *Diagnostic and Statistical Manual* (1994), the book referred to by mental health professionals when determining psychiatric diagnoses. While some may argue that this diagnosis offers legitimacy to women's complaints (much like the diagnosis of "postpartum depression"), the danger in this diagnosis is the potential for exploitation of women based on how the diagnosis could be used. Table 7-8 contains a list of symptoms of PMS, and Table 7-9 contains a list of common treatments.

Pregnancy Complications and Loss

Pregnancy presents a woman with multifaceted experiences. For many women, pregnancy is a welcome condition that is associated with long-awaited joy and anticipation. For others, pregnancy is unwelcome, depending upon particular circumstances. The physical aspects of pregnancy can be quite benign for many women, who view and experience their pregnancies as a normal part of life and who do not suffer from complications of pregnancy. Other women, however, experience complications from pregnancy that range from nuisances to disruptions to major threats to health. The scope of these problems lends itself to an entire text on this issue. For the purposes of this book, the major point to emphasize is that pregnancy, while a normal process that is experienced by many women, can also be a time of complications that can lead to serious physical problems. In addition, psychosocial problems may become manifest as a direct result of, or associated with, or coincidental to, a pregnancy. From a feminist perspective, it is essential

TABLE 7-9   Common Treatments for PMS

It is important to treat each woman individually, following up by assessing how well a particular intervention is working, and modifying the treatment if necessary. The following are suggested treatment approaches:

high–complex carbohydrate and high-fiber diet
decreased (or no) caffeine
decreased sugar
decreased alcohol
vitamin B6, 50 to 100 mg per day
calcium, 1.0 G per day
high-potency multivitamin and mineral per day
stress reduction (relaxation techniques such as meditation, taking time for self)
aerobic exercise at least 4 timers per week
regular sleep, approximately 7 to 8 hours per night

that each pregnant woman is viewed as an individual with individual experiences and perceptions of her pregnancy.

Pregnancy has become medicalized within our society. Before physicians routinely attended at births, it was common practice for midwives to do so. The basis of their practice was care and nurture for a person, not treatment of a disease. The woman was an active participant in her child's birth. However, with the increasing medicalization of pregnancy, and the professionalization of attendants, childbirth itself became an illness, and the pregnant woman a passive host from whom the baby was to be taken/delivered. In the 1950s, women were put to sleep—the ultimate in passivity—with a combination of drugs that included a hypnotic, a narcotic, and an amnesiac called scopolamine; women suffered intense pain in labor, but experienced total amnesia. If women were not grateful, they were certainly supposed to be. In the 1970s, in the midst of the women's consciousness raising movement, a quiet revolution began. Women demanded choice about where and how they would deliver, and insisted on being fully participant. Courses were developed for childbirth preparation, and women were once again encouraged to nurse their babies. Women requested the right to walk during labor, without being tied down, the right to push in the second stage of labor from a more natural and physiologically rational sitting position, and the right to share the birth experience with a loved one of their choice (Ehrenreich & English, 1973; Martin, 1987). Consumerism has been a major pressure behind recent research that rethinks the value of routine ultrasound and routine fetal monitoring. Although it is not clear at the present time what barriers professional midwifery must overcome in order to strengthen their place in the health care system and be able to grow and develop, given competition between physicians and nurses and impending changes in the structure of health care insurance, the contribution that nurse midwives have made to childbirth has been enormous.

Women with serious complications of pregnancy, however, undoubtedly benefit from medical intervention. In this category, of course, belong diabetes, hypertension, exacerbation of cardiac disease, preeclampsia, premature labor and prematurity, postmaturity, and small-for-gestational-weight (SGA) fetuses. There have been some notable successes—the almost complete elimination of Rh disease and development of medications to stop premature labor—and some stubborn failures—inability to reduce prematurity rates or prevent preeclampsia, for example. Yet basic prenatal care is not available early in pregnancy to everyone in our society, and the United States still ranks behind 19 other industrialized nations in perinatal mortality.

Pregnancy loss is also a significant problem for women. It is estimated that approximately 50 percent of pregnancies end in spontaneous abortion (miscarriage) (Speroff, Glass, & Kase, 1994). This number is higher than most people know, because many spontaneous abortions occur before a woman has missed a menstrual period. Causes of reproductive loss include genetic abnormalities, hormonal problems, and anatomical problems. Often, however, the cause is unknown. Many women describe feeling somewhat "dismissed" by others regarding their feelings of loss related to miscarriage, particularly when others view such a loss as intangible and abstract. The women themselves, however, often experience a profound loss and need time to grieve (Swanson-Kauffman, 1986).

Endometriosis

Endometriosis is another women's condition that, similar to PMS, is a chronic progressive and elusive condition. The diagnosis of endometriosis refers to the abnormal growth of endometrial tissue within the pelvic area, on or near the ovaries, within the fallopian tubes, on the bladder, or disseminated to other parts of the body, even as far as the lung, where it can cause spontaneous pneumothorax or lung puncture. This condition causes severe pain for women, but it is asymptomatic in others, and the degree of pain does not correlate well with the severity of the disease. Endometriosis is also a major cause of infertility. The treatment for it, ironically, is pregnancy, because the suppression of ovulation associated with pregnancy retards growth of endometriomas (blood-filled growths or implants), which grow under the influence of ovulatory hormones. Other treatments consist of

TABLE 7-10   Treatments for Endometriosis

Treatments	Side Effects
Oral contraceptives (high progestin)	thrombosis, cardiovascular effects
Danocrine	androgenic side effects, such as hair growth
GnRh agonists	possible bone loss
Surgery	normal risks of surgery
Prostaglandin inhibitors	palliative relief only

danocrine, an androgenic hormone, oral contraceptives, or monthly injections of GnRh agonist, all of which suppress ovulation and, therefore, suppress the growth of the endometriomal implants. Table 7-10 contains a list of the treatments and their side effects.

Endometriosis is important to understand from a feminist perspective because it is a major cause of pelvic pain in women. Women often seek health care because of their pelvic pain, and often, because such pelvic pain is misunderstood, they are dismissed with the notion that the pain is "all in your head." Women report that often others do not understand their pain (Boston Women's Health Collective, 1992). Or, on the other hand, they are often treated medically in extreme ways such as total hysterectomy, when in fact such major surgery is no longer warranted to treat the underlying cause of the pelvic pain (Boston Women's Health Collective, 1992). It is usually the women with greater privilege (upper class, Caucasian) who also are aware of greater choices available regarding treatments, and more able to demand the expensive investigation (diagnostic laparoscopy) that is required in most cases to make the diagnosis.

Dysfunctional Uterine Bleeding

Dysfunctional uterine bleeding (DUB) is sometimes a vague and catchall diagnosis for any kind of irregular uterine bleeding without a specific physiological cause attributed to it. However, the physiological cause is not always as elusive as it appears, in that this irregular bleeding is usually due to a change in the hormonal balance, creating a state of anovulation. Over several months of anovulation, the lining of the uterus (endometrium) builds up, but because there is no (or little) progesterone to oppose the estrogen, this lining is not shed monthly (as in a regular menstrual cycle). The result is that this continuous build-up of endometrial tissue eventually must be shed, and this usually manifests itself as very heavy bleeding on a very irregular basis.

Women on birth control pills may experience breakthrough bleeding, which may or may not be considered significant (often this depends upon the woman's own perception of the bleeding). The treatment for DUB is usually hormonal manipulation (progesterone to induce withdrawal bleeding and then resume a normal menstrual cycle) or in cases of extreme bleeding that does not respond to medical therapy, dilatation and curettage.

Lifestyle-Related Disorders

Sexually Transmitted Diseases

Sexually transmitted diseases (STDs) represent a major health threat to both men and women. Sexually transmitted diseases can be categorized according to vaginal infections (mainly bacterial vaginosis and trichomonas), viral infections (herpes, human papilloma virus, and syphilis), and pelvic infections (chlamydia and gonorrhea). In addition, the human immunodeficiency virus (HIV) is the newest epidemic to be transmitted sexually.

Efforts to eradicate STDs have been aimed at education regarding how these diseases are transmitted, in the hopes that with knowledge persons will change their behaviors. This has worked to some extent, but it certainly does not encompass all the many and complex issues around prevention of STDs. It is essential that health care providers understand the motivations behind women's sometimes unhealthy lifestyle choices. When women have been socialized to believe that they are not complete adults without being in an intimate relationship with a man, it is not difficult to understand why many women continue to risk their health (i.e., through exposure to STDs) so that they can engage in heterosexual relationships in the hope that they will develop a long-term relationship with a man. As practitioners, we need to understand better the psychosocial foundations for women's behaviors, especially self-destructive behaviors, and learn to communicate empathy, develop relationships of trust, and refrain from criticizing or creating self-criticism.

Substance Abuse

Substance abuse refers to the continued ingestion of psychoactive substances, despite one's awareness of the problems and risks related to such ingestion. The primary substances involved include alcohol, sedatives, cannabis (marijuana), and cocaine, among others (Harris

& Seimer, 1994). Several theories exist regarding the etiology of substance abuse; among them are factors related to gender, age, race, physiology, and genetics (Harris & Seimer, 1994). Treatment involves some form of counseling, and often medication with its inherent side effects and risks. An understanding of the woman's perception of why she abuses substances as well as an understanding of her social context and how that context likely contributes to such abuse is essential. Often medical literature portrays substance-abusing women as morally inferior to others. This is particularly so in the case of substance-abusing pregnant women because of the often dire effects of such abuse on the developing fetus. While this is a complicated and complex issue, a feminist perspective includes an understanding of the circumstances of a woman's life, as these circumstances have influenced her substance abuse behavior. Kearney (1993) provides poignant perspectives of crack-abusing mothers who struggle with their substance abuse while wanting to provide a loving, nurturing home to their infants. Superimposed on the complexity and often lack of understanding of women's circumstances that may lead to substance abuse is the lack of treatment facilities for women, particularly facilities that address family and child care needs while specifically providing treatment for substance abuse. Effective substance abuse treatment must address the myriad issues confronting women in their daily lives.

Abuse and Self-Abuse

Violence against women is a major health problem, with most violent acts being performed by intimates (domestic violence). Such violence crosses all ethnic and class lines. Research has shown that the stereotypical image of the kinds of women who are abused is unfounded (Pagelow, 1992). Violence can occur in the form of physical and/or emotional abuse. Rape and incest are common in United States society—no one knows exactly how common—and can impair a woman's self-respect and ability to develop relationships of intimacy throughout her life span.

As with women substance abusers, women who are victims of violent abuse by others, especially domestic abuse, are often blamed for the abuse, and the women often blame themselves. A feminist perspective of this situation includes understanding and appreciating the woman's social context and the meaning that the relationship, albeit an abusive relationship, has to her (Landenburger, 1989).

Abuse of self is often related to abuse by others in that a cycle of violence seems to exist in which women who have been abused begin to see themselves as lacking self-worth, and they may, in turn, be abusive to themselves (physically and/or emotionally). Suicide is a significant health hazard to women, as this is closely related to depression, a condition for which women are at increased risk.

Stress, Role Strain, and Coping

The primary stressor of women during the midlife years is the loss of relationships and relationship potential through death, divorce, geographic moves, and loss of friendship networks because of competing demands on time. Cook (1985) found that women aged 35–44 are especially vulnerable to both somatic and psychological symptoms. Another stressor, which is also a limiting factor on relationships, is the increase in female participation in the labor force (see Figure 7-1). The largest increase since 1960 is among those women likely to have competing responsibilities to children and parents.

Stress is pervasive in the lives of many persons, and women experience stress in many ways. Stress may result from the constant strain of juggling multiple roles (McBride, 1988), or from constantly striving for goals that are blocked by barriers. Many women believe that they are expected to perform as "superwomen," conjuring the image of a breathless woman, briefcase in one hand, child in the other hand, running to a meeting via the day care center to drop her child off, working a full day, doing all her housework until every surface gleams, spending "quality time" with children, and still being interested in sex at bedtime. Figures 7-2 and 7-3 provide the data to back up such a picture of very little assistance with tasks that fall into the domain of the traditional role.

Such an image, while perhaps accurate for some women, has an underlying message that is detrimental to many women, because most women, while experiencing this much stress and strain, have not been able to attain the beautiful appearance, beautiful career, beautiful house, and perfect children portrayed in the superwoman image. Aspiring to this unrealistic image causes even more distress and role strain, and may contribute to ill health (Baruch & Barnett, 1986). Some women adapt, learn to limit role expectations and demands, and find that multiple roles can bring multiple benefits and enrichment (Froberg, Gjerdingen, & Preston, 1986). Both flexible hours and social support appear to be key factors in coping (Norbeck & Resnick, 1986; Pugliesi, 1988). In *Women's Two Roles*, Moen (1992) describes working women according to four categories: the captives, the conflicted, the copers, and the committed, and sets them on a continuum that corresponds to degree of life satisfaction:

Captive	Conflicted	Coping	Committed

least satisfied .... most satisfied

The literature on employed women indicates that, overall, employed women describe the most satisfaction and the fewest symptoms of illness (Jennings, Mazaik, & McKinley, 1984).

Nutrition

Women's nutrition has received increasing attention in recent years due to the recognition that eating disorders are much more prevalent in women than they are in men. Specifically, anorexia nervosa and bulimia pose particular problems for women, especially in the early reproductive years. These conditions are discussed in more detail later in the chapter, with emphasis on prevention of such conditions. However, even in the absence of an actual diagnosis of an eating disorder, many women have subclinical eating disorders, such as compulsive overeating, compulsive dieting, and less severe disorders such as iron-deficiency anemia or calcium deficiency.

Women's nutritional problems, and in particular the prevalence of eating disorders among women, have been analyzed from a feminist perspective. Chernin (1981, 1985) describes what she refers to as the "tyranny of slenderness" that profoundly influences women to become obsessed with dieting and to achieve an unrealistically thin and unhealthy body. Eating disorders in women represent women's confrontation with a profound contradiction in their lives: trying to meet the social image of women as slender (or even "skinny") while simultaneously trying to meet the health needs of mature women who require a certain amount of fat to maintain a healthy estrogen level.

Psychiatric Illness

Mood Disorders: Unipolar and Bipolar

Unipolar mood disorder refers to depression without the reverse or other end of the continuum, which is mania. Bipolar mood disorder refers to manic depression. Depression in women is pervasive, with considerable controversy regarding its causes or explanations. Theoretical beliefs about depression can be categorized according to psychodynamic, cognitive, interpersonal, and biochemical explanations. Recent feminist literature has suggested that women's depression may be explained by women's constant suppression of their authentic selves, usually for the sake of maintaining a relationship with a male partner/ spouse (Jack, 1991; Miller, 1986). Women's voices and women's authenticity have been negated and/or suppressed within the social context of patriarchy. For many women, sadness that is unattended to becomes transformed into clinical depression. Which theoretical notion, or combination thereof, to which a health care professional ascribes regarding the cause of depression directs the choice of treatment. Treatment can consist of various kinds of psychotherapy, from psychodynamic to cognitive to behavioral, in combination with or without antidepressant medication. Some professionals prescribe antidepressants without concurrent psychotherapy, though the prevailing belief is that antidepressants work best in combination with psychotherapy. Again, this is dependent upon the theoretical beliefs of the therapist.

Personality Disorders
Persons who have what is considered a very rigid or maladaptive organization of attitudes, beliefs, values, and patterns of adaptation may fall within the category of personality disorders (Godfrey, 1991). Three main clusters of personality disorders exist, as follows: (a) odd and eccentric, (b) dramatic and emotional, and (c) anxiety and fear based. Such a diagnosis must be clearly understood, and the reasons for determining such a diagnosis as well as the implications of the diagnosis for each individual woman must be carefully considered.

Schizophrenia
Schizophrenia is a very complicated diagnosis that includes several different types. It includes severe deterioration in personality, affect, and intellectual functioning, and this deterioration is often irreversible (Lohr, 1991). Schizophrenia is a condition of both men and women. The relevance for women, however, often is related to the fact that social and gender issues may contribute to both the onset and the treatment of this disorder.

Psychosis
Psychosis refers to psychotic disorders which include disorders that are not classified elsewhere, including brief reactive psychosis, schizoaffective disorder, induced psychotic disorder, and schizophreniform disorder. In addition, a fifth category includes psychotic disorders that do not meet the criteria for any of the four above-mentioned categories or disorders for which not enough information exists to make a specific diagnosis (Whitley, 1991). Here again, as in schizophrenia, psychosis

is a condition of both men and women, but particular social and gender issues for women may contribute to women being diagnosed with such disorders, as well as to the way such disorders are treated in women.

Health Promotion and Illness Prevention

From a nursing perspective, it is appropriate to emphasize health promotion for women. From a feminist perspective, the women's health movement of the 1960s, as part of the second wave of the women's movement, succeeded in encouraging women to engage in self-help and to learn about their bodies and how to promote optimum health. The Boston Women's Health Collective, which produced *Our Bodies, Ourselves* and triggered an entire self-help movement, was instrumental in this process. Thus, a chapter on women's health during the reproductive years would not be complete without attention to health promotion and illness prevention.

While certain illnesses, diseases, and conditions occur because of a genetic predisposition to them or because of other risk factors that cannot be reversed, most conditions are exacerbated or ameliorated by certain lifestyle changes. It is in this arena that practitioners, health educators, health services researchers, and public health specialists can assist women to make changes that result in better health outcomes.

Nutrition

In the interests of approaching women's nutrition from a health promotion perspective, the thrust of this section is on how to encourage optimum nutrition for women. A low-fat, low-cholesterol, high-fiber diet is the optimal diet for most people. It is believed that this kind of diet may prevent heart disease and some forms of cancer, such as colon cancer. The American Heart Association recommends that one should eat a diet composed of no more than 30 percent fat, with saturated fats being reduced as much as possible. Recently, others (Ornish, 1990) have advocated a diet even lower than 30 percent fat (closer to 10 to 20 percent), and this issue is currently being debated.

True obesity (as measured by age-related weight ranges, not ideal weights) is a major contributor to illness in the United States, playing a role in gallbladder disease, cardiovascular disease, diabetes, arthritis, reproductive disorders, and possibly some cancers. Genetic inheritance and learned behaviors are both involved.

Many women are attracted to the various diet programs that are offered commercially. While these programs usually are successful in assisting women to lose weight, they have been found to be unsuccessful in achieving maintained weight loss for about 95 percent of persons. Regular physical activity and permanent alteration of eating habits are the only proven methods of weight reduction.

Exercise

Exercise for women has received increasing attention as more and more women are becoming and staying physically active. However, much of the attention in this area is directed toward women who excel in physical arenas, such as marathon runners, body builders, and Olympic Games participants. Often this media attention sets up a model to which women aspire and then, more often than not, which they fail to achieve. In the interests of women's health, health care providers need to encourage their women clients to exercise in moderation, achieving cardiovascular and optimum weight maintenance through aerobic exercise. Such exercise includes 20 minutes of sustained increased cardiac output (within the training range) at least three times a week. This is sufficient to increase blood flow—and nutrient and oxygen delivery—to muscles and skin. Exercise depletes glycogen stores (the muscle nutrient "warehouse"), but stimulates enzyme activity to replenish glycogen levels, and contributes to maintenance of bone density. Exercise may also aid in the release of natural neuroendocrine mood elevators such as beta endorphins. Steptoe, Edwards, Moses, and Mathews (1989) were able to demonstrate that women who had elevated anxiety and depression scores on psychometric testing returned to normal levels after getting involved in programs of moderate but regular exercise.

Exercise is important during pregnancy, assuming no risk factors exist that contraindicate the safety of exercise. The current recommendations regarding exercise during pregnancy are that pregnant women should continue routine physical activity that does not have inherent risks (such as skydiving, that has a risk of falling; or high-altitude climbing, that has a risk of low oxygen consumption). In fact, pregnant women who have not exercised previously are advised to take up mild to moderate exercise in the form of walking regularly (Hancock, Olshansky, Abrums, & McCarthy, 1994).

Exercise is particularly important in reducing risk factors for cardiovascular disease. The majority of research on cardiovascular disease and risk factors has been on males, with much of the findings from that research extrapolated to females. Because women are believed to be protected from cardiovascular disease because of estrogen, most women of reproductive age are considered to be at low risk for heart attacks. Unfortunately, this belief often leads to the omission by health care providers of teaching women how to reduce their risks. The fact that women experience a decrease in estrogen during the menopausal transition and beyond is evidence enough that women need to make lifestyle changes before that time, because lifestyle changes are successful only if they occur over time. In addition, it is incorrect to believe that cardiovascular disease is not a concern for women during their reproductive years. Cardiac mortality in males has decreased so significantly, and women's stress and cigarette consumption have increased so significantly that women now exceed men in risk for cardiac events. The value of exercise in diminishing the ratio of the LDL to HDL cholesterol fraction cannot be underestimated.

Stress Reduction

Stress is a pervasive problem in our fast-moving society. Women, especially, are prone to stress due to overload of responsibilities and expectations. In recent years, programs of stress reduction have been developed. These programs include techniques such as biofeedback, meditation, exercise, massage, and psychotherapy. While many of these programs are very effective, individual women must be encouraged to choose the program(s) with which they feel most comfortable.

Smoking Cessation

Lung cancer, the major cause of cancer death in women, has been found to be caused by smoking in about 95 percent of cases. The issues surrounding women and smoking are complex. Historically, when women began to smoke, it was a symbolic gesture of freedom, of liberation, of "You've come a long way, baby." Advertisements for smoking portray women who smoke as sexy and as free thinkers. While many adult women are beginning to understand the direct correlation between smoking and lung cancer, there are still many women who deny this or who truly are uninformed. In addition, many adolescent girls smoke due to peer pressure and due to the belief that smoking is sophisticated.

Lung cancer is the number one cause of cancer mortality in women and men (Petersen, 1994). In addition, recent research (Risch et al., 1993) indicates that women are more susceptible than men to the risk of lung cancer, which may be explained by the fact that more men than women have recently stopped smoking, but may also be explained by a higher biological susceptibility in women, or later stage of diagnosis because of lack of recognition of the risk by physicians. Education about the dangers of smoking must take place in a format that is not self-righteous, but that conveys an understanding to women about the many complex and ambiguous messages that they receive and process in our society.

Breast Health
Clinical breast exam and yearly mammography are recommended for all women over 50 years of age, and for women ages 40–50 who have a family history of breast disease or other risk factors. There is currently controversy about the effectiveness of mammography for low-risk women in the 40–50 age range. In women under 40, mammography is not effective because of tissue density in the youthful breast; for these women, self-exam on a regular basis is the best protection.

The potential sensitivity of breast self-exam (BSE) may be greater than that currently achieved (34 percent of all breast cancers). The thoroughness of a self-exam improves after training (Lauver, 1990).

Safe Sex
The issue of safe sex, or, more appropriately, safer sex, has received increasing attention in the media. Before the AIDS epidemic, sexually transmitted diseases certainly existed and were feared by both women and men, and herpes, in particular, was a dreaded infection because a cure does not exist for this viral disease. With the advent of the AIDS epidemic, the urgency of teaching people to engage in safer sex practices was increased. However, due to many myths and denial on the part of many people, as well as heterosexism in believing that AIDS was a gay male disease, safer sexual practices were ignored by many. Slowly, over time, AIDS began to be recognized for the nondiscriminatory disease that it is, and safer sexual practices received more attention. Controversy continues to surround this topic. Nurses play a key role in teaching persons about safer sex, but also in becoming politically active to ensure that safer sex is discussed and taught in schools and that condoms are made available to everyone.

Safer sexual practices consist of methods by which the exchange of infected bodily fluids (specifically blood, semen, and vaginal fluid) is prevented. The sure method of doing this is through abstinence, and the next best way is by engaging in a mutually monogamous sexual relationship with an uninfected (HIV-negative) person. Beyond that, certain precautions are necessary to prevent the transmission of infections, particularly HIV. Barrier methods of contraception are considered very useful, though the diaphragm, while a barrier method, does not prevent contact between sperm and the vagina. The male condom is considered the only barrier method that is effective, though newer methods such as a female condom have been developed and are currently being tested. The condom must be used from start to finish during sexual relations (i.e., used during foreplay, during oral-genital contact, during anal contact, and during penile-vaginal intercourse).

Use of Seatbelts

Seatbelts have been found, according to several studies, to save lives in case of an automobile accident. In addition, car seats for infants and small children have been found to be effective in saving lives in such cases as well (McCarthy & Hancock, 1994).

Summary

This chapter has presented an overview of common women's health issues during the reproductive years. It highlights the need for emphasis on primary care and, particularly, the role of the nurse clinician in understanding women's experiences of their health issues. A feminist perspective underlies the approach to care outlined by this chapter.

References

Baruch, G., & Barnett, R. (1986). Role quality, multiple role involvement, and psychological wellbeing in midlife women. *Journal of Personality and Social Psychology, 51,* 578–585.

Belenky, M. F., Clinchy, B. M., Goldberger, N. R., & Tarule, J. M. (1986). *Women's ways of knowing.* New York: Basic Books.

Boston Women's Health Collective (1992). *The new our bodies, ourselves.* New York: Touchstone.

Chernin, K. (1981). *The obsession: Reflections on the tyranny of slenderness.* New York: Harper and Row.

Chernin, K. (1985). *The hungry self: Women, eating and identity.* New York: Harper and Row.

Chodorow, N. (1978). *The reproduction of mothering: Psychoanalysis and the sociology of gender.* Berkeley: University of California Press.

Cook, D. J. (1985). Social support and stressful life events during midlife. *Maturitas, 7,* 303–317.

Dalton, J. (1990). Chronic musculoskeletal symptoms and sexuality. In C. I. Fogel & D. Lauver (Eds.), *Sexual health promotion* (pp. 325–336). Philadelphia: W. B. Saunders Company.

Diagnostic and Statistical Manual of Mental Disorders (4th ed.). Washington, DC: American Psychiatric Association.

Ehrenreich, B., & English, D. (1973). *Witches, midwives and nurses: A history of women healers.* Old Westbury, NY: Feminist Press.

Erickson, E. H. (1950). *Childhood and society.* New York: Norton.

Falludi, S. (1991). *Backlash: The undeclared war against American women.* New York: Doubleday.

Froberg, D., Gjerdingen, D., & Preston, M. (1986). Multiple roles and women's mental and physical health: What have we learned? *Women and Health, 11,* 79–96.

Garner, C. H. (1991). *Principles of infertility nursing.* Boca Raton, FL: CRC Press.

Gilligan, C. (1982). *In a different voice.* Cambridge, MA: Harvard University Press.

Godfrey, M. (1991). Clients with personality disorder. In G. K. McFarland & M. D. Thomas (Eds.), *Psychiatric mental health nursing: Application of the nursing process* (pp. 587–594). Philadelphia: J. B. Lippincott.

Hancock, L. A., Olshansky, E. F., Abrums, M. E., & McCarthy, A. M. (1994). The prenatal period. In C. L. Edelman & C. L. Mandle (Eds.), *Health promotion throughout the lifespan* (3rd ed.) (pp. 367–406). St. Louis: C. V. Mosby.

Harris, N., & Seimer, B. (1994). Psychosocial health concerns. In E. Q. Youngkin & M. S. Davis (Eds.), *Women's health: A primary care clinical guide.* Norwalk, CT: Appleton & Lange.

Hauser, S. L. (1994). Multiple sclerosis and other demyelinating diseases. In K. Isselbacher, E. Braunwald, J. D. Wilson, J. B. Martin, A. S. Fauci, & D. L. Kasper (Eds.), *Harrison's principles of internal medicine* (13th ed., Vol. 2). New York: McGraw Hill.

Heilbrun, C. (1988). *Writing a woman's life.* New York: Ballantine Books.

Hooks, B. (1982). *Ain't I a woman? Black women and feminism.* Boston: South End Press.

Jack, D. (1991). *Silencing the self: Women and depression.* Cambridge, MA: Harvard University Press.

Jennings, S., Mazaik, C., & McKinley, S. (1984). Women and work: An investigation of the association between health and employment status in middle aged women. *Social Science and Medicine, 19,* 423–431.

Kearney, M. H. (1993). Salvaging the self: A grounded theory study of pregnancy on crack cocaine. Unpublished doctoral dissertation, University of California at San Francisco.

Keleher, K. C. (1991). Occupational health: How work environments can affect reproductive capacity and outcome. *Nurse Practitioner*, *16*(1), 23–37.

Landenburger, K. M. (1989). The process of entrapment in and recovery from an abusive relationship. *Issues in Mental Health Nursing*, *10*, 209–227.

Lauver, D. (1989). Instructional information and breast self-examination practice. *Research in Nursing and Health*, *12*, 11–19.

Levy, B., & Wegman, D. (1988). *Occupational health: Recognizing and preventing work-related diseases*. Boston: Little Brown.

Lohr, M. A. (1991). Clients with schizophrenia. In G. K. McFarland & M. D. Thomas (Eds.), *Psychiatric mental health nursing: Application of the nursing process*. Philadelphia: J. B. Lippincott.

Love, S. L., & Lindsey, K. (1990). *Dr. Susan Love's breast book*. Reading, MA: Addison-Wesley.

McBride, A. (1988). Mental health effects of women's multiple roles. *Image*, *20*(1), 41–47.

McCarthy, A. M., & Hancock, L. A. (1994). School-age child. In C. L. Edelman & C. L. Mandle (Eds.), *Health promotion through the lifespan* (3rd ed.) (pp. 449–539). St. Louis: C. V. Mosby.

Martin, E. (1987). *The woman in the body*. Boston: Beacon Press.

Miller, J. B. (1986). *Toward a new psychology of women*. Boston: Beacon Press.

Mitchell, E. S. (1991). The elusive premenstrual syndrome. *NAACOG's Clinical Issues in Perinatal and Women's Health Nursing*, *2*(3), 294–303.

Moen, P. (1992). *Women's two roles: A contemporary dilemma*. New York: Auburn House.

Mullan, R. J., & Murthy, L. I. (1991). Occupational sentinel health events: An updated list for physician recognition and public health surveillance. *American Journal of Industrial Medicine*, *19*, 775.

Norbeck, J., & Resnick, B. (1986). Balancing career and home: How the OHN can relieve stress to improve employee health. *American Association of Occupational Health Nursing Journal*, *34*, 20–25.

Olshansky, E. F. (1987a). Identity of self as infertile: An example of theory generating research. *Advances in Nursing Science*, *2*(2), 54–63.

Olshansky, E. F. (1987b). Infertility and its influence on women's career identities. *Health Care for Women International, 8*(2,3), 185–196.

Olshansky, E. F. (1988). Responses to high technology infertility treatment. *Image, 20*(3), 128–131.

Ornish, D. (1990). *Reversing heart disease.* New York: Ballantine Books.

Pagelow, M. D. (1992). Adult victims of domestic violence: Battered women. *Journal of Interpersonal Violence, 7*(1), 87–120.

Paul, M. (1993). *Occupational and environmental reproductive hazards: A guide for clinicians.* Baltimore: William & Wilkins.

Petersen, G. M. (1994). Epidemiology, screening, and prevention of lung cancer. *Current Opinion in Oncology, 6*(2), 156–161.

Phipps, W., Long, B., Woods, N. F., & Cassmeyer, V. (1991). *Medical surgical nursing* (4th ed.). St. Louis: C. V. Mosby.

Pugliesi, K. (1988). Employment characteristics, social support and the wellbeing of women. *Women's Health, 14,* 35–58.

Risch, H. A., Howe, G. R., Jain, M., Burch, J. D., Holowaty, E. J., & Miller, A. B. (1993). Are female smokers at higher risk for lung cancer than male smokers? A case-control analysis by histologic type. *American Journal of Epidemiology, 138*(5), 281–293.

Sandelowski, M. J. (1990). Failures of volition: Female agency and infertility in historical perspective. *Signs: Journal of Women in Culture and Society, 15*(3), 475–499.

Speroff, L., Glass, R. H., & Kase, N. G. (1994). *Clinical gynecologic endocrinology and infertility* (5th ed.). Baltimore: Williams & Wilkins.

Steptoe, A., Edwards, S., Moses, J., & Matthews, A. (1989). The effects of exercise training on mood and perceived coping ability in anxious adults from the general population. *Journal of Psychosomatic Research, 33,* 537–547.

Swanson-Kauffman, K. M. (1986). Caring in the instance of early pregnancy loss. *Topics in Clinical Nursing, 2,* 37–46.

Whitley, G. (1991). Clients with psychotic disorder not elsewhere classified. In G. K. McFarland & M. D. Thomas (Eds.), *Psychiatric mental health nursing: Application of the nursing process* (pp. 559–564). Philadelphia: J. B. Lippincott.

8

Perimenopause

Ruth M. Barnard
Nancy Reame

Introduction

Menopause is a marker of reproductive transition. This natural "change of life" is neither a disease nor a syndrome connoting a disease process (Voda, 1992). Natural menopause is not an endocrine deficiency disease, resulting from an estrogen insufficiency, contrary to the view of some practitioners. Rather, it is a milestone of continuing maturation. Natural menopause refers to the natural cessation of menses at the completion of the reproductive years, usually defined retrospectively after 12 consecutive months of amenorrhea. Some women have troublesome responses to the accompanying hormonal changes, while others make little note of these events. Women's reactions to menopause are as different as their premenopausal responses to the menstrual cycle or to pregnancy.

Perimenopause is a term used to identify the life period surrounding menopause. Another term, commonly used to describe this entire period of transition to the postreproductive years, is *climacteric*. Perimenopause begins with physiological changes which mark the transition between the reproductive and traditional postreproductive years. Two early perimenopausal changes include shortening of the follicular phase of the menstrual cycle and elevation of blood levels of the pituitary hormone (follicle-stimulating hormone [FSH]). Some researchers restrict the definition of perimenopause to the 1 or 2 years preceding and following actual menopause. Shaver, Giblin, Lentz, and

Lee (1988) defined perimenopause as the time of menstrual cycle irregularities and elevation of FSH greater than 20 mIU/ml until 2 years after the last menstrual period. Others define it as the period between 3 months of menstrual irregularity until eleven months of amenorrhea (McKinlay, Brambilla, & Posner, 1992). Speroff, Glass, and Kase (1989) describe the climacteric beginning about age 40, when there is a decrease in ovulation frequency due to waning ovarian function, and extending as long as 20 years. Thus, the endocrine changes and characteristic signs and symptoms associated with natural menopause extend over a period of years. Although women may not identify themselves as perimenopausal because of the lack of definitive signs of this gradual transition in reproductive capability until there is menstrual irregularity, in this chapter, the broadest definition of perimenopause will be used, covering ages 40 to 60.

Age at Menopause

The average woman now lives about one third of her life after reaching menopause. In the past, most women did not live long enough to experience menopause. In fact, women born in the United States in 1900 had a life expectancy of only 48.3 years (United States Bureau of Census, 1975), compared to 79.1 years for women born in 1991 (United States Bureau of Census, 1993). Although the median age for menopause is considered to be between 50 and 51 (Jaszmann, van Lith, & Zaat, 1969; McKinlay et al., 1992; Thompson, Hart, & Durno, 1973), there is some variation in age of menopause reported worldwide. In Yoruban Nigerian women, the mean age of menopause is 48.4 years (median 48 years; Okonofua, Lawal, & Bamgbose, 1990); in women living in Hawaii, the mean age for all ethnic groups is 49.9 years with no differences observed among Caucasian, Japanese, Chinese, and Hawaiian women (Goodman, Grove, & Gilbert, 1978); in Thai women in Bangkok the average age for menopause is 47.9 years; and in Karachi, Pakistan, the mean age is approximately 47 years with no differences in age among poor, middle class, and privileged women (Wasti, Robinson, Akhtar, Khan, & Badaruddin, 1993). Although life expectancy is increasing, women from third world countries still have significantly shorter life expectancies than women in the United States or most European countries. Because of the smaller proportion of women reaching menopause in the third world, its significance as a health issue may not yet be appreciated there.

In a large cross-sectional population sample of Finnish women aged 45 to 64 years, the median age at natural menopause of smokers and nulliparous women was 50 years; the median age for nonsmokers and women whose first full-term pregnancy occurred before the age of 25 years was 52 years (Luoto, Kaprio, & Uutela, 1994). In a large prospective study in the United States [Massachusetts Women's Health Study], the median age of menopause for smokers was 50.2 years, while the median age of nonsmokers (and of ex-smokers) was 52 years (McKinlay et al., 1992). Although the age of menopause has remained relatively constant over the past several decades, the average age for onset of menses in girls has continued to decline. This is thought to be due to improved environmental factors, especially ante- and post-natal nutrition (Zacharias, Rand, & Wurtman, 1976). Thus, the length of time of potential reproductive capability has gradually increased.

This chapter will review psychosocial and physical changes that occur during the perimenopause as well as highlight common health concerns of this phase. There are clinical care texts available to guide nursing care during perimenopause. These include *Gynecology: Well-woman Care,* edited by Ronnie Lichtman and Susan Papera (Lichtman & Papera, 1990).

Historical Perspectives

Some of the earliest descriptions of the perimenopausal experience date back to the 1700s. In the 18th century, aging peasant women were thought to be unaffected by menopause, but "sensitive, refined" women of the upper classes needed help in managing the decline in estrogenic function with the subsequent body image changes and lost social status (Wilbush, 1988). With the threat of losing their sexual attraction, these women were treated with emmenagogues, leeches, phlebotomy, or other means to promote excretion of toxins that were thought to be retained when menstruation ceased or became irregular (Wilbush, 1988). Even in the 18th century there was disagreement over the treatment of menopause. In 1776 Fothergill (as cited in Wilbush, 1988) reported some physicians believed that menopause was a natural event, needing minimal treatment while physicians Roussel in 1775 and Longrois in 1787 (as cited in Wilbush, 1988) expressed great sympathy for women during menopause and tried to improve their situation.

One of the first significant studies of the menopausal experience was conducted in the late 1920s and published in 1933 by the Council of the Medical Women's Federation (CMWF) in Great Britain. Personal interviews were conducted with about 1200 women aged 29 to 91 whose menses had ceased for at least 5 years. Fifteen percent of the women claimed to have had no symptoms when they passed through the menopause, with single women being significantly less affected (CMWF, 1933). Among those recalling symptoms, the most frequent symptom cited was flushing by 62.3 percent. No relationship was found between age of onset of menstruation and age of menopause. The results of this study must be treated with some caution because of the length of time between interview and last menses; it is likely that some of these women may have forgotten some of their experiences.

Over the years clinicians tried to ease some of the symptoms women experienced. Using fresh animal ovaries, ovotherapy became popular for clinical use at the turn of the century, primarily for hot flashes (Quirk & Wendel, 1983). When the lay book, *Feminine Forever*, was published thirty years ago, the daily use of estrogen supplements was touted to be the answer to the fountain of youth for maturing women (Wilson, 1966) and probably was the major factor that spurred estrogen treatment in the 1960s and 1970s. Robert Wilson, a physician, claimed that menopause was curable and could be prevented. He wrote, ". . . thanks to recent medical advances, it is possible for any woman to retain her sexual appeal along with her sexual vitality throughout later life. By retaining these functions she also safeguards the less direct and more elusive aspects of her total femininity" (p. 16). Many clinicians and others agreed with him; however, many women, as well as other clinicians, strongly disputed his assertions. Perhaps, because his views were so outrageous in focusing on women's sexual appeal and looking young, Wilson aided development of the feminist movement.

Traditionally in American culture, menopause has been dreaded by many women as a time of mystery, an age of instability, or an ending of usefulness. Little research had been done on menopause. Physicians' advice, if offered, was based on case study reports or their own clinical experiences with patients presenting with significant problems. In 1963, supported by a grant from the National Institute of Mental Health, Neugarten, Wood, Kraines, and Loomis (1963) studied women's attitudes toward menopause. They found that women were eager to talk about menopause, wanted more information, and generally did not believe the "old wives' tales" which had been passed on to them. The recent surge in popularity of self-help books (Borton, 1992; Sheehy, 1992) related to menopause as well as books and televised talk shows with personal testimonials of menopausal experiences has contributed to a new openness in sharing information.

The medical literature in the 1970s and 1980s shows a significant increase in case studies and research reports related to menopause. For example, although incorrect, it was commonly believed there was an increase in body temperature with a hot flash, and that hot flashes only occurred from the chest up. However, no systematic research had been conducted on this common troublesome menopausal symptom until Molnar (1975) published extensive documentation from one subject (his wife) of physiological changes occurring during menopausal hot flashes. Besides an increase in heart rate during a hot flash, he reported that skin temperature of toes as well as fingers increased following a hot flash, and that core temperature decreased slightly (Molnar, 1975). During the 1970s, researchers began to examine changes in other hormones and neurotransmitters as well as to search for the trigger of hot flashes. In 1979, Casper, Yen, and Wilkes (1979) found that a pulse of luteinizing hormone (LH) *always followed* the occurrence of a hot flash. This finding sparked further studies, especially on the physiological changes associated with menopause.

Neuroendocrine Regulation of the Perimenopausal Transition

It is widely believed that the hallmark change in the menstrual cycle before menopause is an increase in follicle-stimulating hormone (FSH) levels in the face of normal basal LH, presumably due to declining estrogenic influence on the hypothalamic-pituitary-ovarian axis (Sherman & Korenman, 1975; Sherman, West, & Korenman, 1976). This view is based mainly on data from cross-sectional studies and single daily hormone measures and thus is not reflective of neuroendocrine dynamics. In one longitudinal study (Sherman et al., 1976) of six women ages 46–51 with regular cycles in which daily hormone measures were collected across the cycle, basal levels of FSH were elevated during the follicular phase, mean LH was similar, and estradiol (E2) *was* lower during the luteal phase compared to women aged 18–30. No differences were noted for the two women aged 40–41. The authors took these findings to mean that endocrine changes occur rather late in the premenopause. A more recent study (Lee, Lenton, Sexton, & Cooke, 1988) with a larger sample size has shown that the rise in FSH secretion occurs as early as age 35, but no aging effects were observed in LH secretion until age 45. Thus, the current view of the transition to the post-reproductive years is that the regulation of LH secretion is more resistant to the decline of ovarian function, with little change in secretory patterns until just prior to menopause. In a recent review by Speroff (1993) of dysfunctional uterine bleeding, the author reports that "the rise in FSH [in normal women] is not apparent until age 40, and there is no change in LH levels until menopause" (p. 2).

Using a longitudinal design with intensive blood sampling across an 8-hour day during the follicular, mid luteal and late luteal phases of women in their 20s, 30s, and 40s, Reame, Kelch, Beitins, and Yu (1993) recently confirmed the gradual rise in FSH with age, and also discovered subtle rises in pulsatile LH secretion. In women over 40, the size of the LH pulses was larger in the follicular and late luteal phases and smaller in the mid luteal phase, resulting in a flattening of the cyclic rise and fall in pulsatile LH secretion typically seen in young women, despite similar levels of ovarian estradiol and progesterone across groups. This evidence of altered gonadotropin secretion in women over 40, long before regular ovulatory cycles have ceased, supports the view that impaired negative ovarian feedback is a normal part of aging and is independent of ovarian sex steroids.

Recently, it has been discovered that the ovary also produces protein hormones—inhibin, activin, and follistatin—that play a role in the regulation of FSH. As their names imply, inhibin and follistatin act to inhibit FSH secretion, while activin stimulates FSH release (Findlay, 1993). They also may serve as local hormones in the ovary, regulating LH-induced androgen production. During the perimenopause, it is believed that the aging ovary gradually loses its ability to secrete inhibin, thus causing the differential rise in FSH (Burger, 1993). However, the model of these ovarian proteins as circulating hormones with a single site of action has undergone significant revision. It is now clear that they have a wide tissue distribution, where they may play a variety of roles that remain to be fully defined (Findlay, 1993).

Signs and Symptoms of Menopause

In many women, the decrease in ovarian production of estradiol and progesterone that heralds the climacteric and eventual menopause is accompanied by signs and symptoms, most notably hot flashes, sleep disturbances, genitourinary complaints, and changes to skin, muscle strength, and memory (Anderson, Hamburger, Liu, & Rebar, 1987; Greene, 1976). These changes are believed to be the direct biologic consequences of estrogen withdrawal from target organs as the ovary becomes depleted of follicles capable of responding to pituitary FSH and production of estrogen (Jaffe, 1991). More than 7 million women visit health care practitioners each year for hormone replacement therapy (HRT) prescriptions (U.S. Congress Office of Technology Assessment, 1992). Thus, a widely held medical view has emerged that menopause is an estrogen-deficiency disease with long-term health sequelae.

Critics of this theory point to epidemiologic studies of healthy, menopausal women drawn from community samples who report minimal symptoms which do not require medical management (Sherman & Korenman, 1975; Sherman et al., 1976), suggesting that the menopause experience is highly variable from woman to woman. Evidence from international, cross-cultural studies of symptomatology also supports a heterogeneous etiology for menopausal symptoms (Lee et al., 1988). Sociodemographic factors such as social class, employment status, and reproductive history have not been predictive (McKinlay & Jeffreys, 1974; Sherman, Wallace, Bean, Chang, & Schlabaugh, 1981), thus suggesting that other biobehavioral influences on symptomatology may account for this variability in symptom severity.

Other reasons for variability in responses are suggested by results from previous ecologic and laboratory investigations. These studies indicate that several nutritional factors, such as obesity and dietary components (energy, fat, fiber, micronutrients, and phytoestrogens) may affect hormonal status and reproductive health, notably breast cancer (Kemmann, Pasquale, & Skat, 1983; Martin–Du Pan, Hermann, & Chardon, 1990; Pirke et al., 1989; Reichman et al., 1992; Rose, Goldman, Connolly, & Strong, 1991). See Table 8-1 for a listing of common phytoestrogens, plant substances which mimic estrogen in humans.

A further caveat about the true impact of menopause on women's health relates to the failure to attend to the experiences of non-White women. The majority of the clinical and epidemiologic investigations of menopause have systematically excluded women of color. Thus, the biologic, psychosocial, and epidemiologic constructs that have emerged to inform the clinical management of menopause-related health problems cannot be generalized to a large and growing segment of the United States population.

TABLE 8-1 Examples of Phytoestrogens

Fruits	apples, cherries
Grains	alfalfa, barley, oats, rice, rye, wheat
Soybean products	miso, tofu
Vegetables	cabbage, carrots, chickpeas, green beans, peas, potatoes, yams
Miscellaneous	coffee, garlic, yeast

Hot Flashes

One of the most troublesome changes commonly reported by women in the perimenopause is the occurrence of hot flashes (some women use the term "hot flushes"). In fact, hot flashes are the most frequently reported menopausal symptom which brings women to health care providers (Judd, 1983; Kronenberg, 1990). Hot flashes which occur during sleep are usually referred to as *night sweats*. Because hot flashes and night sweats often begin prior to the cessation of menstrual cycling, women do not always recognize this symptom associated with impending menopause. Women may deny that they are experiencing hot flashes when questioned by clinicians because they are still menstruating and have not yet labeled the symptom as such.

Hot flashes are experienced by approximately 75 percent of women around the time of menopause, and about 15 percent of these women experience severe hot flashes that significantly decrease their quality of life (Kronenberg, 1990). Hot flashes may be experienced for a few months or may continue into old age. Some women have hot flashes at regular intervals, ranging from 45 to 90 minutes, while others notice them more frequently at one time of the day or night. In a large cross-sectional study, two thirds of the women reported experiencing hot flashes, and over 90 percent of these reported discussing them with their physician (Hemminki, Brambilla, McKinlay, & Posner, 1991). A telephone survey of 594 perimenopausal women in Minnesota showed the prevalence of hot flashes to be 88 percent; women with surgical menopause (removal of ovaries) had a hot flash prevalence of 92 percent (Feldman, Voda, & Gronseth, 1985). In one community in Sweden, a survey of all women in specific age groups (ages 65, 59, 57, and 55) found that 51 percent of the women reported hot flashes, 10 percent were using hormone replacement therapy, and another 10 percent had abandoned hormone therapy for various reasons (Lindgren,

Berg, Hammar, & Zuccon, 1993). Large prospective studies are needed to document the onset, occurrence, and timing of signs and symptoms in relation to hormonal changes. Recall of menopausal experiences may not be accurate. Just as the discomforts of childbirth are not remembered, the discomforts of menopause probably are forgotten over time.

Hot Flash Physiology

A hot flash is a sudden, transient feeling of warmth which is usually accompanied by flushing and sweating. Some women report a momentary aura 30 to 60 seconds prior to the start of a hot flash. The current theory to explain the symptom of hot flashes is that the temperature *set point* is lowered for a short period of time by some factor yet to be determined (Tataryn et al., 1980). This lowering of the thermostat causes the body's thermoregulatory system to start the cooling mechanism of marked vasodilatation, sweating, and a motivation to remove clothing, similar to what is experienced when a fever breaks (see Figure 8-1).

Upon the occurrence of a hot flash, the marked increased blood flow to the extremities causes a rise in finger (and toe) temperature, followed by sweating, which in turn cools the body and decreases core temperature slightly. Women often have a great urge to remove jackets, sweaters, or coats during this time. Shortly after the initial lowering of the setpoint, it is theorized that the setpoint returns to the original point. Probably because core temperature has decreased slightly due to the marked vasodilatation and sweating, women often report feeling chilled at the end of hot flashes.

Hot flashes can vary in intensity between women as well as in the same woman, being modulated by factors such as time of day, ambient temperature, interpersonal situations, and food and drink. Some women report very mild flashes that are just a warm feeling that lasts for less than 5 minutes, while others report a very intense feeling of heat with sweat running down their bodies. Recently, the role of ambient temperature in relation to hot flashes has shown that cool ambient temperatures can dramatically decrease the frequency and perceived intensity of hot flashes (Kronenberg & Barnard, 1992). Just turning down the room thermostat moderately can relieve the discomfort of hot flashes.

The central trigger for hot flashes is still unknown. Certainly estrogen withdrawal has a role in the occurrence of hot flashes, but

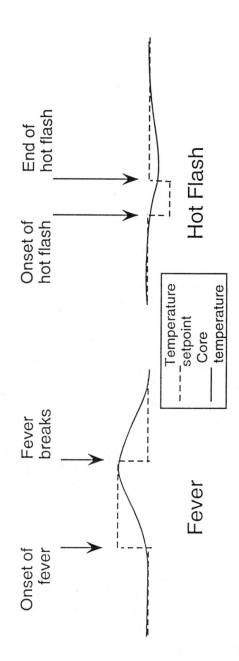

FIGURE 8-1 Hypothesized thermoregulatory setpoint changes with a hot flash and with a fever. Similar physiological responses (peripheral vasodilatation, sweating, and lower core temperature) occur with onset of a hot flash and at the time a fever breaks.

its specific mechanism is not known. No acute change in estrogen levels prior to a hot flash has been found (Meldrum et al., 1980). However, when estrogen supplements are taken by women having hot flashes, the frequency and intensity of hot flashes are decreased and may even be completely eliminated. If women have been experiencing hot flashes for some time, it usually takes from 3 to 6 weeks for supplemental estrogen to have an effect.

Women perceive excessive heat with a hot flash. Although it has been proposed that a hot flash is a burst of excessive heat, there is no evidence to support this. Skin and extremity temperatures do not quite reach core body temperature. The feeling of excessive heat is most likely explained by the shift of the warmer trunk blood to the surface and extremities.

Although it may be hard to believe in this era of enlightenment, some clinicians still have the mistaken belief that hot flashes are only a psychiatric manifestation. In 1991, Tait proposed, "It is time that women and health professionals understood that the hot flushes of the menopause are due to the activation and resuppression of the strong emotion [resentment]" (Tait, 1991, p. 455).

There are some documented hormone and neurotransmitter changes that occur following a hot flash, but no precipitating changes have been found that are causally linked. A hot flash is followed by increased pulsatile secretion of LH (Casper et al., 1979); adrenocorticotropic hormone and cortisol (Genazzani et al., 1984; Meldrum et al., 1980); and dehydroepiandrostenedione, androstenedione, and growth hormone (Meldrum et al., 1980). Epinephrine levels have been reported to increase (Kronenberg, Côté, Linkie, Dyrenfurth & Downey, 1984; Mashchak, Kletzky, Artal, & Mishell, 1984) or remain stable (Casper, Yen, & Wilkes, 1979; Cignarelli et al., 1989). Beta endorphin has been reported to increase (Genazzani et al., 1984) and to decrease (Tepper, Pardo, Ovadia, & Beyth, 1992). No differences have been found in estradiol, estrone, and thyroid-stimulating hormone (Meldrum et al., 1980); dopamine (Casper et al., 1979; Cignarelli et al., 1989); prolactin (Casper et al., 1979; Meldrum et al., 1980); and glucose, glucagon, insulin, and free fatty acid (Cignarelli et al., 1989). Norepinephrine has shown mixed results: increased (Cignarelli et al., 1989), decreased (Kronenberg et al., 1984), and no change (Casper et al., 1979; Cignarelli et al., 1989; Lightman, Jacobs, Maguire, McGarrick, & Jeffcoate, 1981). Some measurement difficulties of these hormones and neurotransmitters may account for the conflicting results (e.g., short half-life of the substance and an inadequate blood sampling schedule, or deterioration of sample a collection/storage temperature). In addition, sample sizes may have been too small to detect significant changes in hormone concentrations.

Low estrogen levels are not a sufficient condition for hot flashes to occur. Prepubertal girls have low estrogen and do not have hot flashes. Women who had experienced menses but developed hypothalamic amenorrhea following emotional stress or weight loss and had postmenopausal levels of estrogen do not have hot flashes (Gambone et al., 1984). Pulses of LH are not essential for women to have hot flashes. Women with isolated gonadotropin deficiency do not have hot flashes until they have been treated with estrogen, and then it is withdrawn (Gambone et al., 1984).

Although estrogen levels are significantly lower in menopausal women, they are even lower in symptomatic women. Estradiol, estrone, percent non-sex-hormone–binding globulin-bound estradiol, and total non-sex-hormone–binding globulin-bound estradiol were significantly lower in women with hot flashes compared to women matched on age, years since menopause, and presence or absence of ovaries (Erlik, Meldrum, & Judd, 1982). The symptomatic women also had a significantly lower percent ideal body weight (Erlik, Meldrum, & Judd, 1982). Higher levels of estrogens in heavier women are thought to be due to an increased conversion of androstenedione to estrone by the greater amount of fat tissue (Speroff et al., 1989). The increased aromatization of androgens and the decrease in sex hormone binding globulin (which increases the amount of free estrogen) is thought to be the basis for the well-known association between obesity and endometrial cancer (Speroff et al., 1989).

Vaginal and Urogenital Changes

Aging and the decrease in estrogen cause tissue changes that are quite significant. The vulva begin to lose subcutaneous fatty tissue, and the epidermis thins. The vaginal epithelium becomes thin, and the vagina shortens, is less elastic, loses its rugae, and decreases in both general and arousal lubrication (Brown & Hammond, 1987). A decrease in vaginal glycogen, which is acted on by lactobacilli resulting in lactic acid, leads to a less acidic pH vagina. This less acidic environment is more susceptible to infection (Milsom, Arvidsson, Ekelund, Molander, & Eriksson, 1993).

Some perimenopausal women report discomfort with intercourse and often report that they can no longer participate due to pain. This dyspareunia and pruritus is due to vulvar, introital, and vaginal atrophy (Speroff et al., 1989). Even women who are not sexually active may have discomfort from vaginal dryness. Regardless of hormone levels and type of activity, whether coitus or self-stimulation, continued sexual exchange appears to play a role in the maintenance of overall vaginal health (Bachmann, 1993). A recent small study reported desirable results from one vaginal moisturizer (Nachtigall, 1994). Astroglide® and Replens® are the two most commonly recommended. Many clinicians recommend them as substitute moisturizers, but many women do not find them satisfactory.

Topical or systemic treatment with an estrogenic compound dramatically improves the vaginal tissue, increasing the cellular depth and lubrication (Semmens & Wagner, 1985). Even without estrogen replacement, sexually active older women have less vaginal atrophy than older women who are not sexually active (Speroff et al., 1989). However, the vaginal relaxation with cystocele, rectocele, and uterine prolapse that may occur is not a consequence of lowered estrogen (Wilson et al., 1987).

The urethral meatus may develop a caruncle that may be painful. Even though estrogen preparations are frequently prescribed for urinary complaints, there is some evidence that long-term estrogen use may be associated with an increased risk of urinary tract infection (UTI). Analysis of data from a general practice automated database showed that women with intact uteri who were long-term users of estrogen had a twofold increase in risk of an UTI (Orlander, Jick, Dean, & Jick, 1992). A recent study showed that regular consumption of 300 cc of cranberry juice cocktail per day significantly reduced the frequency of bladder infections in older women. The effect was not fully realized until the women had been drinking the cranberry juice daily for 4 to 8 weeks (Avorn et al., 1994). It is believed that a component of cranberry juice prevents bacteria from adhering to the mucosal lining of the bladder.

Midlife women report some urinary incontinence, primarily stress incontinence. A study of 522 women 45 years of age in Denmark showed that 22 percent of the women stated they experienced incontinence (Hording, Pedersen, Sidenius, & Hedegard, 1986). Pelvic exam revealed that women with incontinence also exhibited a significantly higher incidence of cystocele, uterine prolapse, or impairment of levator muscles. Incontinence was not related to size of uterus, parity, or menopausal state. Stress incontinence may be alleviated to some extent by strengthening the urethral sphincter with Kegel's exercises (Brink, Sampselle, Wells, Diokno, & Gillis, 1989). Genuine stress incontinence will not be affected by treatment with estrogen (Wilson et al., 1987). Recent reports of injecting collagen tissue near the urinary sphincter show encouraging results in persons with stress incontinence (Appell, 1994; Herschorn, Radomski, & Steele, 1992; Kieswetter, Fischer, Wober, & Flamm, 1992).

Health Concerns

Sexuality

Women do not lose their sexuality at menopause and are capable of sexual functioning throughout their lifetime. The presence of a sexual partner seems to be much more of an indicator of sexual activity, rather than any mental or physical state (Youngs, 1990). In one community in Sweden, a survey of all women in specific age groups (ages 65, 59, 57, and 55) found that 62 percent of the women reported sexual activity, with those women who had been postmenopausal for more than 10 years reporting the lowest activity (Lindgren, Berg, Hammar, & Zuccon, 1993). With the decrease in estrogen levels, there is tissue atrophy and decreased vaginal lubrication that become troublesome to women during intercourse. This is especially true for women after the onset of precipitous menopause by surgery or chemotherapy. The lack of vaginal lubrication and subsequent discomfort for the woman may lead to problems with partner performance, and hence lead to a deteriorating relationship.

Masters and Johnson (1966) described sexual responses of 152 women over age 50 indicating that the uterine contractions occurring with orgasm frequently were painful in older women. They also observed that women beyond the mid-50s may take up to 3 minutes to produce vaginal lubrication. However, they observed three women over age 60 who responded to sexual stimulation with rapid production of vaginal lubrication. These women had maintained active sexual relations once or twice a week throughout their adult lives. Masters and Johnson (1966) indicated that women 5 to 10 years postmenopause who experience infrequent intercourse and who do not masturbate with regularity will have difficulty having sexual relations because of inadequate lubrication and vaginal changes.

Fear of embarrassment may be the reason for the largely unreported but high prevalence of sexual problems in the menopausal woman (Downes, 1992). Hormone replacement therapy may relieve the symptoms, but may not be sufficient to manage a psychosexual problem. Health practitioners should include a sexual database while obtaining histories to identify areas that require intervention. A guide to assessment of older women's sexual role and sexual needs is presented by Morrison-Beedy (Morrison-Beedy & Robbins, 1989).

Lesbian Concerns

The literature is beginning to address the health needs of lesbians. A recent review of lesbian health care research reported that most research has focused on attitudes of health care providers or on beliefs and experiences of lesbians who are White middle class women between the ages of 20 and 40 (Stevens, 1992). The importance of identity as a lesbian, including emotions, behavior, and cultural system rather than only sexual orientation, is not recognized or considered by most health care providers (White & Levinson, 1993). The standard interview questions (e.g. "What method of birth control do you use?") assume heterosexuality and can set up barriers between the lesbian and the health care provider (White & Levinson, 1993). Some questions require disclosure of lesbian identity, the person may not be ready to disclose herself, and thus will not answer accurately (Hitchcock & Wilson, 1992).

Studies show that lesbians tend to avoid routine screening, such as Pap smears, possibly due to fear of negative judgment and homophobic responses by the health care provider (Buenting, 1992). Deevey (1990) surveyed health behaviors of 78 lesbians over the age of 50. She reported that a majority indicated experiencing discrimination because of being lesbian and did not trust mainstream health care. Although the health care needs of perimenopausal lesbians may differ little from needs of nonlesbians, the interaction between lesbians and health care providers may discourage these women from preventive health care screening as well as treatment. Research to determine the needs of older lesbian women is just beginning to be undertaken.

Fertility Needs

Some women have not finished having children at the time they enter the perimenopause. In the past, women who had not conceived had only the option of adoption. In recent years, in vitro fertilization–embryo transfer (IVF-ET) has permitted ova to be harvested from a woman's own ovary (or a donor's ovary), fertilized with sperm outside of her body, and then implanted in her uterus, which has been hormonally prepared for pregnancy. The success rate of clinical pregnancy from IVF-ET is approximately 22 percent, and 77 percent of these result in live deliveries (Medical Research International, 1992). The success rates are difficult to compare because of the varying methods used to define success (Wilcox, Peterson, Haseltine, & Martin, 1993). Because of the depletion of ova in older women's ovaries as well as the higher incidence of children with birth defects born to older natural mothers, ova donations from younger women have been solicited recently and used with IVF, with the older woman serving as the gestational carrier (Check, Nowroozi, Barnea, Shaw, & Sauer, 1993; Sauer, Paulson, & Lobo, 1993). (As of this writing, a 62-year-old from Italy is the oldest woman to have a baby by the egg donation and IVF method.) Recently, there have been reports of later development of ovarian cancer following hormonal stimulation for follicle development to be used in IVF (Reynolds, 1993).

Dual career parents often put off having children until later in life when careers are established. Because pregnancy rates decline dramatically after age 40, the extra stress of attempting late pregnancy or undergoing infertility workups and treatment can be detrimental to partnerships. A woman's awareness of approaching the end of her normal reproductive years can cause mixed reactions. She may be pleased that the chances of an unplanned pregnancy are decreased, or she may regret that soon she will be unable to have children. The loss of fertility was not considered a misfortune 30 years ago. In a study of 460 women, Neugarten, Wood, Kraines, and Loomis (1963) reported that only 4 (of 100) women in the age group 45 to 55 indicated "Not being able to have more children was the worst thing in general about the menopause" (p. 149).

Contraception Needs

Although fertility declines progressively with age and coital frequency usually is reduced at perimenopause, pregnancy is still possible when women are ovulating periodically. Most women in the perimenopause are not interested in becoming pregnant and are concerned about contraceptive practices. Timing of heterosexual intercourse, either to continue or to begin the rhythm method, may become difficult because of irregular periods. Fortunately, oral contraceptives may be used by many perimenopausal women. In

1989 the Fertility and Maternal Health Drugs Advisory Committee of the FDA recommended to the FDA that there should be no upper age limit for combined oral contraceptive pill use by healthy, nonsmoking women. Women who continue to take contraceptive pills that induce a monthly withdrawal "period" may not even recognize they are in menopause until they discontinue their use of the pills.

Depending on what the partners are accustomed to, other means of contraception may be used. Barriers, such as the diaphragm, may be continued, but initiation of diaphragm use in perimenopause may enhance the urethral syndrome. Condoms, like diaphragms, are not popular because they require specific intercourse-related planning and may reduce sensual pleasure. Because older heterosexual women are a growing segment of the population who are contracting HIV infections, condoms continue to be recommended as a barrier to transfer of HIV during sexual relations (Stein, 1993). Condoms have also been shown to be effective in preventing other sexually transmitted diseases (STDs) (Feldblum & Fortney, 1988). Rather than depending on condoms to protect themselves, women of any age must practice prevention of STDs by wisely screening and choosing sexual partners as well as by avoiding sexual practices involving anal contact. A helpful summary of methods women could use for HIV prevention was recently published (Stein, 1993).

For women who choose not to use condoms, intrauterine devices (IUDs) are effective contraceptives, with most IUDs now of the copper-releasing type. The other commonly used type of IUD is medicated with progestins (Jones, Wentz, & Burnett, 1988). All IUDs should be removed before uterine atrophy occurs. Spermicides or sponges are thought to be adequate after age 50 for women who are still cycling (Bachmann, 1993; Hollingworth & Guillebaud, 1991). Use of GnRh antagonistic analogs for contraception, which result in inhibition of the LH midcycle surge, may be difficult in perimenopausal women because of the need for precise timing relative to the cycle, and this may be impossible in women with irregular cycles (Jones et al., 1988). The antiprogesterone RU-486 can be used for contraception at several points in the menstrual cycle: at midcycle to suppress the LH midcycle surge; in late luteal to induce menstruation; or when menses are delayed to induce an early abortion (Jones et al., 1988). Use of RU-486 has not been described specifically in perimenopausal women. Because of the risk to the mother, abortion should not be used as a method of birth control, but rather as a backup procedure when there is contraception failure.

Menstrual Dysfunction and Hysterectomy

Some women experience precipitous menopause by surgical removal of the ovaries. The changes, which usually occur with natural menopause at a gradual rate, happen in a much shorter period of time in precipitous menopause. Women respond differently to surgically induced menopause: some observe relatively little discomfort and symptoms, while others have severe problems. The vast majority of hysterectomies for irregular bleeding are performed in women between the ages of 35 and 44. Surgical menopause (hysterectomy with oopherectomy) occurs in 30 percent of White women in this age group. In one study, those women choosing surgery had undergone multiple episodes of curettage for irregular heavy bleeding, had less education, and had a poorer health status compared to those with natural menopause (McKinlay, McKinlay, & Brambilla, 1987a; McKinlay, McKinlay & Brambilla, 1987b).

For African American women, surgical menopause rates approach 50 percent. This is especially troublesome given the well-documented increased risk for coronary artery disease and osteoporosis in premenopausal women after hysterectomy. In the single epidemiologic study conducted on the climacteric status and health symptoms of African American women (Jackson, Taylor, & Pyngolil, 1991), rates of premature menopause were remarkably high in young women: 23 percent of those reporting postmenopause were between 35 and 44 years of age, and 15 percent were under 34 years. While information on surgical procedures was not collected, the authors speculated that menopause in these age cohorts was most likely caused by hysterectomy and pointed to the unmarried, undereducated, underemployed, and relatively poor status of the sample as a possible reason for this observation (Jackson et al., 1991). This study also confirmed the findings of other studies that White women with premature menopause experience more physical and emotional symptoms compared to their same-age peers (McKinlay et al., 1987a). Thus, United States midlife African American women are at increased risk for dysfunctional uterine bleeding, and in turn, hysterectomy and premature menopause with poor consequences for health. Low socioeconomic status, depression, obesity, diet, and psychosocial stress have been implicated as sociocultural antecedents for pathological menstrual bleeding.

Women who are treated by ovariectomy or with the use of antiestrogens, such as tamoxifen, as adjuvant therapy for breast cancer can have accentuated troublesome menopausal symptoms such as increases in the frequency and intensity of hot flashes, marked vaginal dryness, and increases in urinary problems (Love, Cameron, Connell, & Leventhal, 1991). Other drugs used as chemotherapy treatment of various cancers, such as cyclophosphamide (Cytoxin®), can also cause chemical castration and all the subsequent menopausal changes (Koyama et al., 1977).

Late Parenting

Parents who have children in their late childbearing years are confronted with many unique issues (O'Reilly-Green & Cohen, 1993). They may have less in common with parents of their children's playmates due to age differences with other parents, making it more difficult to share experiences and seek advice. Parental energy, agility, and emotional flexibility to keep up with the activities of young children may be lacking in parents nearing 50 years of age. The typical support that grandparents, aunts, and uncles provide for new parents may be unavailable or compromised by illness of these persons. Children born to older parents may not have the opportunity to know their grandparents or may know them only as elderly and ill.

Although pregnancy due to IVF in women over 40 is not common at the present time, the number of older parents could significantly increase as this technique is further perfected and becomes part of mainstream options. In addition to the stresses of the IVF procedure, all the unique issues related to late parenting apply to these couples. Recently, IVF has permitted the crossing of generational lines—mothers can serve as gestational carriers of children that are genetically their grandchildren. New models of family dynamics may have to be developed to guide the interrelationships among family members. Other issues of responsibility, accountability, liability, and obligations should be discussed and negotiated prior to the IVF.

Considerations of Stamina and Capacities

Many studies compare strength and endurance between young and old adults. Therefore, little documentation of these measures is available for perimenopausal women. Women typically notice a change in physical strength in the perimenopause. For some time it has been known that a decline in grip strength related to increased age appears earlier in women than in men. Women begin to find it more difficult to open jars or doors. This marked decline in grip strength occurs in women about age 45 (Phillips, Rook, Siddle, Bruce, & Woledge, 1993). The decline is more gradual in men, starting about age 60. It is interesting to note that women on hormone replacement therapy (HRT) do not show this decline in muscle strength.

If women want to maintain or regain strength and endurance, changes in muscular strength can be reversed with progressive resistance training, provided it is of sufficient intensity and duration (Rogers & Evans, 1993). This exercise training produces improvements in metabolic and force-producing capacity, such that declines in capacity can no longer be considered an inevitable consequence of the aging process (Rogers & Evans, 1993). Exercise has been useful in assisting women with life-threatening conditions to overcome losses due to disease or due to treatment for disease. Functional capacity in breast cancer patients significantly improved with an interval-training exercise intervention (MacVicar, Winningham, & Nickel, 1989).

There is an increase in falls by women at perimenopause, which may be due to weakening leg muscles. The rapid decline in muscle strength may account for some of the tendency for falls; however, changes in balance have not been ruled out. Appropriate exercise would strengthen leg muscles, but other interventions would have to be found if balance is a problem. It has long been known that distal forearm fractures (Colle's fracture) increase at perimenopause (Winner, Morgan, & Evans, 1989).

Psychosocial Domain: Midlife Changes

Some of the psychosocial changes occurring in lives of women in the middle years are related to stages of family or personal development, such as the changing family constellation and work/career changes. The changing family constellation includes both positive and negative changes. An increase in the divorce rate in the United States from 2.6 per 1,000 in 1950 (United States Bureau of Census, 1975) to 4.7 per 1,000 in 1988 (United States Bureau of Census, 1993) and a decrease in the marriage rate from 11.1 per 1,000 in 1950 (United States Bureau of Census, 1975) to 9.7 per 1,000 in 1988 (United States Bureau of Census, 1993) suggests that there is less support for women in nuclear families, resulting in more stress and jeopardizing women's health. The loss by death of parents and grandparents may give a sense of new vulnerability when one's own generation becomes the oldest generation.

For childbearing women, midlife is an age when children leave home to start their careers. The reactions of women to the fact that they no longer have children to care for has been named the "empty nest" syndrome. Research on this issue has provided mixed results. Some of the conclusions, based on clinical populations of women seeking treatment, showed greater rates of depression in those who had been very involved in parenting compared with subjects whose children were still living at home (Bart, 1971). In contrast, other studies show a majority of women viewing midlife as a "time of freedom" (Deutscher, 1968; Lowenthal, 1975). Women with multiple roles (worker, spouse, parent) reported better health than women with single roles (Verbrugge, 1986). In a study of 47 predominantly White women ages 46 to 59 who were chosen from a metropolitan diploma school of nursing alumni directory and who lived in reasonable proximity to the investigators, Wilbur and Dan (1989) reported neither work pattern (stable working, double-track, interrupted, and unstable) nor nest status (full, empty, and transitional) showed any relationship to measures of psychological well-being. Apparently using a narrow definition of perimenopausal women, they reported that perimenopausal women had decreased life satisfaction compared to premenopausal and postmenopausal women from the same sample (Wilbur & Dan, 1989).

Midlife is also a time when women and spouses may be challenged by becoming grandparents. Because over 95 percent of women in the work force within the perimenopausal age groups are employed (United States Bureau of Census, 1993), traditional roles and responsibilities of grandparenting may not be met, which may lead to disappointment, sadness, and stress. However, this employment may also lead to satisfaction. Having an income may allow an opportunity to travel to visit distant grandchildren as well as facilitate other opportunities that require financial support.

There are an increasing number of grandparents raising grandchildren. Often because of parental substance abuse and child maltreatment, grandparents are assuming the responsibility of caring for their grandchildren, giving additional stress to these midlife persons (Kelley, 1993; Minkler, Roe, & Robertson-Beckley, 1994).

This life stage has been described as the "sandwich" generation, caring for or launching their children as well as caring for their parents. In fact, caring for aging parents is reported to be a major source of life stress in middle age (Lieberman, 1978). Primarily, the caregivers are women. Often these women have been employed and have to give up their jobs or at least reduce to a part-time schedule. These changes, along with the physical and psychological load of caring for parents, often lead to excessive stress on the caregiver. This excessive stress may lead to an increase in health problems. A reduction in immune function has been found in persons undergoing severe life stress and in patients with a major depressive disorder (Irwin et al., 1991).

A study of stress and rewards in women occupying the roles of caregiver, mother, and wife indicated that while an accumulation of role stress was associated with poorer well-being, an accumulation of role rewards was also related to better well-being (Stephens, Franks, & Townsend, 1994). Mental and physical health may be improved in caregivers by finding interventions that increase rewards from the variety of roles women play.

Although our society in essence is still a partner-oriented society, women without partners are more accepted than at times in the past. Never-married, childless women, whose responsibility in the past was to take care of ill or elderly family members, are not available to continue these traditional roles. The lack of availability of these "maiden" aunts to assist their married sisters with the management of cross-generational families has added to the burdens of society.

The occurrence and sequencing of life events may have a significant impact on coping with or responding to them. Neugarten (1979) emphasized that "individuals develop a concept of the normal expectable life cycle, a set of anticipations that certain life events will occur at certain times, and a mental clock telling them where they are and whether they are on time or off time" (p. 888). She argued that normal and expectable life events are not crises. Rather, these events are more likely to produce a crisis when they do not occur on time, such as "when children do not leave home on time" (p. 889).

Memory and Cognition

Two common symptoms of women seeking medical treatment during menopause are memory problems and difficulty concentrating. Impairments in cognitive function have been linked to both the biologic and psychosocial transitions that occur in women during midlife (United States Office of Technology Assessment, 1992). Despite intriguing evidence from animal and clinical studies of a role for estrogen in memory function (Honjo et al., 1993; McEwen et al., 1991; Ohkura, Isse, Akazawa, Hamamoto, & Yao 1993), little research using objective psychometric measures has been undertaken on cognitive changes in women experiencing a natural (nonsurgical) menopause.

Most work on cognitive status in women has focused on menstrual cycle effects and gender differences among younger populations for visuospatial/verbal abilities and sensory/perceptual-motor tasks (Broverman et al., 1981; Hampson, 1990; Hampson & Kimura, 1988; Komnenich, Lane, Dickey, & Stone, 1978; Parlee, 1983; Silverman, 1981; Wickham, 1958; Wuttke et al., 1975). The few studies performed to date assessing the effects of sex steroids on memory have predominantly used women before and after surgically induced menopause (i.e., bilateral ovariectomy) who show abrupt symptom onset and severity (Rauramo, Lagerspetz, Engblom, & Punnonen, 1976; Sherwin, 1988), and subjects well beyond their menopausal years (Hackman & Galbraith, 1976). Thus, little is known about the status of cognitive function, especially memory, during the natural perimenopausal transition.

A recently published Japanese study of memory function in 200 women treated at a gynecological outpatient clinic showed significant mean decreases in performance on 10 paired hard associates, a test of memory function (Ohkura et al., 1994). The women were divided into 5-year age groups from age 31 to 65, 30 women in the six youngest groups and 20 women in the 61 to 65 age group. Scores in the two youngest groups (ages 31–35 and 36–40) were significantly higher than any of the older groups (p< .01) (Ohkura et al., 1994). The mean score of the youngest group was 8.0 (SD 2.0), and the mean score of the oldest group was 3.3 (SD 1.6). It was not possible to determine whether change in performance on the memory function test was related to other aging processes or specifically related to hormone changes in women as they age. These data suggest significant memory changes occurring during the perimenopause.

In humans, it is well documented that cerebral perfusion declines with age, with women having higher blood flow values than men until after the menopause. In elderly women with mild cerebrovascular disease, cognition improved with estrogen replacement therapy (ERT) and was associated with a trend toward increased cerebral perfusion (Mortel & Meyer, 1993). In a recent survey of 8,879 women in a California retirement community, those who used ERT were 40 percent less likely to have Alzheimer's disease than women who died of other causes (Cotton, 1994). This finding contradicts an earlier report of a study using a smaller sample of 800 subjects in which no consistent evidence of an effect on cognitive function was found (Barrett-Connor & Kritz-Silverstein, 1993).

Despite intriguing findings from animal studies and impaired patient groups and the widely held popular view that cognitive impairments, especially in memory, are a natural by-product of menopause, there is a paucity of human studies that have attempted to empirically define the relationship between menopause and cognitive status. With respect to the study of memory, only a small number of investigations in the last 20 years have employed objective psychometric instruments to assess the effects of ERT on memory in postmenopausal women, with conflicting results (Ditkoff, Crary, Cristo, & Lobo, 1991; Fedor-Freybergh, 1977; Hackman & Galbraith, 1976; Phillips & Sherwin, 1992; Rauramo et al., 1976; Sherwin & Phillips, 1990; Sherwin, 1988; Vanhule & Demol, 1976).

The strongest evidence confirming a role for estrogen decline in cognitive impairment at menopause comes from the work of Barbara Sherwin (Phillips & Sherwin, 1992; Sherwin & Phillips, 1990; Sherwin, 1988). Using a double-blinded, placebo-controlled cross-over design, Sherwin has studied premenopausal subjects undergoing bilateral oopherectomy as a clinical model for hormone-behavior relationships before and after ERT. With this paradigm, she has demonstrated that injections of estradiol, the most biologically active form of estrogen, maintained short-term verbal memory (Sherwin & Phillips, 1990; Sherwin, 1988) and enhanced the capacity for new learning (Phillips & Sherwin, 1992) compared to placebo. During placebo treatment, short- and long-term memory scores declined after surgery coincident with a dramatic fall in plasma estradiol (Sherwin, 1988). The investigators caution that although statistically significant, the effects on memory were modest and placebo-treated women were able to function normally in their daily activities, although daily measures of perceived cognitive functioning were not employed to confirm this view. To what extent these findings in women after surgical menopause, when changes in the endocrine milieu are sudden and dramatic, can be applied to the situation of spontaneous menopause remains unclear.

Studies of menopausal women fail to assess the cognitive effects of progestogens, which are widely used in contemporary HRT to oppose estrogen's effects on the endometrium in women with an intact uterus. Given the well-documented PMS-like side effects of bloating, breast tenderness, and emotional lability associated with the progestogenic component of the common HRT regimens (Dennerstein & Burrows, 1986; Holst et al., 1989; Sherwin & Gelfand, 1989), it could be argued that any beneficial estrogenic effect on memory and concentration may be attenuated during the progestogenic phase of treatment.

As a way to begin to clarify the influence of ovarian sex steroids on cognitive status during the perimenopause transition, longitudinal studies are needed to measure memory and other cognitive functions. In addition, measures are needed of the effectiveness of non-pharmacological interventions on reducing memory impairment and other cognitive symptoms in women during the midlife transition.

Common Health Problems

Sleep Changes

Given the many demands of work and family, it is not surprising that one of the particular complaints of midlife women is a feeling of "tiredness." However, three conditions sometimes overlooked by clinicians may be associated with this common complaint: night sweats, obstructive sleep apnea syndrome, and psychological distress. Relatively few studies have compared sleep characteristics in women of different ages and health status. It is well established that hot flashes disrupt sleep. Shaver et al. (1988) reported women with hot flashes tended to have lower sleep efficiencies (the ratio of total sleep time to total time in bed) than those not experiencing hot flashes. They also reported significantly longer rapid eye movement (REM) latency (i.e., longer time interval until beginning the first REM stage sleep) in symptomatic women than in nonsymptomatic women (Shaver et al., 1988). Electroencephalographic records show arousal, if not awakening, at the time of a hot flash. The lower sleep efficiency and longer REM latency are indications of poorer sleep, inferring less restful nights for the women with hot flash symptoms. These periodic sleep disruptions can lead to women's complaints of being tired. Estrogen therapy has been shown to improve sleep indirectly by decreasing the number of hot flashes experienced (Erlik et al., 1981).

Obstructive sleep apnea is beginning to be recognized as a women's health problem. Data from the Wisconsin Sleep Cohort Study using a random sample of 602 middle-aged adults from a healthy population showed that undiagnosed sleep-disordered breathing, although lower than in men, is much higher than previously suspected in women (Young et al., 1993). From the study data, Young et al. (1993) developed estimates that 2 percent of women and 4 percent of men in the middle-aged work force meet the minimal diagnostic criteria for the sleep apnea syndrome (an apnea score of 5 or higher and daytime hypersomnolence). This apnea, due to blockage of the air passage during sleep, causes arousal in order for the person to breathe, thus interrupting sleep. Obstructive sleep apnea is frequently associated with obesity, especially of the upper body. Symptoms of obstructive apnea—excessive daytime sleepiness, persistent tired feeling, loud snoring at night with gasps—can be missed without a careful health history.

Psychological distress has been shown to be associated with poor sleep. A study of midlife women found that women who classified themselves as poor sleepers had significantly higher psychological distress scores, higher somatic symptoms, and higher menopausal symptom scores compared to women who classified themselves as good sleepers (Shaver, Giblin, & Paulsen, 1991).

Cardiovascular Disease

The age-specific death rates for women dying from cardiovascular disease prior to age 60 are significantly lower than for men. Cardiovascular disease increases in women following menopause, and the incidence rate in women reaches that in men. For this reason, it has been proposed that ovarian hormones are responsible for this protective effect. A review article summarizing studies conducted on the development of cardiovascular disease in relation to estrogen found that most studies show a 50 percent reduction in risk of a coronary event in women using unopposed oral estrogen (Barrett-Connor & Bush, 1991). However, the authors point out that no studies in women have looked at endogenous estrogen levels as predictors of cardiovascular disease, that is, prospectively measuring the level of estrogens produced within women's bodies in relation to occurrence of cardiovascular disease (Barrett-Connor & Bush, 1991). Only recently was a study funded to examine the effect of HRT (estrogen and progestins) on risk factors. No long-term research has been conducted to measure whether HRT serves to *prevent* cardiovascular disease.

Changes associated with a greater incidence of cardiovascular risk occur in women who experience a natural menopause and do not take hormone replacement therapy; the levels of low-density lipoprotein (LDL) increase and those of high-density lipoprotein (HDL) decline (Matthews et al., 1989). Normal premenopausal levels of estrogen or hormone replacement therapy in peri- or postmenopause appear to decrease the risk of cardiovascular disease by reversal of this LDL/HDL ratio. Although hormone replacement therapy may protect against the increase in LDL levels, there is a marked increase in triglyceride levels associated with estrogen therapy (Manolio et al., 1993).

A follow-up study using a sample of 1,944 White menopausal women over 54 years of age who were participants in the National

Health and Nutrition Examination Survey started between 1971 and 1975 showed that the use of hormones was linked to a significantly lower risk of dying from cardiovascular disease (Wolf, Madans, Finucane, Higgins, & Kleinman, 1991). A history of diabetes, previous myocardial infarction, smoking, and elevated blood pressure was a strong predictor of cardiovascular disease deaths in the same cohort (Wolf et al., 1991).

Cancer

There is an increase in the occurrence of reproductive cancers at midlife, including breast, ovarian, and uterine cancers. Some progress has been made in understanding the development of cancer and its treatment. Certain types of breast and ovarian cancers can be identified and targeted by antibodies and immunotoxins. Eventually, genetic analysis of individual cancers will guide the application of specific gene therapies to inhibit activated oncogenes or to restore function of tumor-suppressor genes (Bast, 1993).

The increased use of estrogen therapy for menopause symptoms, prevention of cardiovascular disease, and possibly osteoporosis has raised the question of an increase in cancer occurrences. Estrogen is a known promoter of cell growth. The risk of endometrial cancer triples after a few years of unopposed estrogen therapy (Palinkas & Barrett-Connor, 1992). The relationship of estrogen therapy to other cancers is not clear. In a review article, Zumoff (1993) summarized studies of estrogen replacement therapy and the risk of breast cancer. He noted that there seemed to be agreement that women were not at risk for breast cancer with hormone use of less than 10 years. He concluded that the benefits of HRT (diminished coronary disease, diminished osteoporosis, prolongation of life span, and relief of menopausal symptoms) are so overwhelming that all postmenopausal women should receive HRT unless they themselves have had breast cancer or have a mother or sister who has had premenopausal breast cancer (Zumoff, 1993). A prospective analysis of dietary questionnaires obtained as part of the Nurses' Health Study showed that there was an elevated risk of breast cancer in women who drank at least 30 g of alcohol per day (at least 2 drinks) relative to cohort nondrinkers (Giovannucci et al., 1993). Women receiving HRT should be informed of the risk.

Mammograms and breast exams reduce the mortality from breast cancer from 90 percent to 60 percent in women 50 years of age and older, and possibly in women ages 40 to 49 (Shapiro, Venet, Strax, &

Venet, 1988). Current recommendations limit screening of asymptomatic women to those over age 50 (Shapiro, 1994). Many women's groups are urging that screening mammograms be encouraged starting at age 40. The numbers of women receiving screening mammograms has significantly improved between 1987 and 1990 (Breen & Kessler, 1994), but many women are still not being referred by their physicians on a regular basis.

Cancer treatments can propel women into menopause or exacerbate their existing menopausal symptoms similar to surgical menopause. Because the treatment of the cancer has been the priority, the menopausal side effects of some of these treatments have not been appreciated by clinicians.

Lifestyle Issues

Even though there is a greater risk of falling and a decrease in strength starting at perimenopause, activity can have a positive effect on signs and symptoms experienced. In fact, Wilbur & Dan (1992) reported that "leisure energy expenditure may have a positive effect on symptom reduction and that occupational energy expenditure may have a negative effect" (p. 275). Although it may not be a conscious effort, the attitude toward activity may make a significant difference.

Many women attest to the increase in body weight at menopause. It is not clear whether this typical change is associated with menopause per se or to other factors. De Aloysio et al. (1988) reported an increase in women's body mass index was associated with aging rather than with menopausal state and that "the pre-menopause is a weight-gain inducing state" (p. 365). There have been a number of theories proposed as to why women tend to gain weight in the middle years, such as a change in metabolism or a decrease in activity, but as yet there has been no definitive support for any of them.

Aging African American women have higher rates of hypertension, diabetes, cancer, cardiovascular disease, and abnormal uterine bleeding leading to surgical menopause (Dicker et al., 1982). The increased predisposition to disease has been linked to higher body weight, specifically central adiposity compared to White women, particularly in middle age (Adams-Campbell et al., 1990; Folsom et al., 1989). In their recent review, Kumanyika and Adams-Campbell (1991) note that nutritional and dietary factors may contribute to increased risk of chronic diseases in African American women. Weight-related attitudes and dieting behaviors of African American women also appear to differ from those reported in studies of the general population or other groups (Kumanyika, Wilson, & Guilford-Davenport, 1993). In spite of many similarities in the nutritional content of diets of African Americans and Whites, evidence from survey studies suggests that some aspects of diet may differ by race (Block, Rosenberger, & Patterson, 1988). For example, lower consumption of potassium, calcium, fiber, carotenoids, and preformed vitamin A in African American women may affect both health risk and endocrine status (Kumanyika & Adams-Campbell, 1991).

Psychosocial stress may also play an important role in mediating these higher rates of physical ills as well as underlying the emotional problems that disproportionately affect African American women, including depression, and drug and alcohol use (Regier et al., 1984). It has been documented empirically that African American midlife women are more likely to be subjected to a number of stressful life events due to a lack of economic resources, such as job and marital instability, lack of male companions as head of households, erratic income, and infrequent changes and relocations (Jackson, 1985). Clearly, low socioeconomic status would further amplify the incidence of disease morbidity, perhaps by increasing the potential for health risk behaviors and barriers to health care.

The effect of exercise in addition to an energy-restrictive diet was studied in randomly assigned healthy overweight postmenopausal women (Svendsen, Hassager, & Christiansen, 1993). Comparing diet-only and diet-plus-exercise intervention groups to the control group showed significant weight loss and a decrease in cardiovascular risk factors. The resting metabolic rate was significantly increased in the exercise group compared with the control group. When the two intervention groups were compared, the exercise group lost significantly more fat (but no lean tissue mass) than the diet-only group. There were no major differences in bone mineral densities or collagen and bone turnover.

Bone

Bone density decreases as part of the aging process. This loss accelerates at menopause for about 5 years and then resumes the premenopausal loss rate. Typically, between the ages of 50 and 80 years, women's bone density decreases about 30 percent (Ettinger, Genant, & Cann, 1985). When entering menopause, Asian and White women tend to have less bone mass than African American women. Thus, Asian and

White women are more affected by the loss that is accelerated at menopause. In addition, women develop problems with bone loss earlier than men, because they have less bone mass initially, and thus are more vulnerable to fractures. This decreased bone density leads to fragility fractures, especially of the upper femur, vertebrae, and distal forearm. Calcium is constantly being exchanged within bones to provide the needed amount for cellular exchanges. Estrogen acts to delay the resorption of calcium, promoting greater bone density. Both an adequate intake of calcium and adequate supply of estrogen are essential in maintaining healthy bones. When there is a decrease in estrogen, such as at menopause, the rate of bone loss increases significantly. Estrogen administration at menopause slows bone density loss from 2 percent per year for the 5 years following menopause and 1 percent for subsequent years to a rate of only 0.5 percent. However, the effect of estrogen dissipates after therapy is stopped. Treatment with estrogen started later in life, such as at 70 years, increases bone density 10 percent and then slows the loss to about 0.5 percent, suggesting that estrogen for bone loss need not be initiated until well past menopause (Christiansen & Riis, 1990; Lufkin et al., 1992).

Osteoporosis is associated with spine and hip fractures, which are comprised of trabecular bone. The increase in fractures following menopause is partly due to bone loss and partly due to bone architecture. Risk of hip fracture decreases with greater bone density. Estrogen therapy has been found to play a significant role in preventing hip fracture by increasing the bone density in women who are currently taking it (Kiel, Felson, Anderson, Wilson, & Moskowitz, 1987). However, the median age for hip fracture among postmenopausal women is 80 years, and most women of 80 years are not taking estrogen.

Recent data from the Framingham Study (Felson et al., 1993) suggested that at least 7 years of estrogen therapy were necessary for a persistent effect on bone density, but, even then, the effect may not persist in women after age 75. In the past, most women treated with postmenopausal estrogen therapy did not take it for more than 5 years. In fact, Ettinger and Grady (1993) state that the bone loss rate stabilizes in women 80 years of age between groups who have taken estrogen replacement for 10 years immediately following menopause and those who never took estrogen; the former group will have lost approximately 27 percent of initial bone density, and those never taking estrogen will have lost approximately 30 percent. Other estrogen administration schedules should be considered, such as having women take estrogen from time of menopause for the rest of their lives; starting estrogen after an osteoporotic fracture has occurred;

or starting estrogen at age 70 and continuing it for the rest of their lives (Ettinger & Grady, 1993).

Psychiatric Illness

Much controversy exists in the psychological literature about the contributions of psychiatric morbidity, hormonal status, and psychological variables such as self-concept, stressful life events, and coping styles to the broad spectrum of behavioral signs and symptoms observed at menopause (Ballinger, 1990; Matthews, 1992; McKinlay et al., 1987b). To date, no studies have properly delineated the hormonal events and their relations to the changes in mood; rather, these studies have relied on subject self-report of irregularity or cessation of menses as biological landmarks to define the climacteric and the menopause. Thus, it is not clear to what extent menopause *per se* plays a role as a biologic trigger for the onset of psychiatric illness. Although in the past perimenopausal women have been described as experiencing marked depression, a review of contemporary epidemiological and clinical studies found lack of support for this belief (Youngs, 1990).

In a double-blind, placebo-controlled clinical trial of perimenopausal women without significant vasomotor symptoms presenting with depression, subjects received 1 week of placebo patch, then 3 weeks of an estradiol patch or a placebo patch with cross-over at 1 month of placebo subjects to estradiol. Both groups continued on the estradiol patch for a second month. The preliminary analysis suggested that estradiol, but not placebo, was associated with significant improvement in several symptoms of depression (Rubinow & Schmidt, 1994).

Health Promotion and Prevention

The current emphasis, especially by the nursing profession, on preventing illness and promoting health appears to have increased the awareness of the public about the control people have over their own health. Participative sports, gyms, jogging, and activities are more available than previously to midlife women to increase health and prevent certain illnesses.

Prevention of osteoporosis provides good examples of the potency of intervention. In a study of bone mineral density (BMD), women in the 40 to 54 age group who had high physical activity were reported to have significantly higher spine and distal radius BMD than women with lower levels of activity (Zhang, Feldblum, & Fortney, 1992). Thus, these women are less likely to have fractures in these areas. Most clinicians urge that women build up bone mass through activity and good nutrition prior to menopause so that the inevitable losses will cause fewer problems. A large (N=300) controlled study of bone mass in premenopausal women showed no significant aging bone loss, no effect of birth control pills on BMD, and no association of calcium or other nutrient intake on BMD (Mazess & Barden, 1991). Smokers had a lower BMD in certain areas of the body.

Nutritionists encourage perimenopausal women to increase calcium intake in the diet in order to improve bone density. Although there are obvious differences in the typical diet of vegetarian women versus omnivorous women, there is no difference in the trabecular bone density nor the cortical bone density in postmenopausal women following these diets (Tesar, Notelovitz, Shim, Kauwell, & Brown, 1992).

Women should be encouraged to be active, eat balanced meals, eat less saturated fat foods, not smoke, monitor health with health care provider, avoid excessive sun exposure, and live in a safe, healthy environment.

Hormone Replacement Therapy— Making the Decision

Women should collect information on the most recent studies before making a decision whether to take HRT. There is little doubt that some hormone therapy is desirable for women who undergo surgical menopause with removal of ovaries. When women need to have a hysterectomy, there is no scientific basis for removing healthy ovaries. The common practice of removing ovaries in women over age 45 years who are having a hysterectomy needs to be questioned seriously.

Many care providers have diagnosed women at this stage of life as having "estrogen deficiency" and are eager to prescribe some type of hormone therapy to "treat" this problem. In fact, estrogen therapy, which once was given to relieve the uncomfortable symptoms some women experience, now appears to be prescribed primarily for the protective effects of estrogen on bone and cardiovascular systems. The rationale for use has generally been based on comparing cardiovascular problem rates between men and women by age, noting the sharp increase in the rate of cardiovascular problems that occurs after menopause, and based on the increase in hip and spine fractures due to fragile bones. Retrospective studies have shown postmenopausal use of estrogen therapy is associated with less cardiovascular disease, but there is no evidence that this therapy or combined therapy (estrogen and progestogen) has any effect on people who do not have risk factors. Researchers are beginning to conduct prospective studies of women looking at cardiovascular, bone, and other systems along with use of estrogen and other hormone replacement therapy. Questions are being raised about the rationale for replacement with sex steroids designed to prevent osteoporosis and cardiovascular disease while possibly enhancing risk of cancer-producing changes in the uterus and breast. Questions also are being raised as to whether the effect of supplementary estrogen on bone may be overstated for groups of women who are at less risk for osteoporosis.

Barrett-Connor and Miller (1993) advise, based on currently available data, that the prescription of HRT for women primarily to prevent heart disease is not indicated unless they are at high risk by virtue of their LDL/HDL ratio or the presence of manifest coronary heart disease. No data are available that show that estrogen therapy has an effect in women who are not at risk.

Surveys were sent annually for 3 years to 291 mostly perimenopausal women (35 to 55 years old) participating in the Midlife Women's Health Survey from across the United States to study women's patterns of hormone use. Hormone use rose from 9.4 percent to 21.6 percent during these years with only 1 percent stopping each year. Throughout the three years, 75 percent of the women remained nonusers (Mansfield & Voda, 1994). In a large European (N=2,236) cross-sectional study of the use of estrogens, most women reported using estrogens for a relatively short period of time, and those who were users had had a surgical menopause. There was a small gradual increase in use of hormones over a period of 6 years, with those reporting current use rising from 3 percent to 9 percent (Hemminki et al., 1991).

The emphasis on HRT, especially estrogen, as a means of preventing cardiovascular disease and slowing bone thinning may have influenced more women to stay on or start this therapy. It is unfortunate that no studies are available which compare various long-term administrations, dosages, intervals, and combinations of these sex steroid drugs on menopausal women. The prescriptions tend to vary from estrogen days 1–25 with progestogen days 15–25, to low-dose combinations taken daily, and many other combinations. The rationales seem based on the care provider's clinical experience along with the results in a given patient.

Although estrogen replacement therapy has been embraced by the medical community for its effectiveness in treating acute menopausal symptoms and reducing risk of cardiovascular disease and osteoporosis in later life, controversy persists about side effects and possible long-term sequelae, including breast cancer. The high drop-out rates (up to 30 percent) associated with both ERT and HRT (sequential estrogen plus progestogen) attest to the view that other nonsteroidal and nonpharmacological interventions for health promotion of menopausal women are sorely needed (U.S. Office of Technology Assessment, 1992).

Informally, women have expressed two reasons for stopping treatment: first, they are concerned about the risk of developing cancer, and second, they do not like the side effects of the preparations. Some of the side effects of HRT that women dislike include withdrawal bleeding, tender breasts, bloating, irritability, mood swings, and indigestion. The variations in HRT timing and dosage are often altered to eliminate undesired side effects.

Although estrogenic compounds have been the class of hormone assessed by all studies to date, the chemical preparations, dosages, and routes of administration have differed from study to study, primarily as a function of the year of study and the country in which the study was conducted. Thus, differences in potency and metabolism of the estrogenic preparations also limit the ability to compare the findings. However, despite the difficulty in making cross-study comparisons and the inconsistency of the findings, these studies tend to support some beneficial effect of ERT on memory, at least in women after surgical menopause with bilateral ovariectomy.

Many women report using natural substances to manage changes they experience with the menopause. These include combinations of herbs, such as black cohosh, blue cohosh, false unicorn root, sage, motherwort, blessed thistle, licorice, chaste tree, wild yam, and squaw vine. Many of these herbs are known to have hormonal effects just as the phytoestrogens mentioned earlier. Vitamin E is also used by many women, especially for hot flashes. Whether natural substances or artificial hormones are taken, women must be aware that there are side effects of any treatment as well as effects of no treatment.

Summary

Many women find a new sense of freedom and energy to try new ventures during this period of their lives. Others caught in the sandwich generation may not yet feel this freedom. The great increase in the basic information about the menopause experience and the increasing knowledge coming from systematic research should make the public, especially women, more informed about what experiences might occur and what options exist for interventions to relieve or attenuate troublesome ones. Just as exercise helps women improve strength and endurance at any age, other healthy actions can improve other aspects of their lives. Nursing, with its health emphasis, can play a very important role in providing information and in testing new and alternate interventions. Better information about perimenopause should be incorporated into nursing programs.

As more women share menopausal descriptions and experiences with daughters, families, and other women, coming generations should be better informed about menopause, and, hopefully, just as *periods* are now talked about openly by many in our society, women will no longer hide the fact that they are experiencing menopausal changes and symptoms.

References

Adams-Campbell, L., Nwankwo, M., Ukoli, F., Omene, J., Haile, G., & Kuller, L. (1990). Body fat distribution patterns and blood pressure in black and white women. *Journal of the National Medical Association, 82*(8), 573–576.

Anderson, E., Hamburger, S., Liu, J. H., & Rebar, R. W. (1987). Characteristics of menopausal women seeking assistance. *American Journal of Obstetrics and Gynecology, 156*(2), 428–433.

Appell, R. (1994). Collagen injection therapy for urinary incontinence. *Urologic Clinics of North America, 21*(1), 177–182.

Avorn, J., Monane, M., Gurwitz, J., Glynn, R., Choodnovsky, I., & Lipsitz, L. (1994). Reduction of bacteriuria and pyuria after ingestion of cranberry juice. *Journal of the American Medical Association, 271*(10), 751–754.

Bachmann, G. A. (1993). Sexual function in the perimenopause. *Obstetrics & Gynecology Clinics of North America, 20*(2), 379–389.

Ballinger, C. (1990). Psychiatric aspects of the menopause. *British Journal of Psychiatry, 156,* 773–787.

Barrett-Connor, E., & Bush, T. L. (1991). Estrogen and coronary heart disease in women. *Clinical Cardiology, 265*(14), 1861–1867.

Barrett-Connor, E., & Kritz-Silverstein, D. (1993). Estrogen replacement therapy and cognitive function in older women. *Journal of the American Medical Association, 269,* 2637–2641.

Barrett-Connor, E., & Miller, V. (1993). Estrogens, lipids, and heart disease. *Clinics in Geriatric Medicine, 9*(1), 57–67.

Bart, P. (1971). Depression in middle-aged women. In V. Gornich & B. Moran (Eds.), *Women in sexist society* (pp. 163–186). New York: Basic Books.

Bast Jr., R. (1993). Perspectives on the future of cancer markers. *Clinical Chemistry, 39,* 2444–2451.

Block, G., Rosenberger, W., & Patterson, B. (1988). Calories, fat and cholesterol: Intake patterns in the US population by race, sex and age. *American Journal of Public Health, 78*(9), 1150–1155.

Borton, J. C. (1992). *Drawing from the women's well.* San Diego: LuraMedia.

Breen, N., & Kessler, L. (1994). Changes in the use of screening mammography: Evidence from the 1987 and 1990 National Health Interview Surveys. *American Journal of Public Health, 84*(1), 62–67.

Brink, C. A., Sampselle, C. M., Wells, T. J., Diokno, A. C., & Gillis, G. L. (1989). A digital test for pelvic muscle strength in older women with urinary incontinence. *Nursing Research, 38*(4), 196–199.

Broverman, D., Vogel, W., Klaiber, E., Majcher, D., Shea, D., & Paul, V. (1981). Changes in cognitive task performance across the menstrual cycle. *Journal of Comparative and Physiological Psychology* (4), 646–654.

Brown, K. H., & Hammond, C. B. (1987). Urogenital atrophy. *Obstetrics and Gynecology Clinics of North America, 15*(1), 13–32.

Buenting, J. A. (1992). Health life-styles of lesbian and heterosexual women. *Health Care Women International, 13,* 165–171.

Burger, H. (1993). Evidence for a negative feedback role of inhibin in follicle stimulating hormone regulation in women. *Human Reproduction, 8* (Suppl 2), 129–132.

Casper, R. F., Yen, S. S. C., & Wilkes, M. M. (1979). Menopausal flushes: A neuroendocrine link with pulsatile luteinizing hormone secretion. *Science, 205*(24), 823–825.

Check, J., Nowroozi, K., Barnea, E., Shaw, K., & Sauer, M. (1993). Successful delivery after age 50: A report of two cases as a result of oocyte donation. *Obstetrics and Gynecology, 81*(5 (pt 2)), 835–836.

Christiansen, C., & Riis, B. (1990). [17]Beta-estradiol and continuous northisterone: A unique treatment for established osteoporosis in elderly women. *Journal of Clinical Endocrinology and Metabolism, 71*, 836–841.

Cignarelli, M., Cicinelli, E., Corso, M., Cospite, M. R., Garutti, G., Tafaro, E., Giorgino, R., & Schonauer, S. (1989). Biophysical and endocrine-metabolic changes during menopausal hot flashes: Increase in plasma free fatty acid and norepinephrine levels. *Gynecologic and Obstetric Investigation, 27*, 34–37.

Cotton, P. (1994). Constellation of risks and processes seen in search for Alzheimer's clues [news]. *Journal of the American Medical Association, 271*(2), 89–91.

Council of the Medical Women's Federation. (1933). An investigation of the menopause in one thousand women. Report to the Council of the Medical Women's Federation. *The Lancet, 1*(5706), 106–108.

de Aloysio, D., Villecco, A. S., Fabiani, A. G., Mauloni, M., Altieri, P., Miliffi, L., & Bottiglioni, F. (1988). Body mass index distribution in climacteric women. *Maturitas, 9*, 359–366.

Deevey, S. (1990). Older lesbian women. An invisible minority. *Journal of Gerontological Nursing, 16*(5), 35–39.

Dennerstein, L., & Burrows, G. (1986). Psychological effects of progestogens in the postmenopausal years. *Maturitas, 8*(2), 101–106.

Deutscher, M. (1968). Adult work and developmental models. *American Journal of Orthopsychiatry, 38*(5), 882–892.

Dicker, R. C., Scally, M. J., Greenspan, J. R., Layde, P. M., Ory, H. W., Maze, J. M., & Smith, J. C. (1982). Hysterectomy among women of reproductive age. Trends in the United States, 1970–1978. *Journal of the American Medical Association, 248*(3), 323–327.

Ditkoff, E. C., Crary, W. G., Cristo, M., & Lobo, R. (1991). Estrogen improves psychological function in asymptomatic postmenopausal women. *Obstetrics and Gynecology, 78*(6), 991–995.

Downes, E. G. R. (1992). Sexuality of the menopausal woman [Editorial]. *British Journal of Hospital Medicine, 47*(6), 409–410.

Erlik, Y., Meldrum, D. R., & Judd, H. L. (1982). Estrogen levels in postmenopausal women with hot flashes. *Obstetrics and Gynecology, 59*(4), 403–407.

Erlik, Y., Tataryn, I. V., Meldrum, D. R., Lomax, P., Bajorek, J., & Judd, H. (1981). Association of waking episodes with menopausal hot flushes. *Journal of the American Medical Association*, 245(17), 1741–1744.

Ettinger, B., Genant, H., & Cann, C. (1985). Long term estrogen replacement therapy prevents bone loss and fractures. *Annals of Internal Medicine*, 102, 319–24.

Ettinger, B., & Grady, D. (1993). The waning effect of postmenopausal estrogen therapy on osteoporosis [Editorial]. *New England Journal of Medicine*, 329, 1192–1193.

Fedor-Freybergh, P. (1977). The influence of oestrogens on the wellbeing and mental performance in climacteric and postmenopausal women. *Acta Obstetricia et Gynecologica Scandinavica Supplement*, 64, 1–91.

Feldblum, P., & Fortney, J. (1988). Condoms, spermicides, and the transmission of human immunodeficiency virus: A review of the literature. *American Journal of Public Health*, 78(1), 52–54.

Feldman, B. M., Voda, A., & Gronseth, E. (1985). The prevalence of hot flash and associated variables among perimenopausal women. *Research in Nursing and Health*, 8, 261–268.

Felson, D. T., Zhang, Y., Hannan, M. T., Kiel, D. P., Wilson, P. W. F., & Anderson, J. J. (1993). The effect of postmenopausal estrogen therapy on bone density in elderly women. *New England Journal of Medicine*, 329(16), 1141–1146.

Findlay, J. (1993). An update on the roles of inhibin, activin, and follistatin as local regulators of folliculogenesis. *Biology of Reproduction*, 48(1), 15–23.

Folsom, A. R., Burke, G. L., Ballew, C., Jacobs Jr., D. R., Haskell, W. L., Donahue, R. P., Liu, K. A., & Hilner, J. E. (1989). Relation of body fatness and its distribution to cardiovascular risk factors in your blacks and whites. The role of insulin. *American Journal of Epidemiology*, 130(5), 911–924.

Gambone, J., Meldrum, D. R., Laufer, L., Chang, R. J., Lu, J. K. H., & Judd, H. L. (1984). Further delineation of hypothalamic dysfunction responsible for menopausal hot flashes. *Journal of Clinical Endocrinology and Metabolism*, 59(6), 1097–1102.

Genazzani, A. R., Petraglia, F., Facchinetti, F., Facchini, V., Volpe, A., & Alessandrini, G. (1984). Increase of proopiomelanocortin-related peptides during subjective menopausal flushes. *American Journal of Obstetrics and Gynecology*, 149(7), 775–779.

Giovannucci, E., Stampfer, M. J., Colditz, G. A., Manson, J. E., Rosner, B. A., Longnecker, M. P., Speizer, F. E., & Willet, W. C. (1993). Recall and selection bias in reporting past alcohol consumption among breast cancer cases. *Cancer Causes and Control*, 4, 441–448.

Goodman, M., Grove, J., & Gilbert, F., Jr. (1978). Age at menopause in relation to reproductive history in Japanese, Caucasian, Chinese and Hawaiian women living in Hawaii. *Journal of Gerontology*, *33*(5), 688–694.

Greene, J. G. (1976). A factor analytic study of climacteric symptoms. *Journal of Psychosomatic Research*, *20*(5), 425–430.

Hackman, B. W., & Galbraith, D. (1976). Replacement therapy with piperazine oestrone sulphate ('Harmogen') and its effect on memory. *Current Medical Research and Opinion*, *4*(4), 303–306.

Hampson, E. (1990). Estrogen-related variations in human-spatial and articulatory-motor skills. *Psychoneuroendocrinology*, *15*(2), 97–111.

Hampson, E., & Kimura, D. (1988). Reciprocal effects of hormonal fluctuations on human motor and perceptual-spatial skills. *Behavioral Neuroscience*, *102*(3), 456–459.

Hemminki, E., Brambilla, D. J., McKinlay, S. M., & Posner, J. G. (1991). Use of estrogens among middle-aged Massachusetts women. *DICIP, The Annals of Pharmacotherapy*, *25*(April), 418–423.

Herschorn, S., Radomski, S., & Steele, D. (1992). Early experience with intraurethral collagen injections for urinary incontinence. *Journal of Urology*, *148*(6), 1797–1800.

Hitchcock, J. M., & Wilson, H. S. (1992). Personal risking: Lesbian self-disclosure of sexual orientation to professional health care providers. *Nursing Research*, *41*(3), 178–183.

Hollingworth, B. A., & Guillebaud, J. (1991). Contraception in the perimenopause. *British Journal of Hospital Medicine*, *45*(April), 213–215.

Holst, J., Backstrom, T., Hammarback, S., & von Schoultz, B. (1989). Progestogen addition during oestrogen replacement therapy—Effects on vasomotor symptoms and mood. *Maturitas*, *11*(1), 13–20.

Honjo, H., Ogino, Y., Tanaka, K., Kashiwagi, H., Okada, K., & Hayashi, K. (1993). Senile dementia (Alzheimer's type) and estrogen—double blind study and combination with gestagen. In *Fourth Annual North American Menopause Society* (p. 186). San Diego: North American Menopause Society.

Hording, U., Pedersen, K. H., Sidenius, K., & Hedegard, L. (1986). Urinary incontinence in 45-year-old women. *Scandinavian Journal of Urology and Nephrology*, *20*, 183–186.

Irwin, M., Brown, M., Patterson, T., Hauger, R., Mascovich, A., & Grant, I. (1991). Neuropeptide Y and natural killer cell activity:

Findings in depression and Alzheimer caregiver stress. *FASEB Journal*, 5(15), 3100–3107.

Jackson, B. (1985). Role of social resource variables upon life satisfaction in black climacteric hysterectomized women. *Nursing Papers*, 17(1), 4–22.

Jackson, B. B., Taylor, J., & Pyngolil, M. (1991). How age conditions the relationship between climacteric status and health symptoms in African American women. *Research in Nursing and Health*, 14(1), 1–9.

Jaffe, R. (1991). The menopause and perimenopausal period. In S. Yen & R. Jaffe (Eds.), *Reproductive endocrinology: Physiology, pathophysiology and clinical management* (pp. 406–423). Philadelphia: W. B. Saunders Co.

Jaszmann, L., van Lith, N. D., & Zaat, J. C. A. (1969). The perimenopausal symptoms: The statistical analysis of a survey, Part A & B. *Medical Gynaecology and Sociology*, 4, 268–277.

Jones, H. W. I., Wentz, A. C., & Burnett, L. S. (1988). *Novak's textbook of gynecology* (11th ed.). Baltimore: Williams & Wilkins.

Judd, H. L. (1983). Pathophysiology of menopausal hot flushes. In J. Meites (Ed.), *Neuroendocrinology of aging* (pp. 173–202). New York: Plenum Press.

Kelley, S. (1993). Caregiver stress in grandparents raising grandchildren. *Image—the Journal of Nursing Scholarship*, 25(4), 331–337.

Kemmann, E., Pasquale, S., & Skat, R. (1983). Amenorrhea associated with carotenemia. *Journal of the American Medical Association*, 249(7), 926–929.

Kiel, D., Felson, D., Anderson, J., Wilson, P., & Moskowitz, M. (1987). Hip fracture and the use of estrogens in postmenopausal women. The Framingham Study. *New England Journal of Medicine*, 317(19), 1169–1174.

Kieswetter, H., Fischer, M., Wober, L., & Flamm, J. (1992). Endoscopic implantation of collagen (GAX) for the treatment of urinary incontinence. *British Journal of Urology*, 69(1), 22–25.

Komnenich, P., Lane, D., Dickey, R., & Stone, S. (1978). Gonadal hormones and cognitive performance. *Physiological Psychology*, 6, 115–120.

Koyama, H., Wada, T., Nishizawa, Y., Iwanaga, T., Aoki, Y., Terasawa, T., Kosaki, G., Yamamoto, T., & Wada, A. (1977). Cyclophosphamide-induced ovarian failure and its therapeutic significance in patients with breast cancer. *Cancer*, 39, 1403–1409.

Kronenberg, F. (1990). Hot flashes: Epidemiology and physiology. *Annals of the New York Academy of Science*, 592, 52–86.

Kronenberg, F., & Barnard, R. M. (1992). Modulation of menopausal hot flashes by ambient temperature. *Journal of Thermal Biology*, *17*(1), 43–49.

Kronenberg, F., Côté, L. J., Linkie, D. M., Dyrenfurth, I., & Downey, J. A. (1984). Menopausal hot flashes: Thermoregulatory, cardiovascular, and circulating catecholamine and LH changes. *Canadian Journal of Physiology and Pharmacology*, *6*, 31–43.

Kumanyika, S., & Adams-Campbell, L. (1991). Obesity, diet and psychosocial factors contributing to cardiovascular disease in blacks. In E. Saunders (Ed.), *Cardiovascular Diseases in Blacks* (pp. 47–73). Philadelphia: F. A. Davis.

Kumanyika, S., Wilson, J., & Guilford-Davenport, M. (1993). Weight-related attitudes and behaviors of black women. *Journal of the American Dietetic Association*, *93*(4), 416–422.

Lee, S., Lenton, E., Sexton, L., & Cooke, I. (1988). The effect of age on the cyclical patterns of plasma LH, FSH, estradiol and progesterone in women with regular menstrual cycles. *Human Reproduction*, *3*, 851–855.

Lichtman, R., & Papera, S. (1990). *Gynecology: Well-Woman care*. Norwalk, CT: Appleton & Lange.

Lieberman, G. (1978). Children of the elderly as natural helpers: Some demographic differences. *American Journal of Community Psychology*, *6*, 489–498.

Lightman, S. L., Jacobs, H. S., Maguire, A. K., McGarrick, G., & Jeffcoate, S. L. (1981). Climacteric flushing: Clinical and endocrine response to infusion of naloxone. *British Journal of Obstetrics and Gynaecology*, *88*, 919–924.

Lindgren, R., Berg, G., Hammar, M., & Zuccon, E. (1993). Hormonal replacement therapy and sexuality in a population of Swedish postmenopausal women. *Acta Obstetricia et Gynecologica Scandinavica* *72*, 292–297.

Love, R. R., Cameron, L., Connell, B. L., & Leventhal, H. (1991) Symptoms associated with tamoxifen treatment in postmenopausal women. *Archives of Internal Medicine*, *151*, 1842–1847.

Lowenthal, M. F. (1975). Psychosocial variations across the adult life course: Frontiers for research and policy. *Gerontologist*, *15* 6–12.

Lufkin, E., Wahner, H., O'Fallon, W., Hodgson, S. F., Kotowica M. A., Lanc, A. W., Judd, H. L., Caplan, R. H., & Riggs, B. L (1992). Treatment of postmenopausal osteoporosis with transderma estrogen. *Annals of Internal Medicine*, *117*, 1–9.

Luoto, R., Kaprio, J., & Uutela, A. (1994). Age at natural menopause and sociodemographic status in Finland. *American Journal of Epidemiology, 139*(1), 64–76.

MacVicar, M. G., Winningham, M. L., & Nickel, J. (1989). Effects of aerobic interval training on cancer patients' functional capacity. *Nursing Research, 38*(6), 348–351.

Manolio, T. A., Furberg, C. D., Shemanski, L., Psaty, B. M., O'Leary, D. H., Tracy, R. P., & Bush, T. L. (1993). Association of postmenopausal estrogen use with cardiovascular disease and its risk factors in older women. *Circulation, 88*(part 1), 2163–2171.

Mansfield, P. K., & Voda, A. M. (1994). Hormone use among middle-aged women: Results of a three year study. *Menopause: The Journal of the North American Menopause Society, 1*(2), 99–108.

Martin–Du Pan, R., Hermann, W., & Chardon, F. (1990). Hypercarotinemie, amenorrhee et regime vegetarien [Hypercarotenemia, amenorrhea and a vegetarian diet]. *Journal de Gynecologie, Obstetrique et Biologie de la Reproduction, 19*(3), 290–294.

Mashchak, C. A., Kletzky, O. A., Artal, R., & Mishell, D. R. J. (1984). The relation of physiological changes to subjective symptoms in postmenopausal women and without hot flushes. *Maturitas, 6,* 301–308.

Masters, W., & Johnson, V. (1966). *Human sexual response.* Boston: Little Brown.

Matthews, K., Meilahn, E., Kuller, L. H., Kelsey, S., Caggiula, A. W., & Wing, R. R. (1989). Menopause and risk factors for coronary heart disease. *New England Journal of Medicine, 321*(10), 641–646.

Matthews, K. A. (1992). Myths and realities of the menopause. *Psychosomatic Medicine, 54*(1), 1–9.

Mazess, R. B., & Barden, H. S. (1991). Bone density in premenopausal women: Effects of age, dietary intake, physical activity, smoking, and birth-control pills. *American Journal of Clinical Nutrition, 53,* 132–142.

McEwen, B., Coirini, H., Westlind-Danielsson, A., Frankfurt, M., Gould, E., Schumacher, M., & Woolley, C. (1991). Steroid hormones as mediators of neural plasticity. *Journal of Steroid Biochemistry, 39*(2), 223–232.

McKinlay, J., McKinlay, S., & Brambilla, D. (1987a). Health status and utilization behavior associated with menopause. *American Journal of Epidemiology, 125*(1), 110–121.

McKinlay, J., McKinlay, S., & Brambilla, D. (1987b). The relative contributions of endocrine changes and social circumstances to depression in mid-aged women. *Journal of Health and Social Behavior, 28*(4), 345–363.

McKinlay, S. M., Brambilla, D. J., & Posner, J. G. (1992). The normal menopause transition. *Maturitas, 14*, 103–115.

McKinlay, S. M., & Jeffreys, M. (1974). The menopausal syndrome. *British Journal of Preventive and Social Medicine, 28*, 108–115.

Medical Research International, Society for Assisted Reproductive Technology (SART), The American Fertility Society. (1992). In vitro fertilization–embryo transfer (IVF-ET) in the United States: 1990 results from the IVF-ET Registry. *Fertility and Sterility, 57,* 15–24.

Meldrum, D. R., Tataryn, I. V., Frumar, A. M., Erlik, Y., Lu, K. H., & Judd, H. L. (1980). Gonadotropins, estrogens, and adrenal steroids during the menopausal hot flash. *Journal of Clinical Endocrinology and Metabolism, 50*(4), 685–689.

Milsom, I., Arvidsson, L., Ekelund, P., Molander, U., & Eriksson, O. (1993). Factors influencing vaginal cytology, pH and bacterial flora in elderly women. *Acta Obstetricia et Gynecologica Scandinavica, 72*, 286–291.

Minkler, M., Roe, K., & Robertson-Beckley, R. (1994). Raising grandchildren from crack-cocaine households: Effects on family and friendship ties of African-American women. *American Journal of Orthopsychiatry, 64*(1), 20–29.

Molnar, G. (1975). Body temperatures during menopausal hot flashes. *Journal of Applied Physiology, 38*(3), 499–503.

Morrison-Beedy, D., & Robbins, L. (1989). Sexual assessment and the aging female. *Nurse Practitioner, 14*(12 December), 35–45.

Mortel, K., & Meyer, J. (1993). The role of estrogens in vascular dementia. In *Fourth Annual North American Menopause Society* p. 67. San Diego: North American Menopause Society.

Neugarten, B. L. (1979). Time, age, and the life cycle. *American Journal of Psychiatry, 136*(7), 887–894.

Neugarten, B. L., Wood, V., Kraines, R. J., & Loomis, B. (1963). Women's attitudes toward the menopause. *Vita Humana, 6*, 140–151.

Ohkura, T., Isse, K., Akazawa, K., Hamamoto, M., & Yasi, Y. (1993). Estrogen replacement therapy for dementia of the Alzheimer type in women—short and long term ERT. In *Fourth Annual North American Menopause Society*, p. 109. San Diego: North American Menopause Society.

Ohkura, T., Isse, K., Watabe, H., Segawa, Y., Mitsuya, K., Enomoto, H. Hayashi, M., & Yaoi, Y. (1994). [A clinical study on memory function in climacteric and periclimacteric women]. *Nippon Sanka Fujinka Gakkai Zasshi*. *Acta Obstetricia et Gynecologica*, *46*(3), 271–276.

Okonofua, F., Lawal, A., & Bamgbose, J. (1990). Features of menopause and menopausal age in Nigerian women. *International Journal of Gynaecology and Obstetrics*, *31*(4), 341–345.

O'Reilly-Green, C., & Cohen, W. (1993). Pregnancy in women aged 40 and older. *Obstetrics and Gynecology Clinics of North America*, *20*(2), 313–331.

Orlander, J. D., Jick, S. S., Dean, A. D. & Jick, H. (1992). Urinary tract infections and estrogen use in older women. *Journal of the American Geriatrics Society*, *40*, 817–820.

Palinkas, L. A., & Barrett-Connor, E. (1992). Estrogen use and depressive symptoms in postmenopausal women. *Obstetrics and Gynecology*, *80*, 30–36.

Parlee, M. (1983). Menstrual rhythms in sensory processes: A review of fluctuations in vision, olfaction, audition, taste, and touch. *Psychology Bulletin*, *93*(3), 539–548.

Phillips, S., & Sherwin, B. (1992). Effects of estrogen on memory function in surgically menopausal women. *Psychoneuroendocrinology*, *17*(5), 485–495.

Phillips, S. K., Rook, K. M., Siddle, N. C., Bruce, S. A., & Woledge, R. C. (1993). Muscle weakness in women occurs at an earlier age than in men, but strength is preserved by hormone replacement therapy. *Clinical Science*, *84*, 95–98.

Pirke, K., Schweiger, U., Strowitzki, T., Tuschi, R., Laessle, R., Broocks, A., Huber, B., & Middendorf, R. (1989). Dieting causes menstrual irregularities in normal weight women through impairment of episodic luteinizing hormone secretion. *Fertility and Sterility*, *51*(2), 263–268.

Quirk Jr., J. G., & Wendel Jr., G. D. (1983). Biologic effects of natural and synthetic estrogens. In H. J. Buchsbaum (Ed.), *The menopause* (pp. 55–75). New York: Springer-Verlag.

Rauramo, L., Lagerspetz, K., Engblom, P., & Punnonen, R. (1976). The effect of castration and peroral estrogen therapy on some psychological functions. *Acta Obstetricia et Gynecologica Scandinavica Supplement*, *51*, 3–15.

Reame, N., Kelch, R., Beitins, I., & Yu, M. (1993). Intensive sampling studies of gonadotropin and sex steroid secretion in ovulatory premenopausal women across the menstrual cycle. In *North American Menopause Society Annual Meeting*, p. 12. San Diego: North American Menopause Society.

Regier, D., Myers, J., Kramer, M., Robins, L., Blazer, D., Hough, R., Eaton, W., & Locke, B. (1984). The NIMH Epidemiologic Catchment Area program. Historical context, major objectives, and study population characteristics. *Archives of General Psychiatry, 41*(10), 934–941.

Reichman, M., Judd, J., Taylor, P., Nair, P., Jones, D., & Campbell, W. (1992). Effect of dietary fat on length of the follicular phase of the menstrual cycle in a controlled diet setting. *Journal of Clinical Endocrinology and Metabolism, 74*(5), 1171–1175.

Reynolds, T. (1993). Fertility drugs may raise ovarian cancer risk. *Journal of the National Cancer Institute, 85*(2), 84–86.

Rogers, M., & Evans, W. (1993). Changes in skeletal muscle with aging: Effects of exercise training. *Exercise and Sport Sciences Reviews, 21*, 65–102.

Rose, D., Goldman, M., Connolly, J., & Strong, L. (1991). High-fiber diet reduces serum estrogen concentrations in premenopausal women. *American Journal of Clinical Nutrition, 54*(3), 520–525.

Rubinow, D. R., & Schmidt, P. J. (1994). Depression and the perimenopause. *Menopausal Medicine, 2*(2), 5–8.

Sauer, M., Paulson, R., & Lobo, R. (1993). Pregnancy after age 50: Application of oocyte donation to women after natural menopause. *Lancet, 341*, 321–323.

Semmens, J. P., & Wagner, G. (1985). Effects of estrogen therapy on vaginal physiology during menopause. *Obstetrics and Gynecology, 66*, 15.

Shapiro, S. (1994). The call for change in breast cancer screening guidelines [Editorial]. *American Journal of Public Health, 84*(1), 10–11.

Shapiro, S., Venet, W., Strax, P., & Venet, L. (1988). *Periodic screening for breast cancer: The Health Insurance Plan Project and its sequelae, 1963–1986.* Baltimore: Johns Hopkins University Press.

Shaver, J., Giblin, E., Lentz, M., & Lee, K. (1988). Sleep patterns and stability in perimenopausal women. *Sleep, 11*(6), 556–561.

Shaver, J. L. F., Giblin, E., & Paulsen, V. (1991). Sleep quality subtypes in midlife women. *Sleep, 14*(1), 18–23.

Sheehy, G. (1992). *The silent passage.* New York: Random House.

Sherman, B., & Korenman, S. (1975). Hormonal characteristics of the human menstrual cycle throughout reproductive life. *Journal of Clinical Investigation, 55*(4), 699–706.

Sherman, B., Wallace, R., Bean, J., Chang, Y., & Schlabaugh, L. (1981). The relationship of menopausal hot flushes to medical and reproductive experience. *Journal of Gerontology, 36*, 306–309.

Sherman, B., West, J., & Korenman, S. (1976). The menopause transition: Analysis of LH, FSH, estradiol, and progesterone concentrations during menstrual cycles of older women. *Journal of Clinical Endocrinology and Metabolism, 42*(4), 629–636.

Sherwin, B., & Gelfand, M. (1989). A prospective one-year study of estrogen and progestin in postmenopausal women: Effects on clinical symptoms and lipoprotein lipids. *Obstetrics and Gynecology, 73,* 759–766.

Sherwin, B., & Phillips, S. (1990). Estrogen and cognitive functioning in surgically menopausal women. *Annals of the New York Academy of Sciences, 592,* 474–475.

Sherwin, B. B. (1988). Estrogen and/or androgen replacement therapy and cognitive functioning in surgically menopausal women. *Psychoneuroendocrinology, 13*(4), 345–357.

Silverman, E. (1981). Speech fluency fluctuations during the menstrual cycle. *Journal of Speech and Hearing Research, 18*(1), 202–206.

Speroff, L. (1993). Dysfunctional uterine bleeding in older women. *Menopausal Medicine, 1,* 1–4.

Speroff, L., Glass, R. H., & Kase, N. G. (1989). *Clinical gynecologic endocrinology and infertility* (4th ed.). Baltimore: Williams & Wilkins.

Stein, Z. (1993). HIV prevention: An update on the status of methods women can use [Editorial]. *American Journal of Public Health, 83*(10), 1379–1382.

Stephens, M., Franks, M., & Townsend, A. (1994). Stress and rewards in women's multiple roles: The case of women in the middle. *Psychology of Aging, 9*(1), 45–52.

Stevens, P. E. (1992). Lesbian health care research: A review of the literature from 1970 to 1990. *Health Care of Women International, 13,* 91–120.

Svendsen, O. L., Hassager, C., & Christiansen, C. (1993). Effect of an energy-restrictive diet, with or without exercise, on lean tissue mass, resting metabolic rate, cardiovascular risk factors, and bone in overweight postmenopausal women. *American Journal of Medicine, 95,* 131–140.

Tait, M. J. (1991). Hot flushes in women [Letter to the editor]. *New Zealand Medical Journal* (23 October), 455.

Tataryn, I. V., Lomax, P., Bajorek, J. G., Chesarek, W., Meldrum, D. R., & Judd, H. L. (1980). Postmenopausal hot flushes: A disorder of thermoregulation. *Maturitas, 2,* 101–107.

Tepper, R., Pardo, J., Ovadia, J., & Beyth, Y. (1992). Menopausal hot flushes, plasma calcitonin and beta-endorphin. *Gynecologic and Obstetric Investigation, 33,* 98–101.

Tesar, R., Notelovitz, M., Shim, E., Kauwell, G., & Brown, J. (1992). Axial and peripheral bone density and nutrient intakes of post-menopausal vegetarian and omnivorous women. *American Journal of Clinical Nutrition, 56,* 699–704.

Thompson, B., Hart, S. A., & Durno, D. (1973). Menopausal age and symptomology in a general practice. *Journal of Biosocial Science, 5,* 71–82.

U.S. Bureau of the Census. (1975). *Historical statistics of the United States, Colonial times to 1970.* Washington, DC: U.S. Government Printing Office.

U.S. Bureau of the Census. (1993). *Statistical abstract of the United States* (113th ed.). Lanham, MD: Bernan Press.

U.S. Office of Technology Assessment. (1992). *The menopause, hormone therapy and women's health.* OTA-BP-BA-88. Washington, DC: U.S. Government Printing Office.

Vanhule, G., & Demol, R. (1976). A double-blind study into the influence of estriol on a number of psychological tests in post-menopausal women. In P. Van Keep, R. Greenblatt, & M. Albeaux-Fernet (Eds.), *Consensus on menopausal research* (pp. 94–99). London: MTP Press.

Verbrugge, L. (1986). Role burdens and physical health of women and men. *Women and Health, 11*(1), 47–77.

Voda, A. M. (1992). Menopause: A normal view. *Clinical Obstetric and Gynecology, 35*(4), 923–933.

Wasti, S., Robinson, S., Akhtar, Y., Khan, S., & Badaruddin, N. (1993). Characteristics of menopause in three socioeconomic urban groups in Karachi, Pakistan. *Maturitas, 16*(1), 61–69.

White, J., & Levinson, W. (1993). Primary care of lesbian patients *Journal of General Internal Medicine, 8,* 41–47.

Wickham, M. (1958). The effects of the menstrual cycle on test performance. *British Journal of Psychology, 49,* 34–41.

Wilbur, J., & Dan, A. J. (1989). The impact of work patterns on psychological well-being of midlife nurses. *Western Journal of Nursing Research, 11*(6), 703–716.

Wilbush, J. (1988). Climacteric disorders—Historical perspectives. In J. W. W. Studd & M. I. Whitehead (Eds.), *The menopause.* Boston: Blackwell Scientific Publications.

Wilcox, L., Peterson, H., Haseltine, F., & Martin, M. (1993). Defining and interpreting pregnancy success rates for in vitro fertilization *Fertility and Sterility, 60*(1), 18–25.

Wilson, P., Faragher, B., Butler, B., Bullock, D., Robinson, E., & Brown, A. (1987). Treatment with oral piperazine oestrone sulphate for genuine stress incontinence in postmenopausal women. *British Journal of Obstetrics and Gynaecology, 94*, 568.

Wilson, R. (1966). *Feminine forever.* New York: M. Evans in association with J. B. Lippincott.

Winner, S. J., Morgan, C. A., & Evans, J. G. (1989). Perimenopausal risk of falling and incidence of distal forearm fracture. *British Medical Journal, 298*, 1486–1488.

Wolf, P. H., Madans, J. H., Finucane, F. F., Higgins, M., & Kleinman, J. C. (1991). Reduction of cardiovascular disease–related mortality among postmenopausal women who use hormones: Evidence from a national cohort. *American Journal of Obstetrics and Gynecology, 164*, 489–494.

Wuttke, W., Arnold, P., Becker, D., Creutzfeldt, O., Langenstein, S., & Tirsch, W. (1975). Circulating hormones, EEG, and performance in psychological tests of women with and without oral contraceptives. *Psychoneuroendocrinology, 1*(2), 141–151.

Young, T., Palta, M., Dempsey, J., Skatrud, J., Weber, S., & Badr, S. (1993). The occurrence of sleep-disordered breathing among middle-aged adults. *New England Journal of Medicine, 328*(17), 1230–1235.

Youngs, D. D. (1990). Some misconceptions concerning the menopause. *Obstetrics and Gynecology, 75*(5 May), 881–883.

Zacharias, L., Rand, W. M., & Wurtman, R. J. (1976). A prospective study of sexual development and growth in American girls: The statistics of menarche. *Obstetrical and Gynecological Survey, 31*, 325–337.

Zhang, J., Feldblum, P., & Fortney, J. (1992). Moderate physical activity and bone density among perimenopausal women. *American Journal of Public Health, 82*(5), 736–738.

Zumoff, B. (1993). Biological and endocrinological insights into the possible breast cancer risk from menopausal estrogen replacement therapy. *Steroids, 58*, 196–204.

9

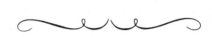

Growing Older

Susan Pfister
Molly Dougherty

The population of persons aged 65 years and over in the United States is growing, both in absolute numbers and in proportion (American Association of Retired Persons & Administration on Aging, 1994). Women comprise the majority of this population. As women age, they face many challenges. Some of these challenges include adaptation to physiological aging changes, resistance to negative stereotyping by society, coping with diminished financial resources, and living with chronic health problems. Most elders encounter one or more chronic health problems during the later stages of their lives which could result in disability and dependence (Schneider & Guralnik, 1990). However, some people maintain their health and functional capabilities well into their later years. These people have achieved successful aging (Rowe & Kahn, 1987).

A major challenge for older women is to discover and utilize strategies that will assist them in aging successfully. Involvement in health promotion activities, development of opportunities for personal growth, exploration of alternative social roles, and utilization of available resources are examples of strategies that may enhance or contribute to the older woman's quality of life. In working with older women, gerontological nurses can formulate "mutual goals" and "priorities" that will assist elders to "attain and maintain the highest level of health, well-being, and quality of life achievable . . ." (American Nurses' Association, 1987, p. 9). These and other issues will be discussed in this chapter. A brief review of physiological aging changes will begin the discussion, followed by psychosocial concerns and common health problems. The final section will describe strategies older women may find helpful in their quest to maintain or improve their health and expand their creative horizons.

Physical Dimension: Physiology of Aging

This section represents an overview of physiological aging changes. Entire texts have been published on this topic, and the reader is referred to these texts for more details regarding specific aging changes. As pointed out by Kenney (1989), changes associated with age are actually representations of a shifting state of normality along the life span continuum. It is difficult at times to distinguish these "normal" changes, resulting from the aging process itself, from those changes occurring due to the presence of pathology. The majority of the aging changes described are found in both men and women. For reproductive system changes, the focus for this chapter will be on older women.

Aging changes can be categorized as reflecting (a) loss of functional cells/tissue, (b) diminished efficiency of an organ or system, or (c) reduction in reserve capabilities of the body. The overall impact of these changes is minimal on the older person's daily existence. However, when faced with additional demands or stressors, elders have less capacity and require more time to meet these demands, physiologically. Examples of aging changes included in each of the above categories will be discussed.

Loss of Mass

Loss of tissue is most apparent in the loss of lean muscle mass with age (Kenney, 1989). Losses are minimized, however, in muscles in which activity has been maintained. The amount of subcutaneous adipose tissue decreases, contributing to alterations in elders' body surface temperature regulation. Hair loss occurs, remaining hair turns gray, and fingernails and toenails become thick and brittle. Bone density decreases and there is degeneration of cartilage. This process results in a loss of height due to vertebral bone loss. There is atrophy of the thymus gland, a component of the immune system, and most endocrine glands lose weight and size (Byyny & Speroff, 1990). Aging also results in losses of functional renal and hepatic tissue.

In the central nervous system, neurons are lost and the brain decreases in size. With age, visual changes include decreased size of the pupil, loss of peripheral retina rod receptors, opacities of the lens, and thickening of the lens. Other sensory losses include decline in number of taste buds, diminished salivary production, decreased moisture in cerumen, and altered vibratory, pain, and thermal sensations. These changes occur linearly with age. Loss of teeth, often noted in older people, is frequently related to dental hygiene practices rather than aging. In older women, the uterus has lost half its mass and there is shrinkage of the fallopian tubes, ovaries, and vagina. The loss of estrogen leads to thinning of the mucosa lining the vaginal wall and bladder, drying of the vagina, decreased size of the labia and clitoris, loss of pubic hair, loss of breast alveoli and adipose tissue, and shrinkage of nipples. Relaxation of pelvic muscles is common.

Diminished System Efficiency

Another category of aging changes is that of diminished efficiency of an organ or system in the body. This decrement in function is reflected in the general impairment of homeostatic mechanisms and the blunted response of the immune system in older persons. The osteoclastic-osteoblastic balance of earlier life is disrupted in all older people, but is most severe in postmenopausal women. Decreased estrogen leads to increased bone resorption and resultant loss of bone density. This process puts the older person at risk of fractures of the vertebra, hip, and wrist. Pulmonary function is altered in elders due to diminished compliance of the chest wall and decreased lung elasticity resulting in increased work to breathe. Cilia are lost from the airways, and remaining cilia are not as active as in younger people.

Cardiac output, stroke volume, and maximum heart rate all decrease with age. Over a period of years, changes occur in blood vessel walls resulting in arteriosclerosis and atherosclerosis (Byyny & Speroff, 1990). Total peripheral resistance and systolic blood pressure increase with age, and perfusion decreases. Glomerular filtration rate is decreased, and the kidneys lose their ability to concentrate urine. Hepatic enzyme activity also decreases with age, affecting many hepatic functions. Altered hepatic and renal functions result in slower drug metabolism and clearance of chemical substances from the body.

Presbyesophagus and atrophic gastritis may occur as a result of degeneration of muscular coordination and motor activity in the upper gastrointestinal system. Loss of muscle tone and diminished motor activity in the colon, plus a higher level of stimulation required for the initiation of defecation, all contribute to the constipation of older persons. Decreased efficiency of vision and hearing commonly occur with increasing age. Presbyopia, or changes in visual accommodation, result from reduced flexibility of the lens of the eye. Presbycusis is the loss of the ability to hear high tones and reflects changes in hair cells and auditory acuity. Both conductive and sensorineural hearing losses may occur in elders. There is an overall slowing of central processing in older people, affecting both the central and peripheral nervous systems. Many homeostatic processes require the participation of conscious behavior, and this participation may be limited in some older people.

Minimal Reserve Capabilities

The third category of aging changes to be discussed involves the reduction in the body's reserve capabilities with age. For older people, everyday activities require more effort. Additional demands on the person, such as exercise, infection, trauma or surgery, can overwhelm the elder's capacity for immediate recovery. In other words, recovery time is slowed. Another example of increased response time is related to balance. Older people have more sway than their younger counterparts. Under usual circumstances, this sway is manageable, with elders having adapted to its effect over a number of years. However, when an older person's path is crossed or the person's trajectory is interrupted unexpectedly, the ability to regain balance or "right" oneself is impaired due to increased response time. This situation may result in an elder falling and possibly sustaining a fracture. Increased reaction time is related to the slowing of central nervous system processing. With fewer neurons, there is decreased functional reserve, resulting in potential information overload and confusion of signals.

In summary, physiological aging changes reflect loss of functional tissue, decreased efficiency, and/or reduction in reserve capacity of some organ systems. These aging changes contribute to alterations in functional capability of the older person. Diminished functional capability may lead to levels of dependence ranging from the need for minimal assistance to the state of frailty. The concept of frailty has both physical and psychosocial connotations.

Psychosocial Domain: Aging with Dignity

Frailty

Two terms commonly linked with older people are *frail* and *vulnerable*. Frail elderly are persons who are usually among the older subgroups of seniors, age 75 and above, who are more than minimally impaired in one or more aspects of functional health. According to one source, frail individuals are "older adults who are medically ill or incapacitated most of the time and, therefore, consume the most health care time, space, and dollars" (Miller, 1990, p. 12). Additional characteristics associated with frailty are low income, certain ethnic origins, female gender, and isolation (Ebersole & Hess, 1985). At the very least, those who are frail are already struggling with some aspect of daily survival. In contrast, older people who are vulnerable are living a somewhat tenuous existence day-to-day, but still are able to manage. A minor decline in their capacity, physical or otherwise, can cause them to become frail and in need of immediate assistance (Atchley, 1990).

Although frail and vulnerable older women and men are not uncommon in American society, the majority of elders by far do not fall into either of these categories. Most elders are active, vigorous individuals capable of enjoying life to the fullest. However, some older people fall victim to an overwhelming fear or dread of becoming frail and disabled. The fear alone can handicap an older person's lifestyle (Atchley, 1983). One source of this fear is the elder's internalization of society's negative view of older people, and especially older women, as ugly, crotchety, and decrepit. These stereotypes of older people are damaging to older individuals and American society as a whole. Stereotypes reflect distorted views and are illustrations of the concept of ageism.

Stereotypes

Ageism is the process of systematic stereotyping of and discrimination against people solely on the basis of age (Lewis & Butler, 1972). Members of the media contribute to ageist thinking by portraying older people as either frail or cantankerous. Ageist thinking attributes the following characteristics to all older people: decline of mental faculties, impairment of physical capabilities, slowness uselessness, and financial dependency. These stereotypes reinforce negative attitudes of society towards older people and contribute to a self-fulfilling prophecy some elders consider inevitable.

Myths of aging are based on stereotypes. Examples of specific myths of aging include the following (Burke & Walsh, 1992; Miller, 1990):

1. Older people can no longer make decisions because they are too old to understand and think clearly.

2. Old people are worthless, nonproductive, and therefore a drain on society.

3. The vast majority of older people are institutionalized.

4. Mental confusion is an inevitable, incurable consequence of old age.

5. Sexual urges and activity normally cease around age 55–60.

6. Families no longer care for older people.

7. As people grow older, it is natural for them to want to withdraw from society.

8. Increased disability in older people is attributable to age-related changes alone.

9. Older adults cannot learn complex new skills.

10. Most old people are depressed.

None of these myths is true. This chapter includes information that exposes many of these misconceptions.

Ageism does not affect women and men equally; for women it is combined with sexist attitudes. Men can age, yet be viewed as attractive on the basis of their achievements, experience in the public world, money, and power. These elements do not generally enhance a woman's desirability. In the United States, a woman's beauty and youth are highly valued. Women are subjected to immense pressure to ward off the signs of aging with cosmetic aids and surgery, reflecting the pressure on women to comply with male standards of desirability and eligibility for marriage (Daly, 1978).

Because medicine reflects society, it is hardly surprising that sexism and ageism are apparent in health care. Older women's experience as consumers in the health care system is marked too frequently by reports of neglect and disrespect. Women's chronic diseases are often ignored or undertreated, as medicine occupies itself with more acute conditions. One study of physicians showed that 65 percent felt women's complaints were influenced by emotional factors, 25 percent felt women were more likely than men to make excessive demands, and 21 percent thought women's complaints were more likely than men's to be psychosomatic (Older Women's League, 1989). A conflicting view is presented by Herzog (1989). She states there is little evidence at present to support the idea that women receive different treatment than men. However, she also suggests further research in this area is needed.

There is little recognition of the value of older women's lifetime contributions to society. Women's work is not considered part of the gross national product. The accumulated wisdom, survival skills, and creativity of women are seldom acknowledged (Lewis, 1985). Women, as well as men, experience role changes related to their daily lives as they age.

Role Changes

Retirement and widowhood are two of the role changes older women commonly experience. Retirement includes cessation of the woman's formal employment, retirement of her spouse, or the end of a structured work life for both. Few older women, compared to their male peers, have maintained long-term, full-time formal employment. At the same time, many older women have frail parents or sick husbands who need their assistance and/or grown children who still require economic or other support. For women in this situation, retirement from compensated employment may not be financially feasible, yet may be necessary to cope with family demands. In other situations the effect of retirement may be quite different. Postretirement years may be a time of freedom from stress-related performance expectations, yet productive for both men and women in each individual's specific area of interest.

Widowhood occurs frequently among older women. Women's greater longevity and the societal norm that men marry women younger than themselves are two factors that contribute to the high number of older widows (Arber & Ginn, 1991). Women who have become accustomed to a more dependent role within the marriage, relying on the husband's handling of their business affairs, etc., may find themselves in a stressful situation as the sole survivor. The older woman may suddenly be confronted with responsibilities for which she is ill prepared. Death of a spouse may mean loss of a long-term partner, friend, lover, and constant companion who was the major source of support for the older woman.

Economic Issues

The role changes discussed above may result in diminished financial resources of the older woman. Retirement of self, retirement of husband, or death of spouse or other "supporting" significant other can lead to a dependency on Social Security as the major payer of day-to-day expenses. Social Security benefits may be minimal due to the woman's lifetime of part-time jobs or low-paying positions, plus interruptions in employment for childbirth or taking care of impaired family members. These diminished funds may barely cover housing costs, heating and cooling expenses, food, and clothing. Little is left for medications, hearing aids, glasses, etc., and none of these items is covered by Medicare.

Older women typically have diminished resources compared to men, and single women are at the highest risk of poverty, because they have had diminished earnings throughout their lifetimes.

For an older woman in this type of situation, it is also difficult to obtain a loan or similar financial assistance. She may not have established a credit line, independent of her husband, earlier in life, and may also have had little experience managing finances. Too many expenses and too few financial resources may result in the older woman's reliance on family members for either monetary assistance or a place to live. For women without family, the end result of this situation of dwindling sources of support may be homelessness.

Although older women are more likely to be poor than are older men (Herzog, 1989), not all women exist in such a stark situation. Many older women do have adequate or above adequate means for financial stability as they age. This financial stability may accrue from long-term savings, investments, retirement benefits, and spousal estate holdings. The security of financial stability can contribute to an older woman's positive outlook on the remaining years of her life. In other words, economic means are an important resource for coping with stress. Another buffer against the stresses of life is a supportive social network.

Social Network

An individual's social network generally consists of immediate and extended family members, friends, co-workers, neighbors, peers, and members of organizational affiliations. Losses and changes occur with age that can affect the size of this network. Retirement from work outside the home terminates the frequent contact with co-workers and may result in permanent loss of socialization with these former network members. The older person may decrease the number of community organizations she volunteers for, in order to concentrate her energy on one or two, limiting her social contacts. As financial resources or functional abilities decline, the older woman may need to change living situations (e.g., from private home to senior citizen apartment or congregate living). This uprooting of the elder may result in her living in an environment far from her circle of friends, thereby severely altering her social network.

The older woman's immediate family social network is altered when adult children leave, or frail parents move into her home. The death of spouses, children, extended family members, siblings, and peers may affect the opportunities available for older women to interact with others in a meaningful and enjoyable way. One factor that helps women to buffer these losses and changes is their ability to establish and maintain close relationships with a few individuals. These confidants are more important to older women psychologically than having a large social network or having frequent contact with family (Grace, 1989; Lee & Ishii-Kuntz, 1988). Even with the buffering effect of a few close friends, the older woman may experience loneliness.

Loneliness

As mentioned earlier, women live longer than men and frequently outlive their lifelong partners. Men who have survived into old age and are single, divorced, or widowed tend to marry younger women, leaving older women with fewer prospects for remarriage. Loss of the family home, with relocation to a new living situation, may also result in loneliness for the older woman. Loss of pets and cherished possessions can contribute to the feeling of being totally alone, with no connection to a past, present, or future. Lack of the feeling of being needed may lead to the elder withdrawing from society. This withdrawal can result in social isolation, and the older woman's loneliness is then compounded.

Social isolation may be self-imposed or imposed by others. An older woman with urinary incontinence may severely limit her forays outside the home due to fear of loss of urine in public and resulting stigmatization. Proponents of ageist thinking would suggest that all old people, especially women with wrinkled skin and gray hair, should be invisible. Older women should spend their days quietly biding their time in rocking chairs, apart from the mainstream of society. In actuality, most older women lead active, vigorous lives even though they may experience one or more health problems in their later years.

Common Health Problems

There are three issues relative to the health care of elders that are important to consider prior to discussing specific health problems. One issue is the difficulty in identifying the underlying disorder causing symptoms an elder may be experiencing. The second issue involves the ignorance of many health care practitioners concerning the health needs of older women. The third issue is the need for comprehensive assessment of the older client in order to differentiate treatable pathologic conditions from changes due solely to aging.

Diagnosis of disease in older people may be difficult at best. Older adults may not respond to diseases with the same signs and symptoms as younger persons, and therefore may present with a variety of nonspecific complaints (Burrage, Dixon, & Sehy, 1991). Symptoms of confusion, urinary incontinence, fatigue, syncope, or complaints of "just not feeling well" are commonly heard by health care practitioners. Elderly clients frequently present with multiple complaints rather than one problem. This is due to the fact that many older people are experiencing more than one chronic disease at any given time. All of this points to the importance of specialized expertise of health care providers caring for older people.

The second issue of concern is the ignorance of many medical personnel regarding health needs of older people, especially older women. Recent research suggests that many health care providers are unaware of important factors impacting women's health, such as differences in symptomatology and treatment response between women and men suffering from the same pathological condition, and the recent advances in diagnosis and treatment of women's diseases (Task Force on Older Women's Health, 1993).

The limited expertise of health care providers pertaining to the care of older women combined with the unusual presentation of disease in the elderly necessitates a comprehensive assessment for each older client presenting with a problem. The assumption that a particular symptom is "a part of the aging process" and that "nothing can be done about it" is common to both the health care professional and the elder. This approach, or non-approach, risks missing conditions that are amenable to treatment (Miller & Kaiser, 1993). A comprehensive, multidisciplinary assessment is the most thorough, accurate approach to meeting the health needs of older women.

The following section is a description of some of the specific health problems older women commonly experience. Although older men and women describe their health relatively similarly, women at all ages report more actual limitations in activities of daily life from the effects of aging and illness. This presentation is not meant to be all-inclusive but focuses on selected problems. The reader is referred to medical texts for further details about these disorders and information on problems not included in this discussion. Health problems have been categorized as physiological disorders, mental health problems, and lifestyle issues. Disorders of reproductive structures have been extracted from physiological problems and entered into a separate category due to their importance for older women.

Chronic Physiological Disorders

The physiological disorders that will be discussed are cardiovascular disease, osteoporosis, arthritis, and urinary incontinence.

Cardiovascular disease

Heart disease is the leading cause of death for women over 65 (Older Women's League, 1989). Despite the risk to women from heart disease, nearly all randomized, controlled studies on risk factors, treatment, and outcomes of cardiovascular disease have exclusively involved men (Barry, 1993). Risk factors for coronary artery disease in women include low levels of high-density lipoprotein cholesterol, smoking, hypertension, postmenopausal state, and the presence of diabetes (Barry, 1993). The onset of coronary artery disease in women is approximately 10 years later than it is in men. The most common manifestations of coronary artery disease in women are angina, myocardial infarction, and sudden cardiac death (Byyny & Speroff, 1990). The occurrence of acute myocardial infarction in women, however, is delayed by approximately 20 years as compared to that in men.

More recent studies that controlled for different age and risk factors in women found that women have tended to be referred for angiography and angioplasty significantly less often than men (Joint

National Committee on Detection, Evaluation, and Treatment of High Blood Pressure, 1993). One study found that women are referred for coronary artery bypass graft later in the course of their disease than men, when they are older, sicker, and have an increased chance of postoperative death (Barry, 1993).

Two substances that have an effect on women relative to cardiovascular status are aspirin and estrogen. Aspirin has an apparent cardioprotective effect for women over age 50. There is a significant reduction in coronary artery disease among postmenopausal women on estrogen replacement therapy (perhaps as high as 50 percent; Barry, 1993); the addition of progesterone to reduce cancer risk, however, reduces the cardioprotective effect of estrogen.

As mentioned earlier, hypertension is a prominent risk factor for cardiovascular disease in older people. Once thought to be controversial, the treatment of hypertension in older people has been shown to have a positive effect. Research has demonstrated fewer strokes and myocardial infarctions in actively treated elders as compared to those receiving placebo (Joint National Committee on Detection, Evaluation, and Treatment of High Blood Pressure, 1993). This is particularly important because women experience twice the rate of stroke as men. Older people can benefit from treatment of diastolic blood pressure elevations as well as systolic hypertension.

Initial treatment of hypertension includes modification of lifestyle factors. These modifications include avoidance of tobacco, weight reduction, moderation of alcohol and dietary sodium intake, and increase in physical activity. Antihypertensive medication therapy in older people should be started with lower doses of the drug and increased in smaller increments and over a longer period of time than with younger people receiving this therapy. Older women with hypertension may still receive estrogen replacement therapy (i.e., for osteoporosis) but will require close monitoring of their blood pressure for possible effects (Joint National Committee on Detection, Evaluation, and Treatment of High Blood Pressure, 1993).

Osteoporosis

Osteoporosis is a change in bone structure characterized by a reduction in mass rather than an alteration in chemical composition. This type of bone reduction is mainly attributable to estrogen deficiency and frequently results in fractures. The vertebral bone is especially vulnerable. Hip and wrist fractures are also common. Risk of fracture depends on (a) peak bone mass achieved at maturity, and (b) rate of bone loss throughout life (Byyny & Speroff, 1990). Fractures, especially hip fractures, are a significant cause of institutionalization, mental deterioration, and mortality among the elderly, because they may require lengthy periods of immobility and diminished stimulation (Herzog, 1989).

Various genetic factors; dietary and lifestyle habits including excess caffeine intake, physical inactivity, cigarette smoking, and use of drugs; and diseases are associated with an increased risk of osteoporosis. Thin, Caucasian women are at highest risk for developing this disorder. In the United States, 25 percent of all White women over age 60 are affected by osteoporosis (Levin, 1993). Symptoms of osteoporosis include pain, functional limitations, and increased feelings of stress (Grace, 1989).

Treatment of osteoporosis may include estrogen replacement therapy (protective effect related to heart disease), calcium, vitamin D, fluoride, and weight-bearing activity (as little as 30 minutes per day, 3 times per week; walking is a good activity; Byyny & Speroff, 1990). Prevention is the hallmark of treatment. Estrogen replacement therapy is the most effective single modality for preventing osteoporosis in postmenopausal women. Research has shown that even 70-year-old women may benefit from estrogen replacement therapy (Levin, 1993). All women taking estrogen should be closely followed with annual mammograms and gynecologic examinations. Estrogen replacement therapy has historically been linked to an increased risk for the development of endometrial and breast cancer in some women. However, recent studies indicate that the risk is minimal except for those women with a familial history and/or prior self-history of breast or endometrial cancer.

Calcitonin is a hormone that inhibits osteoclastic activity and has been used to treat osteoporosis. Calcitonin is costly and requires daily injections, but may be indicated in elderly women (20 years postmenopausal) who are experiencing severe back pain from a recent fracture. Calcitonin has an acute beneficial effect on the bone, plus an analgesic effect as a result of the binding of calcitonin to opiate receptors (Levin, 1993).

Arthritis

Two types of arthritis that affect older women are rheumatoid arthritis and osteoarthritis. Rheumatoid arthritis is a systemic inflammatory disease, possibly autoimmune in nature. This disorder involves inflammation of the synovial membrane lining the distal joints, wrists, fingers, and toes, plus morning stiffness, and sometimes fever and weight loss. Symptomatic treatment includes the use of aspirin, nonsteroidal antiinflammatory drugs (NSAIDs), a balance of rest and exercise, and splinting. Older people are more susceptible to the side effects of aspirin and NSAIDs, so low doses of steroids may be preferred. People with rheumatoid arthritis are subject to disability, reduced mobility, and steroid use, which enhances their risk of developing osteoporosis (Byyny & Speroff, 1990).

Osteoarthritis is a chronic, nonsystemic deterioration of articular cartilage. Pain in the involved joints is increased with weight-bearing activity and relieved by rest. This joint problem may occur in the hands, hips, knees, feet, or vertebra. Management of osteoarthritis includes a balance of rest and exercise, and analgesics, such as acetaminophen. Total hip or knee arthroplasty are common surgical procedures for people with osteoarthritis regardless of age (Byyny & Speroff, 1990).

The characteristic pain, stiffness, and swelling in joints due to arthritis may affect the ability of the older person to walk, climb stairs, bend, lift, reach over the head, or control fine motor coordination. These physical impairments, in turn, are related to the more complex abilities required to function independently, and to lead a full and productive life in today's society (Herzog, 1989).

Urinary incontinence

Urinary incontinence involves the involuntary loss of urine, and it is a significant problem for older women. It has been estimated that the prevalence of urinary incontinence is 15 to 30 percent in community-based populations (Herzog & Fultz, 1990), rising to 50 percent or above in nursing home populations (National Institutes of Health Consensus Development Conference [NIHCDC], 1990). These prevalence rates may actually reflect conservative estimates due to the acknowledged problem of client and health care provider underreporting of the existence of incontinence.

Many people feel urinary incontinence is a concomitant of the aging process and that very little can be done to affect its course (DuBeau & Resnick, 1991; Goldstein, Hawthorne, Engeberg, McDowell, & Burgio, 1992; Mitteness, 1987). Incontinence guidelines released nationally include an emphasis on the need for education of the public and health care providers alike as to the importance of accurate assessment, diagnosis, and treatment of urinary incontinence (Urinary Incontinence Guideline Panel [UIGP], 1992).

The consequences of urinary incontinence in affected individuals can be physical, psychological, and/or social (Ouslander, 1992). Physical effects include skin irritations or infections, decubiti, falls (Herzog, Diokno, & Fultz, 1989), and dehydration with its sequelae. Psychological effects may include depression, insecurity, sensory deprivation (McCormick, Scheve, & Leahy, 1988), and altered or nonexistent sexual activity (Wyman, Harkins, & Fantl, 1990). Socially, the individual may feel stigmatized, with resultant social isolation, whether self-imposed or imposed by others (Breakwell & Walker, 1988). Urinary incontinence leads to increased burden on informal or formal caregivers (Flaherty, Miller, & Coe, 1992) and may be a determinant of nursing home placement (Ouslander, 1990).

Treatment approaches for urinary incontinence, following thorough assessment, include behavioral techniques, pharmacologic agents, surgical procedures, and use of incontinence aids such as absorbent pads (UIGP, 1992). Behavioral techniques include bladder training, habit training, prompted voiding, biofeedback (Hadley, 1986), patterned urge response toileting (Colling, Hadley, Eisch, Campbell, & Ouslander, 1992), and pelvic muscle exercises (Dougherty, Bishop, Mooney, Gimotty, & Williams, 1992). Behavioral therapies involve noninvasive procedures that carry minimal risk, and are, therefore, recommended as initial approaches to treating urinary incontinence in older people.

Disorders of Reproductive Structures

The specific problems to be included in this section are breast cancer, pelvic structure/organ cancer, atrophic vaginitis, abnormal uterine bleeding, and prolapse.

Breast cancer

The longer a woman lives, the greater her risk of developing breast cancer. Among women over age 50, the incidence of breast cancer is 331 per 100,000 (Rosenberg, 1993). Despite being at high risk, elderly women tend not to be screened routinely. When older women do seek medical help, their breast cancer is usually more involved or extensive than that of younger women seeking assistance. Older women with breast cancer are not always treated as aggressively as their younger counterparts. Mastectomy is performed on many older patients, but up to one third do not have an axillary dissection (Rosenberg, 1993). This affects the older woman's chances for survival with additional therapy. Older women are viable candidates, in many cases, for the use of radiation therapy and chemotherapy. Healthy patients in their 70s and 80s should receive the same treatment as someone who is 40. Individual treatment risk is far more important than the patient's absolute age.

Breast conservation treatment is appropriate for the primary treatment of many women with early stage breast cancer. It provides a survival equivalent to total mastectomy and axillary dissection, while still preserving the breast. Most women, regardless of age, are concerned about body image. Cosmetic concerns by women over age 50 are viewed by others in American society as less valid than the image concerns of younger women. Breast conservation and reconstruction procedures should be available to women of all ages unless contraindicated for medical reasons.

Pelvic organ cancer
The risk of reproductive tract cancers increases with age (Older Women's League, 1989). Although this is an established fact, efforts toward prevention and detection of cancer in older women are not as extensive as those directed at younger populations. Women over 60 are the least likely of women of any age group to have annual pelvic exams and Pap smears, or to have ever had this screening. Contributing factors to this situation are attitudes of elders and providers that such tests are no longer needed at their age, limited access of elders to health care facilities, and lack of funds to pay for preventive and screening health care procedures.

When elderly patients develop a gynecologic malignancy, the prognosis is worse than for younger women with the same problem (McGonigle, Lagasse, & Karlan, 1993). After site of origin, the stage of the cancer is the most important determinant of treatment and the most important predictor of survival. It is likely that the failure of the elderly to undergo routine pelvic examinations has influenced the stage at diagnosis of gynecologic malignancy in the elderly and, in turn, increased the mortality rate (McGonigle, Lagasse, & Karlan, 1993).

The Pap smear, even if performed on an older woman, may not provide accurate results. Cervical cytology testing for cervical cancer may have a high false-negative rate for elderly women because physiological aging changes (the squamocolumnar junction is often high up in the endocervical canal) preclude adequate sampling. Furthermore, elderly women may have stenotic cervices, making sampling more difficult (McGonigle, Lagasse, & Karlan, 1993).

Not only are the elderly at an increased risk for the development of cancer, but their relative immunosuppression and concurrent medical problems must be considered in evaluating treatment options. Chronological age is too often the major factor influencing treatment decisions. Advanced age is frequently associated with less aggressive therapy for women with gynecologic malignancies compared with younger women. Elderly women, in one study, were more likely to be treated with single rather than multimodality therapy. Most elderly patients can withstand radical surgery almost as well as their younger counterparts. There are several studies that suggest that the elderly are more likely than younger cancer patients to receive palliative rather than curative therapy (McGonigle, Lagasse, & Karlan, 1993).

The death rate for cervical cancer rises significantly with age and is primarily related to the poor prognosis of cervical cancer in this age group. Older women are more likely to have advanced cervical cancer at the time of diagnosis and are also more likely to have complicating medical factors that interfere with treatment. As mentioned earlier, elderly women are less likely to undergo routine screening exams, which may account for the increased incidence and worse prognosis of this cancer. Treatment modalities include surgery and radiotherapy. In many instances, radiation therapy has been the preferred treatment for older cancer victims. However, radical hysterectomy in older women is not associated with increased complications compared with younger women (McGonigle, Lagasse, & Karlan, 1993).

Uterine cancer is the most common gynecologic malignancy in the United States. When an elderly woman develops endometrial cancer, she is much more likely to die of the disease than younger women. Factors associated with increased risk of endometrial cancer include nulliparity, obesity, diabetes, and hypertension. Unopposed estrogen use in postmenopausal women is associated with an increased risk of endometrial cancer, but this can be prevented by adding a progestin to the replacement regimen. Because 90 percent of women with endometrial cancer present with abnormal vaginal bleeding, all postmenopausal bleeding deserves an endometrial biopsy for diagnosis. Treatment of uterine cancer includes surgical staging, adjuvant radiation therapy, and chemotherapy (McGonigle, Lagasse, & Karlan, 1993).

Of all gynecologic malignancies, ovarian cancer presents the greatest challenge to the older woman and the health care provider. Older women are seen initially in the health care setting at a more advanced stage of the disease. Symptoms associated with ovarian cancer are often vague and nonspecific. Treatment of ovarian cancer includes staging laparotomy, second-look surgery, chemotherapy, and radiation therapy. Elderly patients may be less tolerant of radiation therapy than younger patients and may suffer from more complications (McGonigle, Lagasse, & Karlan, 1993).

Atrophic vaginitis

Atrophic vaginitis is an inflammation of the vagina secondary to physiological changes resulting from lack of estrogen. The vaginal lining becomes thin and dry, and loses its elasticity and resistance to infection. This can result in symptoms such as leukorrhea, pruritus, burning, and discomfort during sexual intercourse (Barber, 1988). Secondary infections may develop including sexually transmitted diseases. Treatment may include topical application of estrogen cream to the vagina or oral cyclic estrogen and progesterone therapy (Goldfarb, 1985). Synthetic water-soluble lubricants are available that can replace moisture and facilitate ease of penile penetration. Education regarding vulvar hygiene can contribute to the prevention of secondary infections. Cleansing of the perineal area post voiding, use of loose-fitting cotton underclothing, and avoidance of vaginal deodorants and hygiene sprays may reduce the older woman's risk of vaginal infections (Barber, 1988).

Abnormal uterine bleeding

Vaginal bleeding that occurs postmenopausally has traditionally been considered a highly significant indicator of the presence of malignancy. More recently, this association has been less marked. In one study, the cause of bleeding in 80 percent of women with recurrent postmenopausal bleeding was benign (Casey, 1985). However, bleeding is still considered a warning sign, and therefore warrants timely investigation. Uterine conditions are commonly the source of bleeding, although bleeding can also occur within the lower genital tract (tumors of the vulva and vagina, urethral caruncles, prolapse, trauma, and atrophic vaginitis) and outside the genital tract (hematuria and rectal bleeding). Uterine conditions include ulcers; tumors; polyps of the cervix, corpus, and endometrium; cervicitis; and endometritis.

Comprehensive assessment of any vaginal bleeding is extremely important. Assessment includes a thorough history and physical examination followed by completion of one or more diagnostic procedures such as Pap smears, biopsies, colposcopy, and cytology and histology of endometrial tissues. Once diagnosis is accomplished, treatment frequently involves local excision of small tumors through cautery, cryosurgery, or laser therapy; or surgical excision of larger tumors and surrounding tissues as indicated. Regular follow-up exams of the woman with a history of bleeding episodes is extremely important in order to detect any changes indicative of further pathological developments (Casey, 1985).

Prolapse

In older women, the loss of adequate pelvic support commonly results in prolapse of the bladder (cystocele), the urethra (urethrocele), the uterus, the peritoneum (enterocele), the rectum (rectocele), or a combination of these structures. Supportive pelvic structures include the fascia, ligaments, muscles, and bony pelvis. The stretching of childbirth, postmenopausal changes in perineal structures, aging, and heredity all contribute to the loss of vaginal wall tone and weakening of the pelvic structures (Karram & Walters, 1993).

The weakening of these structures with resulting prolapse leads to symptoms such as the sensation of bulging in the vagina, pelvic pressure and/or pain, low back pain, and sexual difficulties (Walters, 1993). Voiding difficulties, urinary incontinence, constipation, and/or rectal incontinence may be associated with a prolapse. Obesity, chronic lung diseases, metabolic diseases, and demyelinating diseases also contribute to uterine prolapse (Barber, 1988). Treatment options for pelvic support loss include conservative measures and surgical intervention.

Conservative treatment modalities include weight reduction, the use of bulk foods and stool softeners, the use of estrogens, Kegel's exercises (pelvic muscle exercises), and the use of pessaries (Baden & Walker, 1985). If these approaches are unsuccessful, surgical procedures such as anterior and posterior colporrhaphy may be warranted. Age alone is not a contraindication to surgery. However, a comprehensive preoperative assessment of the older woman is essential for identification of coexisting metabolic problems that could predispose the woman to postoperative complications. Prolapses may recur even though surgically repaired. Factors contributing to the increased risk of recurrence include inadequate initial surgical repair, heavy lifting, smoking, obesity, absence of estrogen replacement after menopause, chronic pulmonary disease, and genetic factors (Walters, 1993).

Common health problems of older women include mental health problems as well as physiological problems. Early mental health research on elders focused on life satisfaction and morale. The majority of studies suggest that physical health is the most important correlate of life satisfaction (Grace, 1989). In a study of 243 elderly community-dwelling women, older age was related to lower levels of purpose in life, personal growth, and positive relationships. Well-being was related to the impact of physical health problems on the ability to function in daily life, rather than the total number of health problems (Heidrich, 1993). Poor health, regardless of age, was associated with more depression and anxiety and lower levels of positive relationships and autonomy.

Mental Health Problems

Up to 25 percent of the elderly manifest symptoms of mental disorder (Grace, 1989). Two major disorders associated with older people are depression, reflecting affective problems, and Alzheimer's disease, reflecting cognitive decline. These disorders will be discussed and a few comments will be made regarding organic brain disease and paranoia.

Depression

Depression affects only 10 percent to 15 percent (Khan, Mirolo, Mirolo, & Dobie, 1993) of older women, but in those affected it is often very serious (Byyny & Speroff, 1990). Women have higher rates of depression than men (Herzog, 1989). Depression may result from losses of loved ones, losses of functional abilities, and the use of certain medications (Byyny & Speroff, 1990). Conditions that are likely to lead to depressive reactions include cardiovascular disease and cancer as well as vision and hearing losses. The assessment of depression is difficult because its symptoms may mimic those of physical illness and dementia while, at the same time, it may coexist with these disorders (Grace, 1989). Depression also often coexists with anxiety disorders such as phobias, panic disorder, and generalized anxiety disorder (Khan, Mirolo, Mirolo, & Dobie, 1993).

The symptoms of depression include loss of appetite, weight loss, decreased energy and motivation, and sleep disturbance. However, depressed women more typically have increased appetite and weight gain (Khan, Mirolo, Mirolo, & Dobie, 1993). Other symptoms may include low self-esteem, difficulty concentrating, or general slowing of response (Herzog, 1989), and expressed feelings of uselessness and hopelessness (Miller, 1990).

The treatment of depression includes tender loving care, touching, listening, self-help books, and antidepressants (Byyny & Speroff, 1990). The good news about depression in older people is that this population is generally amenable to treatment. Antidepressants include tricyclics and the newer selective serotonin re-uptake inhibitors (SSRIs; Khan, Mirolo, Mirolo, & Dobie, 1993).

Suicide

Suicide, particularly among the aged, is thought to be related to depression. Underreporting of suicide may be more substantial for the older age groups, because at this age illnesses are usually present, and may be substituted as a more acceptable cause of death than suicide.

Attempted suicide, or parasuicide (Cattell & Wilkinson, 1992), is thought to be even more closely related to depression among the elderly than completed suicide. Although the rate of completed suicide is higher in men, women attempt suicide more frequently than men (Herzog, 1989).

Risk factors for suicide include advanced age, male gender, alcohol/ drug abuse, living alone, chronic disease, major loss such as loss of home or significant other (through death, divorce, separation), pending nursing home placement, depression, psychosis, previous suicide attempt (Khan, Mirolo, Mirolo, & Dobie, 1993), social isolation, and dementia (Byyny & Speroff, 1990). Suicide can be active, involving the actual commission of a harmful act, or passive.

Two examples of passive suicide are poor nutrition and noncompliance (Byyny & Speroff, 1990). A third example, seen among the elderly in particular, is suicide by inaction. An illustration of the third example is failure of an elder to take prompt action upon noting medical symptoms (Herzog, 1989).

Organic brain disease

Intellectual and cognitive impairments increase with age. Recent evidence suggests that women over 80 may have higher rates of cognitive impairment than men of the same age (Herzog, 1989). These impairments can create hardships for the affected individuals and their families plus enormous financial burdens for families and the public. Some of these cognitive problems are due to potentially reversible organic brain disorders, such as infections and tumors. However, the most common cause of severe cognitive impairment in older age is thought to be Alzheimer's disease, which also involves organic changes in the brain (Herzog, 1989). At present there is no test specific for the diagnosis of Alzheimer's disease. It is essential that the presence of reversible organic problems be ruled out before determining the cognitive deficits of an older woman are due to the irreversible changes associated with Alzheimer's disease.

Alzheimer's disease

Dementia is a progressive loss of intellectual capacity with gradual regression of physical and mental ability to a point of near or absolute helplessness (Byyny & Speroff, 1990). Alzheimer's disease accounts for about 75 percent of dementia among the elderly (Older Women's League, 1989). Symptoms include trouble with memory and cognitive functions. It is difficult to distinguish Alzheimer's disease from normal senescent forgetfulness, especially in the early stages. Alzheimer's disease can also be confused with other organic dementias (multi-infarct) and pseudodementia (Grace, 1989).

The treatment of Alzheimer's disease is symptomatic and includes use of memory aids such as lists and other reminders; correction of poor hearing, vision, nutrition, etc.; day care centers; and art and music therapy. Environmental changes should be kept to a minimum and the client reoriented as frequently as possible in order to avoid increased confusion (Byyny & Speroff, 1990). As a degenerative condition, Alzheimer's has a very high secondary victimization rate, taking an excessive toll on family caregivers, most of whom are women (Older Women's League, 1989).

Paranoia

Another mental health problem, that of paranoia, may be seen in older people as a result of perceptual problems, such as impaired eyesight or hearing, leading to confusion (Byyny & Speroff, 1990). People with hearing losses may state that others are whispering about them, or plotting to get rid of them by murder or by placing them in a psychiatric hospital (Barber, 1988). Elders who exhibit paranoid reactions usually have a pattern of suspiciousness or denial of impairment throughout their lifetimes. However, adequate assessment and correction of visual or auditory defects may be quite helpful in assisting some elders to work through these feelings of paranoia.

Lifestyle Issues

Lifestyle-related factors can also contribute to women's health problems. These factors include nutritional concerns, issues related to mobility and functional capabilities, vulnerability, and substance abuse.

Lifestyle factors that contribute to health problems can affect both men and women. However, some women are more at risk of developing problems because they exist in a state of quadruple jeopardy—being old, female, a minority, and poor (Grace, 1989). The access to resources is severely limited for these women.

Altered nutrition

A substantial part of the health problems experienced by the elderly is a result of poor nutrition throughout their lives. In old age, poor nutrition can take several forms. Insufficient quantity or quality of food may be available to the older person due to poverty or physical difficulty in shopping for and preparing food. The elderly tend to make use of foods that involve little preparation, that require little chewing, and that are cheap. Healthy foods, such as fresh fruits and vegetables, are commonly more expensive than prepackaged or refined foods. As a consequence of an unbalanced diet, food consumption may be too high in calories, leading to overweight and obesity.

Even with an adequate, nutritional food supply, the older person may not eat, or may not eat enough to stay healthy. This may happen when diminished sensations of smell, taste, and vision make food appear less appetizing; when lack of teeth or denture problems make chewing difficult; or when living alone means that the social stimuli for cooking and eating are lacking.

Factors contributing to malnutrition include physical, psychological, and social factors. Physical factors include illness, immobility, alcohol abuse, dementia, obesity or cachexia, multiple medications or laxatives, and edentulous or poorly fitting dentures. Psychological factors include emotional stress, loneliness, isolation, depression, and bereavement. Social factors include inadequate food preparation and storage facilities, limited finances, limited social support, and loss of the family member whose responsibilities included shopping and cooking (Hashizume, 1991).

Poor nutrition in older age must be understood, therefore, in the context of the social, health, and economic conditions of the aged. Women are more likely than men to experience certain of those conditions, notably living alone, being poor, and being impaired by functional problems (Herzog, 1989).

Falls
Approximately 25 percent to 30 percent of community-dwelling older people fall each year. Injury serious enough to require medical attention occurs in 5 percent to 10 percent of all falls (Winograd & Gerety, 1993). About half of fallers experience multiple falls each year. These "multiple fallers" are at greatest risk of fall-related injury.

Factors contributing to falls, slips, and trips may be categorized as either intrinsic or extrinsic (Stone & Chenitz, 1991). Intrinsic factors include (a) age-related changes in vision (especially acuity and depth perception), hearing, posture, and gait; (b) inability to correct loss of balance and slowed reaction time; (c) poor judgment; (d) emotional effects (agitation, depression, distraction, confusion, anxiety, and fear); (e) neuromuscular deficits (difficulty rising from a chair, lower extremity weakness, increased sway, and foot problems); (f) fear of incontinence;

(g) denial of illness, weakness, and dependence; (h) pain; (i) podiatric conditions (ingrown toenails, corns, and bunions); (j) adjusting to a new environment; (k) presence of disorders affecting stability (postural hypotension), mobility (osteoporosis), and cognitive function (transient ischemic attack); and (l) drugs, especially sedative hypnotics.

Extrinsic factors include (a) lighting that is too dim or too bright (glare); (b) walking surfaces that are uneven or wet; (c) stairs with edges unclearly defined or inadequate handrails; (d) furniture that is too low, on wheels, or tips easily; (e) bathrooms without grab rails for toilet, tub, or shower; (f) inappropriate or poor fitting footwear and clothing; (g) equipment that is worn out or used improperly (Stone & Chenitz, 1991); (h) throw rugs; and (i) improper height of beds, chairs, or toilets (Miller, 1990).

Once a fall does occur, approximately 1 in 20 falls produces a fracture, usually of the wrist or hip (Winograd & Gerety, 1993). Almost half of all patients with hip fractures enter nursing homes after hospitalization, one half suffer impairments in basic activities of daily living, one third are impaired in instrumental activities of daily living, and only 60 percent return to baseline ambulatory ability (Winograd & Gerety, 1993). In addition to injury, falls significantly affect the quality of life. Fear of falling may occur, with resultant curtailing of activities.

Functional impairments

Most older persons are capable of carrying on their normal daily routines, and very few are unable to perform basic physical care activities (Herzog, 1989). However, functional impairments do occur. Older women report higher levels of disability than older men. On measures of physical function, older women report higher rates of impairment than older men, and Black older women report the worst impairment of all (Herzog, 1989). As pointed out by Kane and Kane (1981), there are areas in addition to physical status that warrant assessment with regard to adequate functioning in the older person. Two of these areas are the social domain and the mental domain. Other authors include emotional functioning (Applegate, Blass, & Williams, 1990). Deficiencies in any of these functional areas can negatively affect an older woman's health. These impairments can also contribute to her vulnerability.

Vulnerability and abuse

The older woman is vulnerable to potential abuses from people and institutions. Older people are targeted as unsuspecting, incapable of understanding or resisting, and trusting, especially of those in authority.

Frail elders are particularly susceptible to abuse by caregivers. There is the misconception by some elders that caregivers would never harm them. Other elders express difficulty identifying alternatives to their present situation. These older people are at the mercy of whoever is willing to offer assistance, regardless of cost or quality of the assistance rendered.

Abuse may range from overt physical violence to more subtle forms of mistreatment or neglect. In most states, cases of elder neglect exceed cases of elder abuse (Lachs & Fulmer, 1993). Neglect may be active, such as intentional withholding of food and medications, or passive, such as provision of inadequate care of the elder. The inadequacy of care may pertain to direct physical care needed for recovery from an illness or surgical procedure or usual daily care required to maintain optimal physical or emotional health. It is estimated that one million elderly persons may experience elder mistreatment annually (Lachs & Fulmer, 1993).

Although early research described the most frequent victims of abuse as older widows, physically frail, and cognitively impaired, more recent studies suggest there are no differences among victims. Older people are at risk of abuse regardless of age, sex, socioeconomic status, level of physical activity, and degree of cognitive ability (Lachs & Fulmer, 1993). The approach to resolution of an abusive situation includes (a) mandatory reporting of the suspected abuse, (b) on-site investigation of the report by the state elder protective agency, (c) possible removal of the person in danger from the abusive situation (d) easing the caregiver's burden through provision of community-based services (e.g., home health aides, adult day care, and respite programs), and (e) treatment of the abuser (Lachs & Fulmer, 1993).

Specific examples of elder abuse include sexual abuse, abandonment by individuals and institutions (i.e., granny dumping), and abuse from con artists selling services elders do not really need or not following through with services they really do need. Older people are considered easy targets for violence on the street and in the home especially on occasions elders are thought to have money, such as days Social Security checks are received. This social abuse of elders contributes to the fear and resultant self-restriction of activities some older people exhibit outside the home.

Alcoholism

The incidence of alcoholism in community-residing elderly individuals aged 65 and over is estimated to be 10 percent to 30 percent or higher. Estimates suggest 10 percent to 15 percent of women over age 65 suffer from psychiatric, physical, or functional impairment related to alcohol (Szwabo, 1993). The abuse of alcohol may be considered within the broader framework of substance abuse. Substance abuse can be broadly defined as the use of illegal substances, taking too few or too many medications, discontinuing medications without consultation with a physician or other health care provider, alcohol use alone or in combination with drugs to treat symptoms, sharing of medications, hoarding and use of old (expired) prescriptions, and reliance upon over-the-counter medications (Szwabo, 1993).

The older woman is vulnerable to substance abuse because of (a) living alone; (b) isolation, loneliness, and depression; (c) unhappiness with her relationship(s); (d) illness or dependency; (e) lack of money for quality treatment; (f) minority status; and (g) the likelihood she has a prescription for psychoactive medications or is self-medicating (Szwabo, 1993). Substance abuse is a complex, progressive, chronic, and treatable disorder. Some elderly individuals become addicted to illegal substances such as marijuana and cocaine. Although some adults become addicted in later life, many have displayed symptoms of addictions throughout their lives.

Lifelong abstinence of alcohol and addictive drugs or the appropriate use of prescription medications (if those are the drugs of abuse) are the goals of treatment. This necessitates a comprehensive interdisciplinary approach. Older women alcoholics pose a treatment problem. In addition to underdiagnosis of the problem in this group, few services and programs specializing in older female alcoholics and their families exist. Lack of appropriate peer support may feed into the patients' and families' resistance in seeking treatment or may perpetuate old patterns of excuses (Szwabo, 1993).

Polypharmacy

On a per capita basis, medication expenditures exceed all other out-of-pocket expenses for health care by Medicare recipients (Winograd & Gerety, 1993). Older women are prescribed drugs such as sedatives, antihypertensives, cardiac medications, vitamins, analgesics, laxatives, hormones, diuretics, and thyroid supplements at rates 2.5 times higher than for men (Szwabo, 1993). Over-the-counter drugs are also used extensively by older adults (Burrage, Dixon, & Sehy, 1991). This high consumption of medications is accompanied by the increased vulnerability of older adults to medication side effects and drug interactions. In elders, the risk of adverse drug reactions is related to the number of medications, the burden of chronic disease, and prescribing without adjustment for age- or disease-associated changes in drug handling or drug response. Drug-induced illnesses account for higher hospitalization rates.

Examination of family dynamics is an integral component of treatment. In the elderly, the escalation of dose or increasing numbers of drugs added or in combination with alcohol may foster increasing symptoms of intoxication manifested by confusion, falling, sleep disturbance, anxiety, panic, and depression, which may be confused with "aging." As with treatment of alcoholism, treatment of drug abuse occurs in two phases—detoxification and rehabilitation. For older adults, detoxification usually requires hospitalization. Older adults are more prone to the physiologic effects of withdrawal (e.g., seizures, cardiovascular problems, falls, delirium, and agitation; Szwabo, 1993). Several research studies have shown, however, that the risks of drug discontinuation were rarely life threatening. Physicians should prioritize medications and discontinue them one at a time (Winograd & Gerety, 1993).

Prescribing practices among physicians perpetuate drug abuse by older adults (Szwabo, 1993). It is important for the health care provider to obtain a list of both prescription and nonprescription medications during initial evaluation of a client, and to review this list periodically.

In summary, the common health problems of older women include physiological disorders, mental health problems, and related lifestyle issues. It has been said that older women are more likely to be impaired by their health problems, while older men are more likely to die from them. Older women report higher rates of non–life threatening illnesses, symptoms, and depression, and of impairments in physical activity, mobility, or personal care activities than do men (Herzog, 1989). Women, then, are the primary users of long-term care because they have more chronic health problems and live longer than men. Long-term care includes in-home services; adult day care; and care in resident facilities, convalescent homes, intermediate care facilities, and skilled nursing facilities (Older Women's League, 1989).

The chronic health problems older women live with may also be a source of stigma and devaluation by other members of society. Not all women, however, perceive stigma as a major factor in their lives. In one research study, the concept of stigma was of limited value in describing the relevance of chronic illness in the lives of elderly women, while more mundane effects of physical problems on daily tasks and lifestyles as a whole were common (Belgrave, 1960). Alterations of self-concept were not experienced universally. In some instances there were more fears than actual experiences of being stigmatized. Even women who suffered severe physical problems continued to think of themselves as basically healthy if they were able to isolate these problems from the rest of their lives. One indirect effect of age is that because chronic illness is so prevalent among today's elderly, having such an affliction does not set an older woman apart from her peers (Belgrave, 1990).

Many older women do experience one or more of the common health problems described previously. The initiation and course of these disorders, however, is not inevitable with age. Health promotion and disease prevention activities can be utilized with older women as with other populations, with the intent of delaying, minimizing the effect of, or actually preventing the occurrence of certain health problems.

Health Promotion and Disease Prevention

Positive health has become a key concept, yet health research continues to focus primarily on pathology and interventions to facilitate recovery from the pathology. Future research should be directed toward what accounts for vigor, energy, and a high level of functioning among older men and women, and how some elders elude the ravages of time (Herzog, 1989; Rowe & Kahn, 1987). Rather than looking at single events (e.g., retirement, loss of spouse or others, and change in living situation) in people's lives, it is important to look at the accumulation of stress-related factors (Herzog, 1989). Perception and interpretation of symptoms have been proposed as important early steps in the process of preventive health behaviors and of seeking health care (Herzog, 1989). Women already perform better in this area than men. Women report symptoms more often and visit physicians more frequently than men. This may be due in part to a woman's lifelong management of reproductive functions and her role as caretaker of the health of the entire family. Whether this attention to self-health changes has beneficial effects for the woman's longevity in older age is unknown (Herzog, 1989). However, this behavior can be used as a foundation on which to build an understanding of and respect for the value of health promotion activities. Activities to be discussed are in the areas of education, health screening, prevention of specific health problems, psychosocial concerns, coping strategies, and life enhancement opportunities.

Education

Self-care to maintain and/or regain wellness needs emphasis among midlife and older women. Simple measures like sleeping 7–8 hours a night, controlling weight (not more than 10 percent over ideal body weight), eating a well-balanced diet, drinking 6 to 8 glasses of water a day, exercising, limiting alcohol intake, and eliminating smoking can produce significantly better health and lower mortality. The myths of aging, discussed earlier in this chapter, need to be exposed so that older women will recognize there are beneficial effects to caring for oneself even in old age, rather than succumbing to the supposed futility of it all by thinking debility is purely a function of age.

Education as to the normal aging changes is a key component of the myth-exposing program. Once older women are aware of what to expect related to the passage of time versus the presence of disease, they can take responsibility for their own lives and engage in behaviors that will positively impact their future health. Education is an important part of each of the following health promotion topics, although it may not be explicitly stated.

Health Screening

Breast self-examination is especially important for older women because they are less likely to have screening mammograms. Many physicians still do not refer their older patients for mammography, and older patients may lack the health insurance coverage to pay for screening mammography. After age 50, mammograms should be performed annually. It is recommended that this schedule be continued throughout a woman's life, even though the final recommendations on the use of mammography in older patients have not yet been established (Rosenberg, 1993).

Additional screening tests include Pap smears, blood pressure assessment, cholesterol screening, and glaucoma testing. Many of these screening procedures can be obtained at minimal or no cost to the individual. Blood pressure reading and cholesterol and glaucoma testing are commonly available at community health fairs in shopping malls and at community centers, sponsored by various health care organizations. Activities such as these may be specifically targeted to the older population, rendering the event a social occurrence as well as a resource for health screening.

Prevention of Specific Health Problems

Disease prevention activities

Vaccinations against specific diseases are invaluable in preventing these diseases. Older people would be well advised to take advantage of those vaccinations which are available (e.g., influenza, pneumonia, and tetanus; Tilston & Williams, 1992). These vaccines are usually offered at minimal cost to the older individual.

Older women are not immune to the human immunodeficiency virus (HIV). Education concerning the value of HIV testing and the importance of instituting behaviors for prevention is essential for this age group, as for younger age groups.

Osteoporosis prevention/treatment behaviors

Exercise is an important activity for the prevention of osteoporosis. Recommended exercises include walking, dancing, and other weight-bearing exercises for one half hour per day. Shoes with good support are an important component of the exercise program. Quitting cigarette smoking is probably beneficial in reducing the risk for osteoporosis, as is limiting caffeine and alcohol intake (Miller, 1990).

A calcium intake of 1000 mg per day for adults and 1500 mg per day for postmenopausal women is widely recommended. Dietary sources of calcium include milk and milk products, raisins, tofu, canned salmon or sardines, and broccoli and other dark green vegetables. Calcium carbonate, phosphate, and citrate (found in some antacids) are effective and inexpensive sources of elemental calcium, and are used as dietary supplements by some older women (Miller, 1990). Calcium supplements are not recommended for people with poor kidney function, a history of kidney stones, or a predisposition to chronic constipation.

Vitamin D supplements may be necessary for sedentary, home-bound older women who attain minimal exposure to the sun. Although vitamin D is necessary for adequate calcium absorption, more than 400 IU per day can have detrimental effects, including increased calcium excretion (Miller, 1990). Estrogen replacement therapy was discussed previously in the section on osteoporosis.

Fall-prevention guidelines

A comprehensive assessment of the older woman and her home environment is important prior to instituting any fall-prevention techniques. Through this assessment, risks for falling can be identified. These risks should be reassessed whenever there is a change in the functional status of the older person (Miller, 1990). Utilizing information obtained in the assessment, home modifications and/or fall-related behavior changes may be addressed (Winograd & Gerety, 1993). Recent studies indicate that improving lower-extremity strength, balance, and aerobic capacity should be part of a fall-prevention program (Winograd & Gerety, 1993).

Specific suggestions related to the prevention of falls include concerns about proper lighting. Steps, stairways, and entranceways in and around buildings should be well illuminated. Too much illumination can also lead to problems. The glare associated with highly polished floors or large expanses of uncovered glass should be avoided. Older people should be encouraged to allow their eyes more time to adjust to changes in light levels when moving from a light to dark area and vice versa.

It is important for elders to maintain clean eyeglasses and have regular eye exams to identify changes and obtain new glasses when needed. It is also important for elders to concentrate while walking, to look ahead at the ground to spot and avoid hazards such as cracks in the sidewalks. The use of canes, walking sticks, and walkers may be helpful if maintained in good condition. Nightlights in the bedroom and bathroom may provide sufficient light to prevent trips and falls at night. Any change in position should be accomplished slowly to allow for adaptation by the elder. Alcohol and tranquilizers should be used cautiously.

Shoes and slippers should be flat and rubber soled, and clothing such as long robes should be avoided. Scatter rugs and small bathroom mats that can slide are potential hazards, as are slick floors. Nonskid treads on stairs and nonskid mats in the tub may be helpful. Handrails in the bath, shower, and by the toilet are essential. Other suggestions include installing handrails on both sides of the stairs, painting stair edges in bright contrasting colors, watching for pet underfoot and scattered pet food, and avoiding clutter in living area (Chenitz, Kussman, & Stone, 1991).

Psychosocial Support

Many older women are caregivers rather than care receivers. The average age of caregivers of older people is 57, but more than one in three caregivers is over age 65. This illustrates the fact that the informal care system is composed in part of young-old individuals caring for old-old individuals. The average woman today can expect to spend as many years caring for a dependent parent as she does in caring for a dependent child (Older Women's League, 1989).

There are formal community-based services in many cities that can provide assistance and support for these caregivers. Nonprofessional workers including home health aides, home attendants, and personal care workers can spend time in the home with the care recipient, allowing the caregiver free time for grocery shopping, relaxation, or whatever activities she prefers. Day care centers for the elderly provide a different alternative. The elderly care recipient is brought to the center, allowing the caregiver free time in or out of the home environment. Both of these options are forms of respite care. Anything that frees the caregiver from continuous, direct contact with the care recipient can be viewed as respite care.

Another source of assistance for caregivers is that of support groups. Support groups are composed of individuals who have previously been through or are currently experiencing the same type of situation as the caregiver. Examples of support groups include those for people living with Alzheimer's disease victims, those for families of people with alcoholism, and those for caregivers of cancer victims.

Coping Strategies

Coping strategies, or coping responses, are the behaviors, cognitions, and perceptions that persons use when they attempt to deal with their life stresses (Herzog, 1989). Which coping strategies are used may depend on the availability of coping resources. Coping resources can be broadly categorized as sociocultural (personal networks, financial resources, and educational resources) or psychological (personality characteristics, i.e., mastery, self-esteem, and intelligence). A most important source of coping resources is the psychological view of one's inner self, or the self-concept.

Strengths as survivors

Many older women, especially minority older women, have spent their lives as strategists, marshalling scarce resources to cope with everyday demands. Older women are survivors, and that, in itself, is a strength.

As the older population increases in numbers, many more people will be living with various types of chronic ailments and illnesses. More healthy persons will be living longer, as health care providers increasingly emphasize health promotion. Assisting elders to focus on their strengths may help them to achieve goals they never before thought possible. Most people are familiar with the vicious cycle of inability to do something, followed by discouragement and depression, followed by diminished desire and even less success in performance of an activity, and so on. A positive cycle works the same way: goal achievement in activities leads to encouragement, which enhances the possibility of achieving further goals (Burke & Walsh, 1992). The positive approach can be very successful if internalized by the older woman and utilized as she faces the many challenges of daily life.

Exercising control

A personal sense of control, or the ability to influence one's own life by making choices and decisions about one's life, has been shown through research to be associated with positive physical and psychological health among older individuals (Rodin & Timko, 1992). Conversely, a loss of perceived control is associated with poor health outcomes. Many factors can affect a person's sense of control. Ageism can be a major factor in that many in society view an individual's decision-making capabilities as severely reduced or absent once this individual has turned 65 years old. Family members with the best of intentions may begin taking over certain affairs for an elder when the elder is still able and desirous of daily self-management. Health care providers, at times, promote such activities by family members through speaking about the elder and the elder's medical condition directly to the family, bypassing the patient entirely.

Not all older people wish to maintain or actively utilize personal control over their lives. Some may feel that growing old means passing on the burden of decision making to others and thereby experience relief with this shift of control. If asked to assume greater control over their health and other aspects of their lives, these elders may experience stress, worry, and self-blame (Rodin, 1986). Other elders succumb to ageist thinking and exhibit an attitude of "Why try? It's useless." These elders view physical changes as an inevitable part of aging and are less likely to engage in health-protective or health-promotion behaviors (Rodin & Timko, 1992). This variability among older people in preference for amount of control increases with increasing age (Rodin, 1986).

Gerontological nurses can act as advocates for those older women who prefer to maintain or regain control over aspects of their lives. Support and encouragement of their decision-making activities is important for these women. Nurses can function as liaisons between the older woman and her family, and the older woman and the health care system. Once provided with information regarding options for health promotion, health maintenance, and disease treatment, the older woman's decisions should be elicited, considered seriously, and followed as closely as possible.

Utilization of available resources

Health care resources available to the older woman range from services to support independent living in the community to skilled nursing services in acute care institutions. Community-based services include health promotion programs, outreach programs, ambulatory clinics, adult day care, and in-home assistance, including both nonprofessional workers and skilled home health personnel (Burke & Walsh, 1992). Institutions providing health care include nursing homes, inpatient mental health centers, and acute care hospitals and medical centers.

Approximately one third of all people aged 65 and older live alone, and are at risk as their health fails. By 2030, the number of elders in the population will rise from one in nine to one in five (Commonwealth Fund Commission on the Elderly Living Alone, 1988). Eight percent of older women living alone at home currently have significant impairment in activities of daily life (ADL) and cannot function without assistance, and three quarters of nursing home residents are women. Funding levels are inadequate for community-based support that permits elders to "age in place," the preference of the majority (Leutz, Capitman, MacAdam, & Abrahams, 1992).

There are a variety of housing options for older people, depending on their financial resources. Alternatives to privately owned homes or individually rented apartments include congregate living, age-segregated housing, living with family or roommates, residential care facilities (assisted living; Baggett, 1989), and continuing-care retirement communities (Golant, 1992).

Spiritual support

Some elders utilize spiritual beliefs as stress reducers or buffers in everyday life. Religious feelings and attitudes are higher among older adults than among their younger counterparts, and elders report turning to faith more often when faced with adversities. The strength of religious beliefs is related to subjective well-being. Within this age range, women are more likely than men to attend church frequently. Race differences are also notable, with older African Americans being more likely than older Whites to resort to prayer in stressful situations (Herzog, 1989).

Cognitive improvement techniques

Memory skills can be improved in older people. As with other body functions, "if you don't use it, you lose it." Cognitive activities previously taken for granted may no longer occur automatically as one ages. Active use of the mind and focused remembering can minimize functional loss and promote resumption of previously lost abilities. Specific techniques to enhance memory include written reminders such as lists, calendars, and notebooks. Auditory cues (e.g., timers and alarm clocks) are most helpful when used in conjunction with written reminders. Helpful hints related to the environment include maintaining specific places for specific items and keeping the items in their proper places (e.g., keys on a hook near the door).

Additional memory techniques include forming associations between names and mental images, and grouping information into smaller pieces that can be more readily remembered. One form of grouping is to organize information into logically related categories. Other examples of grouping include the use of rhyming cues or cues using the first letter of each information element forming an acronym (Miller, 1990).

Nutritional interventions

Resources are available in many communities to assist older adults in meeting their nutritional needs. With respect to obtaining food, local offices on aging may provide assistance with transportation or grocery shopping. Meals on Wheels programs actually deliver meals to older adults in their own homes at minimal cost. Group meal programs at centralized nutrition centers are available in many communities through the federally funded National Nutrition Program for the Elderly, established under the Older Americans Act. In addition to providing inexpensive and nutritionally balanced meals, the group meal programs provide excellent opportunities for elders to socialize.

Elders who prepare their own food at home may find that activity hindered by environmental barriers. Mid-level storage areas may facilitate access to food preparation containers and implements, and thereby remove what may be the one obstacle an older woman faces in successful food preparation. The enjoyment of eating may be altered by diminished gustatory and olfactory sensations. Good oral hygiene, especially prior to meals, will enhance food enjoyment. The use of low-sodium food additives may also be helpful. Some elders experience satiety with ingestion of small amounts of food. For these elders, smaller, more frequent meals would be preferable to the standard three meals per day (Miller, 1990).

Education regarding nutritional requirements of older people is important, both for the elders themselves and for their caregivers or food preparers. A reduction in calories, to match the reduced metabolism of older people, is appropriate, as well as reduced intake of fat, cholesterol, sugar, and salt. It is recommended that alcohol consumption be restricted to two drinks per day (Hashizume 1991). Another recommendation for elders is an increased intake of fruits, vegetables, and whole grains.

Safety tips

Safety encompasses many areas of daily life. With age, certain activities do not occur automatically as they once did. Slowed processing within the central nervous system limits the capacity to handle numerous incoming stimuli. Maintaining active awareness of one's own environment and preparing in advance for potential adverse events allows the older woman to respond to stressors with minimal effect. Techniques that facilitate safety on a daily basis include being alert to potential risks or dangers, focusing on the activity in which one is currently involved, remaining attuned to one's own body, and approaching life from a proactive rather than reactive stance. Protective behaviors appropriate for individual health problems are described throughout the Health Promotion and Disease Prevention section of this chapter.

Sources of economic support

It is not uncommon for older women to have limited financial resources. A major factor contributing to this situation is the marginal eligibility of many women for retirement benefits due to a lifetime of erratic formal employment. Older women who are close to a point of eligibility for early retirement may experience pressure from their work environment to "get out early." They may also be pressured by their spouses, who have already retired, to leave jobs before the point where they are able to take advantage of the full range of benefits (Rathbone-McCuan, 1985). Other factors contributing to the older woman's minimal financial resources include death of a spouse; minimal personal assets such as savings, home ownership, and car ownership; and out-of-pocket expenses related to the treatment of chronic medical conditions.

The federal Social Security system is the sole source of support for some older people. Others seek part-time employment in minimum wage positions to supplement their Social Security income. There are older women who have planned for their later years in advance through long-term investments, and others who have benefited from a financially successful life with their partners as beneficiaries of their spouses' estates. The necessity for preretirement planning is fostering awareness among younger adults of the importance of arranging for external financial support, such as individual retirement accounts and life insurance programs, as an alternative to total future economic reliance on Social Security funds.

Views on retirement

Retirement has different meanings for different people. It may be viewed as a time of reward for a lifetime of concentrated work-related activity. Elders holding this view may use the additional free time for development of their creative interests. Some elders travel extensively. Others move into active adult communities which offer numerous recreational and personal development activities for residents. Volunteer activities may be of interest to the older woman. Volunteers are an integral part of many health care institutions and civic organizations.

Retirement may also be viewed as the point at which an older person is labelled nonproductive, no longer a contributing member of society. Some elders may internalize this view. However, others may consciously limit their involvement in activities outside the home postretirement to spend more time with families or to enjoy periods of uninterrupted quiet and relaxation. The older woman's personal health, financial status, desires, and interests are major considerations in determining the retirement options available to her. Single, older women who continue to live in their own homes or apartments after retirement may find creative outlets through their local senior citizen organizations. These organizations also provide increased opportunity for socialization among elders.

Strengthening the social network

Many communities offer various activities targeting older adults. These activities can directly or indirectly promote social interaction among elders. Older women may need to be encouraged to take advantage of these opportunities. Specific examples of community programs include adult education classes, health courses, and support groups (Tilston & Williams, 1992). Civic organizations, senior citizen centers, group nutritional programs, interest-related clubs, and exercise classes are additional examples. As with any social activity it is up to the individual to actually become involved. Encouraging older women to seek out and develop new friendships is one intervention nurses could utilize frequently. Older women may need to consider becoming more assertive in initiating contacts with others.

Meeting sexual needs

The single most significant determinant of sexual activity in older women is the availability of partners. Attitudes toward sex and patterns of sexual activity have been shown to be fairly constant throughout an individual's lifetime (McCracken, 1988). For this cohort of older women, many were brought up to believe that sexual activity was a "duty" to perform within the boundaries of marriage, and that they should exhibit very little sexual interest (Greengross, 1992; Rankin, 1989); therefore, no husband, no sex. Sex with a female partner and masturbation have generally not been considered viable alternatives by women in this age group (Gupta, 1990).

The older woman herself, a potential partner, or both may be suffering from one or more chronic diseases which may impact negatively on sexual interest as well as sexual performance. The older person may fear harming her partner post–acute disease (e.g., stroke or myocardial infarction) or even precipitating a new onset of the disease (McCracken, 1988; Rankin, 1989). Education with respect to modification of techniques could allow for continuation of sexual activity even by partners who are victims of disease. Lack of education concerning the meaning of sexuality, physical changes with age, sexual practices, and acceptability has also contributed to the older woman's frustration in trying to meet her sexual needs. When most older women were young, there was very little information available concerning sexuality and it was not as freely discussed in society as it is today. Lack of privacy in the living situation (at home with children and grandchildren or in an institution), body image changes, stress, and medications are a few of the additional factors that can impact the older woman's sexual life in a negative manner (Gupta, 1990).

But there are also factors that may have a positive impact on the sexuality of an older woman. One factor is the increased time available in an older person's life to enjoy a partner's company, both sexually and nonsexually. Also, some people express greater satisfaction with sex when older compared to when they were younger (Rankin, 1989). For older women, the fear of conception is gone. This is important considering that birth control devices and substances were not readily available when this cohort of older women was young, nor was birth control as socially acceptable as it is today. Also, sexual expression can occur in modes other than sexual intercourse. Activities such as touching, holding each other, and just being close provide warmth, companionship, and love.

Life Enhancement Opportunities

Maintaining active involvement in life is one strategy people of all ages can use to enhance their feeling of well-being. The approaches to achieving or maintaining this involvement may be quite diverse. The heterogeneity of the older population is reflected in their varied interests and desires relative to remaining "involved." Joining activist groups such as the American Association for Retired Persons (AARP) or the Older Women's League (OWL) of the National Organization for Women (NOW) (Arber & Ginn, 1991) may allow the older woman a forum for expression that is unavailable in other arenas. Running for political office at the local, state, or national level is no longer unheard of for women. Older women with knowledge and experience accumulated over many years have much to offer society in terms of leadership. Professional organizations, alumni associations, women's clubs, charity organizations, and volunteer activities also provide opportunities for sharing of mutual interests and serving the community at large.

Opportunities for growth and creativity evolve from increased awareness through education, both formal and informal. Once elders are aware of "what's out there," they can actively seek involvement according to their individual goals, such as artistic expression, lifestyle behavioral modification, development of specific interests, or attainment of a college degree. Education for elders may be sponsored by local educational institutions (public schools, colleges, universities, and community and technical colleges), community-based organizations (senior centers, area agencies on aging, public libraries, religious organizations, councils on aging, and AARP), government agencies targeting the needs of elders, and elderhostels. The primary goal of education for elders is the improvement of well-being and quality of life.

Summary

Growing older has both positive and negative consequences for women. As discussed in this chapter, physiological aging changes occur that can affect an older woman's functional capabilities in her later years. These effects are minimal, however, unless accompanied by a pathological process. Psychosocial concepts such as frailty, stereotypes, myths, role changes, and social relationships were briefly reviewed, and common health problems of older women were described. Lifestyle issues related to health were also discussed. The challenge for women is to become more knowledgeable and assertive in dealing with their own lives. Older women can, in many instances, influence the course of their lives and exert a positive impact on their health. Health promotion behaviors and ideas for personal growth were offered to assist women in meeting this challenge.

The numbers of older women in the United States are increasing each year. Their needs, desires, and opportunities (or lack thereof) warrant the focused attention of health care providers, policy makers, researchers, government agencies, and the general public. Historically, research on major health problems such as heart disease have included male participants only, with study results automatically interpreted as pertaining to women, even though not scientifically documented. There is beginning to be a shift in this country to include more women in clinical studies and to provide funding for research targeting women's health issues. It is hoped that this trend will continue and broaden to include social, political, and philosophical issues concerning women in addition to health care issues.

References

American Association of Retired Persons & Administration on Aging. (1994). *A profile of older Americans* PF3049(1294). D996. Washington, DC: American Association of Retired Persons.

American Nurses' Association. (1987). *Standards and scope of gerontological nursing practice.* Kansas City, MO: American Nurses' Association.

Applegate, W. B., Blass, J. P., & Williams, T. F. (1990). Instruments for the functional assessment of older patients. *New England Journal of Medicine, 322*(17), 1207–1214.

Arber, S., & Ginn, J. (1991). *Gender and later life: A sociological analysis of resources and constraints.* London, England: Sage.

Atchley, R. C. (1983). *Aging: Continuity and change.* Belmont, CA: Wadsworth.

Atchley, R. C. (1990). Defining the vulnerable older population. In Z. Harel, P. Ehrlich, & R. Hubbard (Eds.), *The vulnerable aged: People, services, and policies* (pp. 18–31). New York: Springer.

Baden, W. F., & Walker, T. (1985). Management of pelvic support loss in the geriatric female. In F. J. Hofmeister (Ed.), *Care of the postmenopausal patient* (pp. 133–156). Philadelphia: George F. Strickley.

Baggett, S. A. (1989). *Residential care for the elderly: Critical issues in public policy.* New York: Greenwood Press.

Barber, H. R. K. (1988). *Perimenopausal and geriatric gynecology.* New York: Macmillan.

Barry, P. (1993). Coronary artery disease in older women. *Geriatrics, 48*(Suppl. 1), 4–8.

Belgrave, L. L. (1990). The relevance of chronic illness in the everyday lives of elderly women. *Journal of Aging and Health, 2*(4), 475–500.

Breakwell, S. L., & Walker, S. N. (1988). Differences in physical health, social interaction, and personal adjustment between continent and incontinent homebound aged women. *Journal of Community Health Nursing, 5*(1), 19–31.

Burke, M. M., & Walsh, M. B. (1992). *Gerontologic nursing: Care of the frail elderly.* St. Louis: Mosby.

Burrage, R. L., Dixon, L., & Sehy, Y. A. (1991). Physical assessment: An overview with sections on the skin, eye, ear, nose, and neck. In W. C. Chenitz, J. T. Stone, & S. A. Salisbury (Eds.), *Clinical gerontological nursing. A guide to advanced practice* (pp. 27–49). Philadelphia: W. B. Saunders.

Byyny, R. L., & Speroff, L. (1990). *A clinical guide for the care of older women.* Baltimore: Williams & Wilkins.

Casey, M. J. (1985). Postmenopausal bleeding. In F. J. Hofmeister (Ed.), *Care of the postmenopausal patient* (pp. 75–107). Philadelphia: George F. Strickley.

Cattell, H., & Wilkinson, G. (1992). Depressed mood in older women. In J. George & S. Ebrahim (Eds.), *Health care for older women* (pp. 148–159). New York: Oxford University Press.

Chenitz, W. C., Kussman, H. L., & Stone, J. T. (1991). Preventing falls. In W. C. Chenitz, J. T. Stone, & S. A. Salisbury (Eds.), *Clinical gerontological nursing. A guide to advanced practice* (pp. 309–328). Philadelphia: W. B. Saunders.

Colling, J., Hadley, B. J., Eisch, J., Campbell, E., & Ouslander, J. G. (1992). Patterned urge response toileting for urinary incontinence: A clinical trial. In S. G. Funk, E. M. Tornquist, M. T. Champagne, & R. A. Wiese (Eds.), *Key aspects of elder care: Managing falls, incontinence, and cognitive impairment* (pp. 169–186). New York: Springer.

Commonwealth Fund Commission on the Elderly Living Alone. (1988). *Aging alone: Profiles and projections.* New York: Commonwealth Fund.

Daly, M. (1978). *Gyn/ecology. The metaethics of radical feminism.* Boston: Beacon Press.

Dougherty, M. C., Bishop, K. R., Mooney, R. A., Gimotty, P. A., & Williams, B. (1992). Graded exercise: Effect on pressures developed by the pelvic muscles. In S. G. Funk, E. M. Tornquist, M. T. Champagne, & R. A. Wiese (Eds.), *Key aspects of elder care: Managing falls, incontinence, and cognitive impairment* (pp. 214–224). New York: Springer.

DuBeau, C. E., & Resnick, N. M. (1991). Evaluation of the causes and severity of geriatric incontinence: A critical appraisal. *The Urologic Clinics of North America, 18*(2), 243–256.

Ebersole, P., & Hess, P. (1985). *Toward healthy aging: Human needs and nursing response.* St. Louis: C. V. Mosby.

Flaherty, J. H., Miller, D. K., & Coe, R. M. (1992). Impact on caregivers of supporting urinary function in noninstitutionalized, chronically ill seniors. *The Gerontologist, 32*(4), 541–545.

Golant, S. M. (1992). *Housing America's elderly. Many possibilities/few choices.* Newbury Park, CA: Sage.

Goldfarb, A. F. (1985). The estrogen-deficient woman. In F. J. Hofmeister (Ed.), *Care of the postmenopausal patient* (pp. 33–46). Philadelphia: George F. Strickley.

Goldstein, M., Hawthorne, M. E., Engeberg, S., McDowell, B. J., & Burgio, K. L. (1992). Urinary incontinence: Why people do not seek help. *Journal of Gerontological Nursing, 18*(4), 15–20.

Grace, L. (Ed.). (1989). *Women in the later years: Health, social, and cultural perspectives.* New York: The Haworth Press.

Greengross, W. (1992). Women, sex, and ageing. In J. George & S. Ebrahim (Eds.), *Health care for older women* (pp. 130–137). New York: Oxford University Press.

Gupta, K. (1990). Sexual dysfunction in elderly women. *Clinics in Geriatric Medicine, 6*(1), 197–203.

Hadley, E. C. (1986). Bladder training and related therapies for urinary incontinence in older people. *Journal of the American Medical Association, 256*(3), 372–379.

Hashizume, S. (1991). Home health care. In W. C. Chenitz, J. T. Stone, & S. A. Salisbury (Eds.), *Clinical gerontological nursing. A guide to advanced practice* (pp. 557–576). Philadelphia: W. B. Saunders.

Heidrich, S. M. (1993). The relationship between physical health and psychological well-being in elderly women: A developmental perspective. *Research in Nursing & Health, 16*(2), 123–130.

Herzog, A. R. (1989). Physical and mental health in older women: Selected research issues and data sources. In A. R. Herzog, K. C.

234   WOMEN ACROSS THE LIFE CYCLE: THE MATURATIONAL PROCESS

Holden, & M. M. Seltzer (Eds.), *Health & economic status of older women* (pp. 35–91). Amityville, NY: Baywood Publishing.
Herzog, A. R., Diokno, A. C., & Fultz, N. H. (1989). Urinary incontinence: Medical and psychosocial aspects. In M. P. Lawton (Ed.), *Annual review of gerontology and geriatrics. Volume 9* (pp. 74–119). New York: Springer.
Herzog, A. R., & Fultz, N. H. (1990). Prevalence and incidence of urinary incontinence in community-dwelling populations. *Journal of the American Geriatrics Society, 38*(3), 273–281.
Joint National Committee on Detection, Evaluation, and Treatment of High Blood Pressure. (1993). *The fifth report of the Joint National Committee on Detection, Evaluation, and Treatment of High Blood Pressure* (NIH Publication No. 93-1088). Bethesda, MD: National Institutes of Health.
Kane, R. A., & Kane, R. L. (1981). *Assessing the elderly. A guide to measurement.* Lexington, MA: Lexington Books.
Karram, M. M., & Walters, M. D. (1993). Pelvic organ prolapse: Enterocele and vaginal vault prolapse. In M. D. Walters & M. M. Karram (Eds.), *Clinical urogynecology* (pp. 236–260). St. Louis: Mosby.
Kenney, R. A. (1989). *Physiology of aging. A synopsis* (2nd ed.). Chicago: Year Book Medical Publishers.
Khan, A., Mirolo, H., Mirolo, M. H., & Dobie, D. J. (1993). Depression in the elderly: A treatable disorder. *Geriatrics, 48*(Suppl. 1), 14–17.
Lachs, M. S., & Fulmer, T. (1993). Recognizing elder abuse and neglect. *Clinics in Geriatric Medicine, 9*(3), 665–675.
Lee, G. R., & Ishii-Kuntz, M. (1988). Social interaction, loneliness, and emotional well-being among the elderly. *Research on Aging, 9*(4), 459–482.
Leutz, W. N., Capitman, J. A., MacAdam, M., & Abrahams, R. (1992). *Care for frail elders: Developing community solutions.* Westport, CT: Auburn House.
Levin, R. M. (1993). Osteoporosis: Prevention is key to management. *Geriatrics, 48*(Suppl. 1), 18–24.
Lewis, M. (1985). Older women and health. An overview. In S. Golub & R. J. Freedman (Eds.), *Health needs of women as they age* (pp. 1–16). New York: The Haworth Press.
Lewis, M. I., & Butler, R. N. (1972). Why is women's lib ignoring old women? *Aging & Human Development, 3*(3), 223–231.
McCormick, K. A., Scheve, A. A. S., & Leahy, E. (1988). Nursing management of urinary incontinence in geriatric inpatients. *The Nursing Clinics of North America, 23*(1), 231–264.

McCracken, A. L. (1988). Sexual practice by elders: The forgotten aspect of functional health. *Journal of Gerontological Nursing*, *14*(10),13–17.

McGonigle, K. F., Lagasse, L. D., & Karlan, B. Y. (1993). Ovarian, uterine, and cervical cancer in the elderly woman. *Clinics in Geriatric Medicine*, *9*(1), 115–130.

Miller, C. A. (1990). *Nursing care of older adults: Theory and practice.* Glenview, IL: Scott, Foresman/Little, Brown Higher Education.

Miller, D. K., & Kaiser, F. E. (1993). Assessment of the older woman. *Clinics in Geriatric Medicine*, *9*(1), 1–19.

Mitteness, L. S. (1987). The management of urinary incontinence by community-living elderly. *The Gerontologist*, *27*(2), 185–193.

National Institutes of Health Consensus Development Conference. (1990). Urinary incontinence in adults. *Journal of the American Geriatrics Society*, *38*(3), 265–272.

Older Women's League. (1989). The picture of health for midlife and older women in America. In L. Grau (Ed.), *Women in the later years: Health, social, and cultural perspectives* (pp. 53–74). New York: The Haworth Press.

Ouslander, J. (1990). Urinary incontinence in nursing homes. *Journal of the American Geriatrics Society*, *38*, 289–291.

Ouslander, J. G. (1992). Geriatric urinary incontinence. *Disease-a-Month*, *38*(2), 71–149.

Rankin, D. J. (1989, November). Intimacy and the elderly. *Nursing Homes*, 10–14.

Rathbone-McCuan, E. (1985). Health needs and social policy. In S. Golub & R. J. Freedman (Eds.), *Health needs of women as they age* (pp. 17–27). New York: The Haworth Press.

Rodin, J. (1986). Aging and health: Effects of the sense of control. *Science*, *233*(4770), 1271–1276.

Rodin, J., & Timko, C. (1992). Sense of control, aging, and health. In M. G. Ory, R. P. Abeles, & P. D. Lipman (Eds.), *Aging, health, and behavior* (pp. 174–206). Newbury Park, CA: Sage.

Rosenberg, A. (1993). Breast cancer: Options for older patients. *Geriatrics*, *48*(Suppl. 1), 9–13.

Rowe, J. W., & Kahn, R. L. (1987). Human aging: Usual and successful. *Science*, *237*, 143–149.

Schneider, E. L., & Guralnik, J. M. (1990). The aging of America: Impact on health care costs. *The Journal of the American Medical Association (JAMA)*, *263*(17), 2335–2340.

Stone, J. T., & Chenitz, W. C. (1991). The problem of falls. In W. C. Chenitz, J. T. Stone, & S. A. Salisbury (Eds.), *Clinical gerontological nursing. A guide to advanced practice* (pp. 291–308). Philadelphia: W. B. Saunders.

Szwabo, P. A. (1993). Substance abuse in older women. *Clinics in Geriatric Medicine, 9*(1), 197–208.

Task Force on Older Women's Health. (1993). Older women's health. *Journal of the American Geriatrics Society, 41*(6), 680–683.

Tilston, J., & Williams, J. (1992). "Everyone wants to go to heaven, but no one wants to die." Screening women over 75—A health promotion approach. In J. George & S. Ebrahim (Eds.), *Health care for older women* (pp. 205–221). New York: Oxford University Press.

Urinary Incontinence Guideline Panel. (1992). *Urinary incontinence in adults: Clinical practice guideline* (AHCPR Publication No. 92–0038). Rockville, MD: Agency for Health Care Policy and Research, Public Health Service, U.S. Department of Health and Human Services.

Walters, M. D. (1993). Pelvic organ prolapse: Cystocele and rectocele. In M. D. Walters & M. M. Karram (Eds.), *Clinical urogynecology* (pp. 225–235). St. Louis: Mosby.

Winograd, C. H., & Gerety, M. B. (1993). Geriatric medicine. *Journal of the American Medical Association (JAMA), 270*(2), 213–216.

Wyman, J. F., Harkins, S. W., & Fantl, J. A. (1990). Psychosocial impact of urinary incontinence in the community-dwelling population. *Journal of the American Geriatrics Society, 38*(3), 282–288.

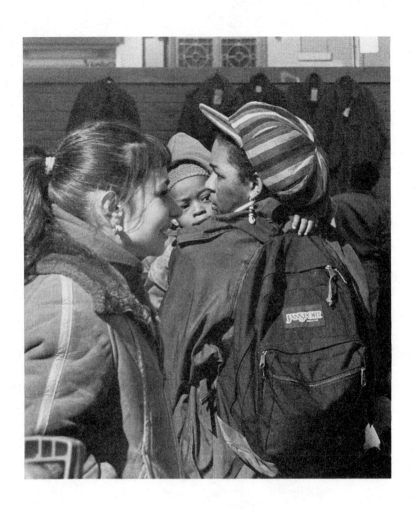

Part Three

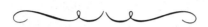

Women's Roles

10

Women as Individuals

Debra E. Lyon

Helmer: Before all else, you are a wife and a mother.
Nora: I don't believe that any longer. I believe that before all
else I am a reasonable human being, just as you are—or, at
all events, that I must try and become one. . . . I can no longer
content myself with what most people say, or with what is found
in books. I must think over things for myself and get to under-
stand them.

Henrik Ibsen, A Doll's House
Used with permission of Everyman's
Library, David Campbell Publishers Ltd.

Even though Ibsen published *A Doll's House* in 1879, Nora's declaration of self is similar in many ways to the search women of today experience as they seek to attain an identity that is comfortable for others yet true to themselves. Female developmental theorists discuss this dilemma as the balance between autonomy and connectedness, with women seeking to obtain their own voice and self-direction without losing their relationships with others. Nora gave up her husband and children in order to find herself; for most women, this is a choice that they wish not to make. But for many, the sacrifices made are sacrifices of self, leading to a diminished or altered personal identity given in exchange for somewhat fragile or tentative relationships with others based on unequal power. The sacrifices of self begin in girlhood and last through the later years. The losses may seem negligible to some, but the loss of voice, autonomy, and self-esteem are real for many women. In O*nBecoming a Person*, Carl Rogers (1991) describes the process of "becoming," the process of discovering who one is, and becoming that person instead of the person that (he) thinks that (he) should be. Although Rogers describes this process using the standard male pronouns of the times, this phenomenon, the process of breaking out and realizing one's true self, is an apt description of a woman's process of finding out who she is and of reaching her potential as an individual. The alternative to becoming one's true self may be understood as the despair as described by the philosopher Kierkegaard. The most common despair is that of not choosing to be oneself, but the deepest despair comes from choosing "to be another than himself" (Rogers, p. 110).

Attaining personhood while housed in a female body is a difficult task for most women. While women have made many gains in this century, including the right to vote, equal employment opportunities, and increased protection by the legal system, female genital mutilation, caning for inciting men to rape, sexual crimes, domestic violence, and surgical alterations to mimic societal ideals of beauty continue. Achieving an identity as a woman continues to be an arduous task, complicated by multiple and conflicting societal expectations. Even though the study of female development has received much attention from female writers such as Carol Gilligan, Jean Miller, and Lyn Mikel Brown, "human" development is still taught in many universities as the stages of development proposed by Erik Erikson (1963). Psychological development of women has been considered an aside, an extra that is better understood outside of the context of human development. Female development has consisted of a study of differences and deficiency, a pathological difference from the masculine norm. Even though Erikson achieved fame and is considered to be the authority of human developmental stages, his work focused on the life events of men, with little outcry from other scientists regarding the lack of generalizability to more than half of the human population: women. Identity formation in women may be better understood as an outgrowth of personal choices, a balance between autonomy plus connectedness, rather than two dichotomous orientations such as generativity versus stagnation, or intimacy versus isolation. Lyn Mikel Brown and Carol Gilligan (1992) state that an "inner sense of connection with others is a central organizing feature in women's development and that psychological crises in women's lives stem from disconnections" (p. 3). Jean Miller (1991) describes the female developmental paradigm as finding a sense of self by making and then sustaining affiliations and relationships with others. It is quite different, in Miller's view, from the masculine model of achieving maturity through separation from others. Miller's model is that of development through mutuality, not development in a void exclusive of relationships with others.

For women, the search to find and become one's true self is often a difficult task. In following the prescribed route, many women may never become who they want or need to be and silence their voices in hopes of reducing conflict within their relationships with others. With assistance from others in trying to counteract the societal pressures to be a "good girl," a woman may take the necessary steps to discover her selfhood. It may be a perilous journey, but the alternative, becoming an inauthentic person, may be a slower demise: the death of selfhood and potential.

The search for self for women combines autonomy and purpose with connectedness, resulting in the dilemma of being true to one's self while achieving connectedness and relationships with others. This dichotomy of autonomy and relationships may be harder to achieve than many have been led to believe, resulting in an age-old struggle for women to find a voice without sacrificing connectedness and relationships. How does one become an autonomous woman without risking alienation from others? Or, in a more common scenario, how does one sustain relationships and connectedness without becoming alienated from one's true self? In *Women's Ways of Knowing*, Belenky, Clinchy, Goldberger, and Tarule (1986) describe "a kind of existential loneliness and despair" that pervaded the interviews of the women who had not found "bridges" back to others (p. 84). For most women, a sense of purpose outside of one's children and partner is necessary for satisfaction. What Betty Friedan described in 1962 in *The Feminine Mystique* as the problem with no name, a sense of dissatisfaction and unhappiness among "housewives" who had achieved the American dream of the 1950s and 1960s, was driven by a lack of control (autonomy) and a lack of selfhood. For many of that era, selfhood was obliterated under the guise of domestic tranquility. Although women have made many gains since that time, declaring recognition as a person is still a risky endeavor for many, a difficult task to tackle. In *Backlash*, Susan Faludi (1991) documented the political and social myths during the last decade that blamed feminism for the problems of women. She cited many examples from the media that implied that feminism was the cause for career women suffering from infertility, burnout, alcoholism, and heart attacks. In the backlash against women's rights, feminists are blamed not only for their own maladies but for such societal ills as no-fault divorce and abortions. The societal problems that have increased in the past three decades may have many causes, but women's seeking gender-based equality is probably the least plausible explanation.

From Butterfly to Caterpillar:
The Retreat to a Cocoon

Women strive to achieve personhood in a process that, in many ways, may be much different from male identity formation. During early childhood, girls and boys have similar levels of self-esteem. At the beginning of adolescence, however, girls' self-esteem begins a precipitous decline that, for most, never returns to the level that is present during the early years. As girls begin the physical maturation process and begin the bodily changes that herald adulthood and the physical transition from girl to woman, the change is antithetical to the metamorphosis of a caterpillar into a butterfly. Many girls narrow their choices, restrict their boundaries, no longer fly free and unencumbered; they retreat to a cocoon that offers security at the expense of freedom and voice of self.

Although girls are faced with Erikson's adolescent challenge of identity versus role confusion, they often resolve identity development differently, because remaining confused about the female role often seems to offer more growth and opportunity than accepting the limits of traditional societal norms. Psychologists have documented the phenomenon within the relational model: the tendency for women to become selfless or voiceless in their relationships and to care for others by diminishing themselves. Brown and Gilligan (1992) noted that this is a paradoxical tendency for women: to give up the relationship with the self for the sake of "relationships" with others.

Before adolescence, perhaps girls are able to be true to themselves without paying as high of a societal or familial penalty. During adolescence, that voice or self may feel too threatening to both the teenaged girl and to others. The retreat from selfhood begins, shrouding the personality and intellect with a denial of self for the sake of building or promoting relationships with others. For many girls who begin life with a free and open mind and physical self, adolescence brings about a constriction of self, a narrowing of self that is socially constructed. The adolescent is no longer unencumbered by the weight of societal restrictions and modifications of her voice. The butterfly no longer flies freely, she crawls slowly towards a socially restricted situation. Some remain in the caterpillar stage; for others, the retreat to the cocoon results. Some incorporate learned helplessness into their daily lives. For most women, however, attaining an identity requires many struggles, beginning within a family and continuing through primary education.

In public schooling, recent attention has been given to the incongruity between the concept of equal education for all and the lack of attention given to girls in American classrooms. In *The Difference: Growing up Female in America*, Judy Mann (1994) details the classroom sexism that begins in the first years of elementary school and continues through college, consisting of girls' receiving much less attention from the teacher and being dominated by boys in classroom discussions. The disparity in the classroom may be one factor in girls' dropping out of higher level math classes in high school, leading to an inadequate preparation for traditional male disciplines such as science and engineering and lower mean SAT math scores than those of boys. Along with having a narrower choice of study, by college age, girls have lower self-esteem and more limited interaction with professors than boys. For many girls, however, socialization in elementary school leads to a premature belief that they are not intellectually able to attain employment outside of the pink-collar jobs that are traditionally delineated for women: jobs that involve cleaning and caring for others, with little autonomy, low pay relative to men's occupations, low intellectual stimulation, and lack of career progression. Economic prospects for the woman who enters the work force after high school are even more dismal, with the average female high school graduate earning less than a male high school dropout. With lower income potential, women enter into a marriage or a committed relationship with a shaky economic foundation, thus creating the dynamics for limited autonomy and a subdued voice. They are thus quieted by financial need and low self-esteem.

While the educational process is influencing the identity formation of women, the influential mass media sends a daily message that sets standards for beauty, family life, and occupational status that cannot be realistically attained by most women. For many women, this dichotomy leads to a sense of "not measuring up." Life's rewards appear to go to those who offer a "better" body with societally desirable attributes to give what Mother Nature could not: large, perky breasts on an otherwise boyish figure; chemically peeled, poreless skin; and a nose that fits societal norms more than it may fit on a woman's face. The messages are neither discrete nor subtle; one can buy this better body on an installment plan, an investment that may pay future rewards of a husband, job advancement, or psychological well-being. For some women, finding an identity involves surgical alteration; unfortunately for the woman whose identity rests on perceived physical attractiveness, the change is temporary. Without further surgical modification, the trajectory of aging takes a toll, sparing no changes that naturally occur. Physical attractiveness is a transient anchor for identity, leading to a loss of self when change occurs through aging, obesity, physical handicap, or any other change to one's perceived ideal self.

A key factor in forming an identity for most women involves the often turbulent process of accepting their bodies as they are. Growing up in a society focused on physical attractiveness and youthful norms of beauty leads many to internalize the value that young and pretty are good, old and ugly are bad. In *The Beauty Myth*, Naomi Woolf (1991) discusses the "beauty backlash," the societal forces that coerce women into starving themselves and undergoing surgery such as breast augmentation that can diminish female sexual responsiveness while providing an image closer to the perceived male ideal of female attractiveness. Woolf (1991) discusses historical societal norms of beauty for women, emphasizing constrictions and limitations to mobility such as foot binding, wearing corsets so tight that internal organs are displaced, and high heels that cause one to teeter unsteadily while the buttocks protrude. Many, if not most, girls in the United States play with "Barbie" dolls. As they squeeze high-heeled shoes on her tiny feet and brush her long hair that falls seductively across her large, pointed breasts, what message does the female child receive? Her brother does not clothe a GI Joe doll with a 10-inch-long penis. At a young age, a girl can look around and see that mommy is not shaped like Barbie. Would mommy look like Barbie if she ate differently, exercised more? A boy may have a realistic chance of growing up and resembling GI Joe; for women, achieving Barbie-like proportions requires surgical alteration.

Even though Americans are increasingly overweight, the media ideal for the standard of female beauty has become thinner, with many models having a pubescent, anorectic appearance. At a very young age, girls begin a lifelong diet (Woolf, 1991; Brown & Gilligan, 1992; Brownmiller, 1984). The obesity rate in the United States has increased, with the average weight of the American woman increasing in the past two decades. At a time when models and media representations of the female ideal body have become 23 percent thinner than the average American woman (Woolf, 1991), the typical woman has become heavier. This dualism may further contribute to the shame and guilt that an obese woman may feel, leading to further coping using food to assuage feelings of "not measuring up." Obese women are discriminated against in employment and lack the societal image that many large men are given of that of "big guy" which has positive implications of strength and virility. There are forces more subtle than the Barbie figurine that hint at a generally unattainable standard. A child's family may be able to counteract some media forces, but the loudest message that many girls hear is that beauty and thinness are the key to female success. As long as beauty pageants require females to appear in swimsuits, evening gowns, and meet a very narrow definition of beauty, the talent contest and money for educational opportunities may be seen as camouflage, hiding a destructive message under the guise of educational opportunity.

Family Connections

For women, family pressures have increased over the past 20 years, with more mothers of young children in the work place. For many women, domestic responsibilities often continue to be a solitary burden, with little assistance from others and a standard for housekeeping that has changed little, even though many women have jobs outside of the home as well as principal responsibility for domestic tasks. Job mobility has decreased the availability of extended family networks to help with the burden of raising small children. Even though women with multiple roles face many challenges in juggling their tasks and allocating their time, studies show that multiple roles can help to promote self-esteem and decrease the rate of depression in women. The answer is not for women to mourn the loss of the fictitious American family of the 1950s—a collective false memory of the "good old days" detailed by Coontz (1992) in *The Way We Never Were*—but to use the independence that the women's movement has achieved to promote goals in both the work place and in the home that are personally meaningful and professionally rewarding.

Along with economic changes that have increased the financial stress on the traditional nuclear family, the increase in divorce has caused hardships for many women, including economic loss and loss of status as a married woman. Bitter custody suits may focus on a working woman as a neglectful mother, using different criteria to decide whether or not someone is a "good" mother or father: the criteria for mother may be stricter and more influenced by societal restrictions on appropriate behaviors for mothers that emphasize family responsibilities more than professional advancement. Economically, divorce has disastrous short-term consequences for many, including a high rate of depression, a loss of income, and social sanctions regarding divorced women as having failed in "keeping a man" and as being threatening to married women. "No-fault" divorce laws have made divorce a simpler legal procedure, leading, in principle, to a quicker marital dissolution and more "equitable" child custody and spousal support agreements.

In reality, women and children have been negatively affected by these changes. The child support system has failed many women and children; in over 50 percent of child support agreements, the required payments are made late or not at all (Sitarz, 1991). Women and children comprise 75 percent of the United States poverty population (American Psychiatric Association [APA], 1990). No-fault divorce laws may take some of the blame for this phenomenon. The welfare system continues to expand, with women and children living on a subsistence income that is inadequate to meet basic needs, yet cannot be supplemented by income earned through work. Although welfare provides for a less than adequate income for most recipients, the prospects of a minimum-wage earner who is responsible for child care and medical insurance are even more bleak. Welfare reform and getting women off of welfare are a political agenda, but the problems of women and children are a societal issue, compounded by gender bias and lack of tolerance.

For the women who have entered into employment outside of the home in record numbers, the nature of the working world mimics many of the societal paradoxes that idealize yet devalue "women's work." *Women's work* is a term used to denote many of the activities performed by women in which there is little status, little indication of a job well done, and an imperceptible beginning and end. These jobs may range from food service worker, beautician, and child care worker to teacher or nurse. Even in professions that require college degrees such as teaching, women who work in traditional "female" occupations earn less than their male counterparts who work in "male" occupations such as business. Women's work involving caretaking of others will likely remain low status and low paying until societal values change to recognize the value of caring in economic as well as societal terms.

Along with the limitations of traditionally female occupations, women who enter into male-dominated fields often face a choice between having children or achieving business success that men in top positions do not face. The "glass ceiling" phenomenon presents another barrier into the higher echelons of the work place. For women who seek top positions, the "old boy" network remains another barrier to hurdle. Women still attain a startlingly low percentage of top management positions, and women with children are even more underrepresented in top positions.

Traditional religions also continue to promote sex-role differentiation between men and women. Even some of the more progressive religions still emphasize the expected role of women as the subordinate to the man of the family. The distinction begins at an early age, with boys having domain in the Catholic church over girls as altar boys, which in fact may lay the basis for the lack of entry of women into the priesthood, and the persistence of fertility mandates of the past. Protestant religions may allow some females into the seminary and jobs as ministers, but congregations remain distinctly divided into women's groups and men's groups, with women responsible for baked goods and domestic responsibilities, and men's groups presiding over outdoor yard sales and the physical maintenance of the church. The woman who would rather participate in outdoor work than baking may take a risk when defying the stereotypical duties assigned to her by gender. In Protestant religions, there is an overt doctrine of the man as head of the household. For single parents and lesbian women, the church may seem out of touch with their lifestyles and condemning of the reality of their lives.

Women in Transition: Losses, Coping, and Growth

According to Maggie Scarf (1980), the first major loss that most females experience in life occurs during adolescence as girls seek to separate from their parents and establish an individual identity. This separation occurs simultaneously with the bodily changes that denote the loss of girlhood. For a girl who perceives adult females as inferior to men and limited by gender-prescribed roles, becoming an adult woman can be a frightening task that offers little consolation for the loss of childhood.

Throughout adulthood, physical changes can signal a loss of status in a society that promotes youthful beauty. The first gray hairs, wrinkles, and changes in body tone herald a change in the ability to rely on one's looks as the basis of power. Theories of aging are biased toward "inevitable" losses and social isolation. Old age has not been seen, until recently, as a period of continued growth and creativity.

There are many conceptualizations of how to age well. But this final developmental phase is based upon successful negotiation of past crises and stages. Without a self-image that includes other means of negotiating power, the aging woman may feel a sense of despair over her perceived losses that is reinforced by media standards of beauty that rarely include discussion of the benefits of aging. Variables leading to successful versus usual aging (see Table 10-1) are complex and often ambiguous. Even though research focusing on the effects of the "empty nest" syndrome is contradictory (Bart, 1971; Deykin 1966; Harkins, 1978), for women who have limited their roles to wife and mother, the termination of childrearing may initiate a crisis of dissatisfaction and lack of meaning in their postchildren lives. Without the role of mother and the responsibility of caring for children, some women are vulnerable to depression and other psychological problems.

For many women, however, menopause also brings a new freedom from menstruation and threat of pregnancy. Aging brings freedom from childrearing responsibilities, and for some, more time to spend in an intimate manner with a partner. In *Ourselves, Growing Older*, Doress and Siegal (1987) differentiate "aging" from "getting old," with the former a biological change, and the latter a social concept, identified and promoted by a particular culture. Aging is a natural, biological phenomenon; getting old is a cultural and self-determined state of mind as well as body.

Maladaptive Behaviors

Legal substance abuse (smoking, overeating, and drinking alcohol among women is reaching epidemic proportions, with side effects such as lung cancer, chronic obstructive pulmonary disease, obesity, and liver disease taking a toll on women's health. Although there are many theories of the origins of substance abuse including the disease model genetic predisposition, and moral weakness, the manifestations of female substance abuse affect not only the individual woman and her family relationships, but also society as a whole in the form of lost work days decreased productivity, and increased health care costs to treat the medical effects of substance abuse. For women, alcoholism exacts a deadlier, swifter blow than for men. Cirrhosis in women generally occurs earlier in the progression of the alcoholism due to the physical differences between men and women. Alcoholism may be more prevalent in lesbians, with some estimates suggesting that 30 percent of lesbians are affected by alcohol problems compared to 10 percent of

TABLE 10-1   Human Aging: Usual vs. Successful

Domain	Contributing Variables
Physiological	carbohydrate metabolism (cardiac risk)
	osteoporosis (mobility and fracture risk)
Behavioral	smoking
	exercise
	nutrition
	stress levels
Genetic	disease risk
Psychosocial	autonomy and control
	bereavement
	geographic relocation
	social supports/relationship network
Cognitive	educational level
	economic resources/supports
	presence of external stimuli

the general population. Although the rate of smoking has dropped dramatically in the past two decades, teenaged girls have the highest rate of smoking of any group. Because smoking is linked with heart disease, lung cancer, and other respiratory ailments, the girl who lights up to fit in with others may make a deadly choice. Along with alcohol intake and smoking, food may become a coping technique or addiction to some women, leading to physical limitation, social stigma, and severe long-term medical effects.

Along with legal substances, illicit substances such as "crack" cocaine have many detrimental effects, with HIV illness adding another potentially fatal consequence for IV drug users and others who use sex work or sexual favors to obtain these drugs. HIV-infected women may be the most stigmatized group in society, due to the additional burden of potential mother-to-fetus transmission. HIV illness is not only a fatal illness; it can also be a "scarlet letter." Even though a woman may have become HIV infected through a sexual relationship with a man, she is stigmatized as a disease vector if her fetus is HIV infected. According to Smeltlzer and Whipple (1991), sexism and lack of empowerment are key factors for women in the AIDS epidemic. Because women contract sexually transmitted diseases more easily than men due to physiological differences, the threat of sexually transmitted disease is an ever present risk, especially for those who lack the power and voice in a relationship to ask a male partner to use a condom.

Although women are instructed to have their male partners wear a condom, unless the woman is educated in a manner that she can understand, is able to voice her needs, and the male is willing to abide by a mutually satisfactory agreement, condoms alone cannot protect vulnerable women from HIV or other sexually transmitted diseases. The stigma associated with drug use is confounded by the spread of HIV in individuals who are now doubly stigmatized due to a status as "HIV-infected substance abuser."

Along with being at risk for substance abuse, women are also at risk for other psychological problems such as depression, anxiety and panic disorders, and gender-stereotyped "personality" disorders. Women experience major depression at twice the rate of men, with female gender being one of the key risk factors for depression (U.S. Department of Health and Human Services, 1993). According to the *Diagnostic and Statistical Manual of Mental Disorders* (4th edition) [DSM-IV], the standard manual used by mental health professionals, the lifetime risk for major depression for women is 10 percent to 25 percent (American Psychiatric Association [APA], 1994). For men, it is much less, from 5 percent to 12 percent. Women of childbearing age have the highest depression rate of any group. The DSM-IV states that the prevalence rate for major depressive disorder appears to be "unrelated to ethnicity, education, income or marital status" (p. 341). For women, gender alone is a key risk factor that surpasses any other socioeconomic variables. Although the number of women taking pre-scription tranquilizers may have dropped since the era of the 1960s, the use of new serotonin re-uptake inhibitors (antidepressants such as Prozac® and Zoloft®) has created a brand new stratum of medicated women. Although these antidepressants may be very effective in treating depression, the long-term side effects are unknown.

Along with major depressive disorder, women have anorexia nervosa and bulimia nervosa at much higher rates than men (APA, 1994). More than 90 percent of cases of anorexia nervosa and bulimia nervosa occur in females, with the incidence increasing in recent decades (APA, 1994). For women, these diseases are both medical and psychological threats to their well-being, with anorexia leading to a loss of menstruation, diminution of secondary sexual characteristics, and severe metabolic and physiological alterations in addition to the psychosocial manifestation of the disease. The roots of anorexia are unknown, although in developmental terms, anorexia can be understood as a rejection of adult female development. Tragically, anorexia has fatal consequences for some who literally starve themselves to death. In bulimia nervosa, frequent vomiting may lead to permanent loss of dentition, with teeth appearing chipped and ragged. Medical complications can arise from esophageal tears, cardiac arrhythmias, and electrolyte imbalances. Both anorexia and bulimia usually occur during late adolescence. While the adolescent girl is focused on controlling her physical being, her mental, social, and developmental growth may be stymied and her coping resources prematurely limited.

Along with the various psychiatric and cultural maladies that affect women disproportionately, a new danger in this decade is for women to become immobilized by a new "victim" mentality made prominent through media talk shows in which individuals cite their inability to overcome genetic or familial "destinies." For women, the danger of this philosophy rests in the eventual conclusion that one's genetics and social circumstances are forces that cannot be overcome. In *Fire with Fire*, Naomi Wolf (1993) differentiates between *victim feminism* and *power feminism*. These terms describe bifurcating paths, one fraught with negativism and stagnation, and the other leading to the discovery and acknowledgment of unrecognized potential. Taken to an extreme, the logical conclusion of the victim stance is that anger, suffering, and a sense of injustice inherently temper all interactions with males. *Webster's* defines a victim as a person or thing destroyed or sacrificed. A philosophy of empowerment seems to be a better starting place for promoting the individualism of women; victimhood can exact an intolerable toll. By following the path of victimhood, women are accepting that due to gender-based genetic "weaknesses," such as menstruation and childbirth, women are not meant to be leaders or to engage in any task that requires mental stability or physical prowess. For those women who suffer abuse as children, physically, emotionally, or sexually, the victim mentality is a verdict that one can never surpass the limitations imposed on one by a cruel other. This may be the most damaging attack of all.

Challenges to Acquiring a Voice

Minority women face an added challenge: attaining culturally compatible womanhood in a Caucasian, male-dominated society. Ethnic and racial minority women who strive to achieve an identity that is culturally as well as personally compatible face a difficult journey to selfhood that is different from that of a member of a majority group. Although women in general fight societal prejudices, minority women may have additional difficulties in seeking connections to others. They fight deeply rooted societal prejudice against "different" expressions of culture, sexuality, and female development that do not mimic the Caucasian, heterosexual, male norm. Assimilation into the dominant culture occurs with a potential diminution of ethnic or racial identity, while retaining membership in a subculture may involve daily struggles to be true to one's group while living in a society that is multicultural yet ethnocentric.

Along with ethnic, racial, and religious minorities, lesbians live in a society that is averse to accepting differences; for lesbians, this reluctance involves accepting sexual differences. As a result of religious and societal reluctance to accept homosexuality as a normal human variant, lesbians are perceived by many as "man hating" instead of "woman loving." Lesbian women face not only rejection from the patriarchal hierarchy, but rejection by heterosexual women who focus on otherness, the perceived deviation of lesbian women from the heterosexual norm.

Lesbians' health care needs may be unique and are likely to be overlooked by a traditional medical system that views every woman of childbearing age as sexually active heterosexuals until proven otherwise. These women are underserved in the health care system. Zeidenstein (1990) found that one half of the lesbians in her sample went for routine gynecological care every 3 to 5 years, or not at all, even though all had completed some higher education. Stevens and Hall (1988) found that three quarters of the women in their sample perceived the interactions that they had with health care providers to be negative due to the stigma associated with being lesbian. Fear and unpleasantness of coming out influenced their failure to access health care. Robertson (1992) in an in-depth study of 10 lesbians, found that the health care concerns of lesbians differ from those of heterosexual women due to the false assumptions of caregivers regarding heterosexuality, reactions to coming out, and the invisibility of lesbians in society. Attitudes towards lesbians by female nurses may contribute to the relative silence of this minority group within the health care system. In a study of female nursing students' attitudes towards lesbians, Eliason and Randall (1991) found a high degree of "lesbian phobia," with 50 percent of students indicating that lesbian lifestyles are not acceptable.

Along with lesbians and religious and ethnic minorities, women with physical or mental challenges face additional tasks as they develop their selfhood. For many, the paradox involves accepting a limitation without accepting the societally deemed limitations that a certain "disability" connotes. Only in the past 20 years have labels such as "cripple," "mongoloid," or "retard" dropped out of our vernacular. Women who are physically or mentally challenged are often perceived by others as asexual or childlike, even as they compensate for their disabilities in many different ways, achieving selfhood despite their additional challenges.

In order to increase the voices of minority women, nursing education focusing on culturally specific health care should include instruction on the needs of sexual minorities, physically and mentally challenged individuals, as well as ethnic and racial minority groups whose needs are often overlooked by the "one-size-fits-all" medical system. Unfortunately for women, and minority women in particular, if they cannot "fit" into the current system, preventative care is delayed, and entry into the system occurs during an acute illness or other event that could have been prevented or minimized by more timely access. For health care workers, the challenge is to be sensitive and not condescending. We are all challenged in some ways, some more obviously than others. Talents and gifts should be assessed as well as limitations. The philosophy of empowerment is a hopeful, growth-oriented way in which to challenge biases and inequalities in education, the work place, and in the health care system.

Growth Through Connection

For many women, coping is a process that involves using strengths along with social support, spirituality, and demographic resources such as education, economic resources, ethnicity, and social class. Individual characteristics may provide some buffer against stress, either inhibiting or promoting coping with environmental stressors. There are many theories of why some people seem to cope better with the circumstances of their lives, including learning theory, sociobiology, and operant conditioning. Variables may include intelligence, personality development, genetic propensity, and a variety of other individual differences as well as social factors such as experience of class, and racial and ethnic discrimination.

Although women have more chronic disease than men, women live longer lives. This physiological hardiness is adequately documented, but there is no clear answer as to why some people survive with one catastrophe after another with strength and grace, and why others seem unable to cope with moderate stressors. One factor is clear, however; for women, a sense of mastery and a sense of connectedness seem to be major variables in coping. As portrayed by Marilyn French (1977) in *The Women's Room*, these were the keys to emotional survival for the female protagonists. Without a sense of autonomy, women juggle multiple demands without a voice to set limits and to plan. Without the ability to plan, a woman reverts to a reactive mode. With autonomy, a woman may become proactive, setting her goals as well as being responsive to those individuals that she has connections to by marriage, through childrearing, or in the work place.

Jean Miller (1986) described power as the capacity to produce a change. Her definition was not limited to power *over* others, a connotation that many women give to the term *power* that implies a destructive force; in her context, power is described as the ability to effect a change, for oneself and for others. Self-abnegation is not compatible with achieving power: using power for others necessitates recognizing and using one's own power to promote a goal.

Along with avenues for self-expression and purposeful activities, connectedness to others or to meaningful causes is a major coping resource for most women. With the demographic changes and the loss of neighborhood, these connections may be harder to achieve as our society has become mobile and average hours worked per week have increased. Friends may be sacrificed as family needs accelerate, and many women mourn the loss of connectedness with other women even though they may live "busy" and "fulfilled" lives as mothers, wives, and workers. Gail Sheehy (1976) described this as "closed-dyad disease," the tendency for a couple to become isolated from lateral supports (friends, neighbors, and extended family) during the early part of a relationship. For a woman, this often involves a loss of sisterhood and platonic male friends in order to expend her energy on her partner. The friendship connection has been overlooked as a requisite for happiness; for women, however, the loss of the friendship groups of adolescence and early adulthood are significant, recognized only through introspection or through more formal therapy. Male developmental theories do not offer an adequate description of the role of connectedness as a part of obtaining a satisfactory and fulfilling existence. Comprehensive health care must include psychosocial assessments of friendship and other social networks.

The Emergent Self

Health care workers can do little to change a woman's self-esteem; acquiring self-esteem is a lifelong process for most individuals, with periods of fluctuation, that cannot be easily modified by external intervention. Self-esteem comes from within, but helping to reframe and modify one's expectations may increase an individual's ability to assess herself differently. What health-care workers can do is to listen, to hear a woman's voice and respond based on *her* needs in a manner that decreases the influence of patriarchal silencing within the health care system. To hear clearly the voice of physically challenged women, minority women, lesbians, or others with special needs, nurses need to be open to various experiences of womanhood. Assumptions related to the "needs" of others must be tempered by our own acknowledgment of our prejudice and limitations; we can only know others if we let them tell us who they are and what their needs are. If we are not open to hearing and respecting what others want to say, then we cannot care for those individuals. Awareness of the voices of women necessitates listening in a manner that supports and encourages an open expression of needs and concerns. Using a caring approach, the nurse enters into the phenomenal world of the other, not only as a nurse, but as a human being. In order to overcome the barriers that separate client from nurse, self-reflection by nurses is essential. This process requires self-evaluation as well as an evaluation of societal forces that reinforce and reward certain behaviors. For female nurses within a patriarchal health care system, this evaluation of professional and personal reality may be a painful process, bringing out an awareness of the tendency for nurses' own voices to be silenced or modified to fit into a gender-based hierarchy that devalues nurses' caring behaviors as worth less than the more easily quantified and societally recognized curing behaviors of physicians. In *Ordered to Care*, Susan Reverby (1987) discusses the mandate to care in a society that does not value caring. In order to help women achieve a voice within this system, nurses must first exert their autonomy and professional selfhood, defining what nursing is in a manner that sets the way for women as patients to declare who they are and what their needs are. Nurses cannot expect women clients in the health care system to achieve a voice unless the voice of women health care workers is clear and loud, emphasizing the value of caring for all. That caring must begin on a horizontal plane, however; nurses cannot care for others from a voiceless and powerless position. Finding a voice will be a process of growth

for nurses as well as other women in the health care system, a chance
to obtain a sense of autonomy and a voice unmuffled by fear and powerlessness.

References

American Psychiatric Association. (1994). *Diagnostic and statistical
manual of mental disorders* (4th ed.). Washington, DC: Author.
Bart, R. (1971). Depression in middle aged women. In V. Gornick
& B. Maran (Eds.), *Women in a sexist society.* New York: Basic
Books.
Belenky, M., Clinchy, B., Goldberger, N. R., & Tarule, J. (1986).
Women's ways of knowing. New York: Basic Books, Inc.
Brown, L., & Gilligan, C. (1992). *Meeting at the crossroads: Women's
psychology and girl's development.* Cambridge, MA: Harvard Uni-
versity Press.
Brownmiller, S. (1984). *Femininity.* New York: Fawcett Columbine.
Coontz, S. (1992). *The way we never were: American families and the
nostalgia trap.* New York: Basic Books.
Deykin, E. (1966). The empty nest: Psychosocial aspects of conflicts
between depressed women and their grown children. *American
Journal of Psychology, 122,* 1422–1426.
Doress, P. B., & Siegal, D. L. (1987). *Ourselves, growing older.* New
York: Simon and Schuster.
Eliason, M., & Randall, C. (1991). Lesbian phobia in nursing students.
Western Journal of Nursing Research, 13(3), 363–374.
Erikson, E. (1963). *Childhood and Society* (2nd ed.). New York: Norton.
Falludi, S. (1991). *Backlash: The undeclared war against American
women.* New York: Crown.
French, M. (1977). *The women's room.* New York: Ballantine Books.
French, M. (1992). *The war against women.* New York: Summit Books.
Friedan, B. (1962). *The feminine mystique.* New York: Dell Publishing.
Gilligan, C. (1982). *In a different voice.* Cambridge, MA: Harvard
University Press.
Harkins, E. (1978). Effects of empty nest transition of self report of
psychological and physical well being. *Journal of Marriage and
Family, 40*(3), 549–556.
Ibsen, H. (1984). *A doll's house* (R. Sharp, Trans.). New York: Ban-
tam Books. (Original work published 1879)

Mann, J. (1994). *The difference: Growing up female in America.* New York: Warner Books.

Miller, J. B. (1986). *Toward a new psychology of women* (2nd ed.). Boston: Beacon Press.

Miller, J. (1991). The development of a women's sense of self. In J. V. Jordan, A. G. Kaplan, J. B. Miller, I. P. Stiver, & J. L. Surrey *Women's growth in connection.* New York: The Guilford Press. pp. 11–26.

Reverby, S. M. (1987). *Ordered to care.* Cambridge, England: Harvard University Press.

Robertson, M. M. (1992). Lesbians as an invisible minority in the health services arena. *Health care for women international, 13,* 155–163.

Rogers, C. R. (1961). *On becoming a person.* Cambridge, MA: The Riverside Press.

Scarf, M. (1980). *Unfinished business.* New York: Ballantine Books.

Sheehy, G. (1976). *Passages.* New York: E. P. Dutton.

Sitarz, D. (1991). *Divorce yourself.* Boulder, CO: Nova Publishing.

Smeltzer, S. C., & Whipple, B. (1991). Women and HIV infection. *Image, 23*(4), 249–255.

Stevens, P., & Hall, J. (1988). Stigma, health beliefs and experience with health-care in lesbian women. *Image, 20,* 69–73.

U. S. Department of Health and Human Services. (1993). *Depression in primary care: Vol. 1* (AHCPR Publication No. 93-0550). Rockville, MD: Agency for Health Care Policy and Research.

Woolf, N. (1991). *The beauty myth.* New York: William Morrow and Company.

Woolf, N. (1993). *Fire with fire.* New York: Random House.

Zeidenstein, L. (1990). Gynecological and childbearing needs of lesbians. *Journal of Nurse Midwifery, 35*(1), 10–18.

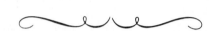

11

Women in the Context of Their Family and Community

Implications for Public and Social Policy

Evelyn Slaght
Catherine Malloy
Ruth E. Zambrana

Introduction

The purpose of this chapter is to provide an overview of the social concerns which influence the lives of women in American society. These concerns involve women's multiple roles, their health and mental health status, and their lack of support, as evidenced by existing policies which do not permit women to fully exercise their rights. Women's lives are significantly influenced by the roles they undertake in the labor force, their families, and the communities in which they live. Their lives are also strongly influenced by the social and public views of their multiple roles and the public policies which are designed to strengthen the roles in which they participate.

Survival Against the Odds:
Historical Discrimination Against Women

Global stereotypes, customs, and norms depict women as inferior to men, dependent, passive, and sometimes as property of men. Historically physicians have supported the view of women as inferior beings, using women's monthly cycle as evidence of their delicate state. They considered women particularly vulnerable to nervous conditions and hysteria. The word *hystero*, from which is derived the word *hysteria*, is the Greek derivative for "uterus" (Jordanova, 1989; Russett, 1989).

The image of women as weak, neurotic, and dependent persists. Women complain that doctors treat men's and women's complaints differently and fail to take women's complaints seriously. Physicians tend to perceive women's problems as "emotional," while male patients are referred for further diagnosis. For example, the problem of interstitial cystitis, a common urological disorder that affects mostly women, was considered a psychosomatic condition for over 100 years. With the development of effective diagnostic equipment, this bladder disease is now better understood, and women are no longer referred for psychiatric help when the disease is identified (Stevens, 1992).

In most societies women bear the burden of family and community responsibility, yet receive few of the benefits. Their contributions to economic, family, and political life have been unrecognized, and as such, remain invisible. Those who are visible and hold power in the major bureaucratic organizations are typically male. As Krieger and Fee (1994) note:

> Simply walk into a hospital and observe that most of the doctors are white men, most of the registered nurses are white women, most of the kitchen and laundry workers are black and Hispanic women, and most of the janitorial staff are black and Hispanic men. Among the patients, notice who has appointments with private clinicians and who is getting care in the emergency room; the color line is obvious. Notice who provides health care at home; wives, mothers, and daughters. The gender line at home and in medical institutions is equally obvious. (p. 12)

Issues of gender and power emerge in the academic disciplines as well, where fundamental conceptions of freedom, equality, and justice are defined in masculine terms. Much of the educational material is male oriented, and health research, with the exception of reproduction, has focused on men (Fee, 1983). The humanities have focused on exploring the experiences of men, and the critics of the works have been male (Sherwin, 1992). Thus, the past is reviewed and reflected through a male lens. Nowhere else is this so dramatically demonstrated than in male metaphors found in the medical literature describing menstruation and menopause. The terms used are not neutral; rather they convey a process of failure, production gone awry, wasted bodily fluids. Using this male framework, the conclusion that ensues is that the female bodily changes are only valuable when they result in pregnancy. Martin (1994) suggests reframing menstruation and menopause, using the positive terms usually reserved for the description of sperm production in medical texts. Although only 1 out of 100 billion sperm fertilizes an egg, the literature does not frame this as a waste product. Reframing the "waste" metaphor in more positive terms might change social attitudes toward menstruation and menopause and contribute to an appreciation of the unique physiology of women.

A bias against women is also seen in the lack of female heroes of historical significance (Sherwin, 1992). This inability to see women persists in contemporary American society. The following example is but one of many to illustrate how women's invisibility is the norm. In the May 15, 1994, edition of the *Washington Post*, a front page article about Vietnam's growing economy was accompanied by a picture and a caption. The picture showed a man and a woman standing in a rice field. The individuals were about the same height, weight, and age. They appeared to be farmers. Yet, the paper's narrative assumed that the farmer was the male. The caption gave the male a name and identified the other person as "his wife." The article was written in a way that assigned the farming accomplishments to the male. With only two people in the picture, the tone of the article suggested that the man was the only important person there. The role of the female was ignored; it was not important enough to discuss. Yet in developing countries, women work the land with the men. In fact, women produce most of the food for their families and do so under unequal conditions of access to land, and in the presence of discriminating legal and cultural practices.

The fabric of the culture is held together by gender-based roles, with men exercising the power. Throughout history, males have held a disproportionate share of the power between the sexes. In the early part of the 20th century, biological explanations justified sex differences in diseases and social roles (Krieger & Fee, 1994). With the discovery and isolation of hormones, researchers began to study the connection of hormones to the reproductive process. Researchers conceived of sex hormones as powerful determinants of gender behavior. The general conception of women was that of genetic limitation and vulnerability to changes in hormonal activity. As a result, much research has concentrated on the physiological connection between chromosomes and hormones, and has failed to take into account environmental factors. Society has blamed everything from our failure to find a cure for uterine cancer to our unwillingness to make certain jobs available on women's biology.

Women still do not have equal access to civil, economic, political, or reproductive rights. In the area of reproductive rights, women's freedom to use family planning varies considerably, and high rates of childbearing and maternal deaths remain a reality for many regions and countries (United Nations, 1991). Women in developed countries often have better access to family planning services, which results in better health status for women and children. They tend to have fewer children, and their years devoted to childbearing and childrearing comprise a smaller time span than occurs for women in developing countries. But pregnancy and childbirth and their complications continue to be a leading cause of death among low-income African Americans in the United States. Unfortunately the statistics often fail to focus attention on women in the lower socioeconomic groups in the United States for whom maternal and infant mortality remains a significant reality, in large part, because of the lack of access to affordable health care (Children's Defense Fund [CDF], 1994). Indicators on health, families, education, economics, and public life suggest that women and men do operate in significantly different worlds (United Nations, 1991).

Political Discrimination Against Women and Children

The United Nations study of the world's women found major gaps in policy investment and earnings, which limit women's full participation in economic, social, and political life (United Nations, 1991). Women continue to lack access to high-paying, high-status positions. The study also found that women were poorly represented in the policy, power, and decision-making process. Of importance is the fact that women do not have a significant high profile in political and professional arenas. Fifty United Nations member states have no woman in any of their top echelon government positions. Although women have made some incursions in the past 20 years in parliaments and at middle management levels, their representation in these areas still averages less than 10 percent and 20 percent, respectively. Their parliamentary representation would have to increase by 35 to 50 percentage points to reach parity with men (United Nations, 1991).

Powerful men in all nations use the authority of institutions to limit women's control over their own lives. Sherwin (1992) sees the subordination of women as an entrenched cultural arrangement supported by many of the institutions of modern society. The courts, legislatures, and medical societies perpetuate the status quo.

Economic Discrimination Against Women and Children

Women and children constitute the majority of the poor in the developed world. This has been referred to as the feminization of poverty (Gimenez, 1994). Worldwide statistics provide evidence that the poor population is increasingly comprised of women and children (Seager & Olson, 1986). Additionally, the elderly who live in poverty are overwhelmingly female. In developing countries, women cannot own property or make decisions about which crops to plant. United Nations (1991) statistics show women represent one half of the global population, one third of the paid labor force, yet receive only one tenth of the world income and own less than 1 percent of the world's property. Women and children under age 5 are most seriously affected by famine (Morgan, 1984).

Sherwin (1992) discusses some of the socially determined obstacles that perpetuate women's inferior status. These include the following facts: women earn two thirds of what men earn; most women's jobs are in the service sector; women's jobs offer few benefits and less job security; there are few positions of authority or political power open to women; and there is limited or no opportunity for advancement for women—the glass ceiling. Women who do advance in the male-dominated professions tend to remain at the lower end of the spectrum. Professional working mothers face expectations to work long hours, to travel out of town on business, and to attend professional meetings in the evening in addition to their childrearing responsibilities. Women working in nonprofessional jobs typically work in factories, in the service sector, in restaurants, or in hospitals with no control over the shift they must work. In all types of employment, women are often regarded as the reserve labor pool, and are the last hired and the first fired during economic downturns and retrenchments (Sherwin, 1992).

The world of work for women is quite different from men's work world. Women enter and leave the work force as a result of economic fluctuations. They work hard for less pay and in work that is not even valued enough to measure as an economic indicator.

Everywhere in the world the work place is segregated by sex. Women tend to be in clerical, sales, and domestic services, and men in manufacturing and transport. Women work in teaching, care giving, and subsistence agriculture, and men in management, administration, and politics. Examination of job categories in more detail reveals even sharper segregation. For example, in teaching, women predominate in elementary or first level education, while men predominate in higher education (United Nations, 1991). In every country where there are data, women's nonagricultural wage rates are substantially lower than men's. In Cyprus, Japan, and Korea, women's wages are the lowest in relation to men's (about half). Most countries report women's wage rates below 75 percent of men's. Even in Canada where women have made inroads into male-dominated jobs, women's earnings are still only 71 percent of men's (United Nations, 1991).

Gender inequity persists in the interpersonal relationships between men and women in the expectations about childrearing and household management. Conflict is a consequence of the tension between the traditional role of the woman and the work role. Women are still considered responsible for the work of the home in many families in a variety of countries. This results in a double work day for the majority of women. Women's sleep and leisure time are sacrificed. In the United States, households are getting smaller; there are fewer children and fewer multigenerational households. Other trends include more single-parent families and more individuals living alone (Cherlin, 1988). An increase in female heads of households has been seen since the 1970s. Women with children are often unsupported by marriage, and the elderly are living independent of their children with inadequate support systems. When elderly individuals need care and assistance, it is the female's role to add that dimension to all of the other multiple roles she is managing. The burden of multiple demands and expectations is increasing for women. Even if a woman has a male partner, she often has to work out of economic necessity. There is a decline in the extended family and the strength of kinship. The end result is that, when unpaid housework and family care is taken into account, women spend more time working than men. In fact, women's nonmarket economic activity takes more than 8 additional hours a week than men's (United Nations, 1991, p. 82), but unpaid housework is excluded from economic measurement. Women's time is not spent in activities that are officially counted or valued as critical to the economy (United Nations, 1991).

Women in the Context of Community and Society

Male bias is implicit in all societies, and the presence of this bias perpetuates existing patterns of attitudes and behavior, and presents serious consequences for women. As discussed earlier, it is through the masculine framework that women come to know art, history, literature, sciences, and philosophy. The academic disciplines are not neutral; they contain masculine presumptions. The result is a biased intellectual focus that perpetuates the oppression of women (Sherwin, 1992).

Gender bias can be seen in the health care field from the way in which women's problems are considered or not considered in the ways that services are delivered. Sherwin (1992) noted that work in bioethics is focused on issues confronting the physician. Yet problems specific to nurses, social workers, and nursing assistants are seldom addressed. The emphasis on physician problems suggests that the work of the physician is the most valued and most important work in health care issues. While other nonphysician health care providers make significant contributions to individuals, families, and communities, they are not accorded the same level of importance. This is reflected in the very questions that are asked in studies, in the control of the health care agenda, and on the operating assumptions. Studies of health care should not be centered solely on outcomes of interest to physician practice. Because health is a dimension of experience transcending merely the physical, questions should address human relationships, values, cultural variations, belief systems, and alternative modalities of healing. Issues of chronic stress and the impact of varying sources of social support should be addressed.

Recently the voices of women (including such groups as the Congressional Caucus for Women's Issues) attracted some attention by demanding fuller participation in their health care and in the major scientific studies being conducted without female representation. It has resulted in the National Institutes of Health giving more attention to cardiovascular diseases, osteoporosis, and cancer, as well as AIDS in women (U.S. Department of Health and Human Services [DHHS], 1991). It was an important step in recognizing that women's health should not focus only on their reproductive capability. The concentration on the reproductive and childbearing aspects of women's lives undervalues the importance of a much broader range of life cycle needs.

Multicultural Factors that Influence Women's Health

There are extensive differences in the quality of women's lives. These differences are influenced by level of education, nature of primary occupation, socioeconomic status, number of children, racial and ethnic group membership, culture and family structure, and living arrangements. Thus, any analysis of women's lives, particularly their health status, must examine the context of their lives to better understand the needs and concerns of diverse groups of women (Baca-Zinn & Dill, 1994). Diversity and multiculturalism in the United States refer to a set of characteristics that distinguish the lives of individuals from the mainstream, dominant culture, middle class lifestyle. These characteristics include language differences, class differences, or different cultural values, either due to place of birth or ethnic background (e.g., Mexican American or American Indian). The interplay between social, environmental, and cultural factors, and gender impact on the health and mental health status of women.

Racial and ethnic minority women, especially women of African American, American Indian, and Hispanic origin, bear a disproportionate burden of poverty, morbidity, and mortality, and consequently have limited access to the social and economic resources required to enhance their quality of life. Discrimination and racism also play a crucial role in affecting the quality of life of many of these women (Leigh, 1994). In a recent study by the Center for Women Policy Studies (1993), the data showed that women of racial and ethnic minority groups experienced subtle but persistent racial, ethnic, and gender biases that affected their mental health status and their ability to balance their work and family roles. In many instances, the result was that they decided to leave current employment positions. For non-Hispanic White women, there are innumerable stressors in the work place, such as sexual harassment and insensitivity of the employer, that are related to gender bias. These stressors negatively influence advancement, economic mobility, and ability to balance work and family roles. The combined effect of racial, ethnic, and gender biases has serious implications for the economic, psychosocial, and health functioning of women of color.

Health represents a complex phenomenon which involves many dimensions of the individual, family system, community environment, and societal resources. In recent years, there has been a growing recognition that health status must be viewed within a familial and socioeconomic context. Moreover, the primary health care needs of women are integrally related to family structure and their multiple roles. Women are responsible for emotional, social, and physical maintenance and caretaking responsibilities associated with their children, partners, and other extended kin. Oftentimes these responsibilities exclude the exercise of self-care practices to maintain their own health and social well-being. Women as health consumers have not been targeted for health maintenance and promotion programs unless there is a specific health problem such as drug addiction, early childbearing, or infertility. At the same time, there has been too little attention paid by researchers to the unique health concerns of ethnically and culturally distinct women and their families.

Health status is also significantly influenced by lifestyle behaviors. Current thinking views lifestyle practices as individual behaviors, with limited recognition of the influence of stress, poverty, environmental conditions, and knowledge and beliefs on health practices and lifestyle behaviors. Among poor and minority women, limited economic means and lack of knowledge and attitudes in these areas, clearly contribute to the potential for unfavorable health practices, poor health status, and overrepresentation in high mortality categories (Table 11-1). Limited attention has been given to the ways in which health behaviors among women and especially low-income women of color are significantly influenced by institutional and societal failures. For example, poverty is highly correlated with poor nutrition, unemployment, and multiple jobs for low pay, which may, in turn, contribute to lower use of preventive health behaviors, and the use of alcohol and drugs. Older minority women, who are far likelier to live at or below the poverty line and in substandard housing, also experience higher levels of chronic illness and disability.

The actual health status of women is an area which has only recently gained prominence in the clinical and research world. The three leading causes of mortality among women are heart disease, cerebrovascular disease, and malignant neoplasms. In examining these rates by race and ethnicity, the data show that Black women are significantly more likely to die from stroke and coronary heart disease, and complications of pregnancy and childbirth than White women; the incidence of breast cancer is higher for White women, but Black and Mexican American women have higher death rates from breast cancer. The survival rate for uterine cancer in 1983–1990 was 84.9 percent for White women, but only 55.2 percent for African American women. Overall, women are more likely than men to experience higher rates of chronic bronchitis, anemia, spastic colon, high blood pressure,

TABLE 11-1 Leading Causes of Death: Females, by Race
Number of Deaths per 100,000 Persons in Population

Causes	White	Black
Cancer	111.1	137.2
Heart disease	103.1	168.1
Cerebrovascular accident	23.8	42.7
Accidents	17.6	20.4
Chronic obstructive pulmonary disease	15.2	10.7
Pneumonia	10.6	13.7
Diabetes	9.5	25.4
Cirrhosis	4.8	11.5
Suicide	4.8	2.4
Septicemia	3.1	8

Source: National Center for Health Statistics, 1992. *Advanced report of final mortality statistics*, 43(6), Washington, DC: Author

immunologic diseases (rheumatoid arthritis, systemic lupus, systemic sclerosis, multiple sclerosis, and diabetes mellitus), and affective disorders (Report of the National Institutes of Health, 1991).

In examining the disease patterns in women, there are distinct differences by socioeconomic status, and by racial and ethnic group status. Poor women and women of color are more likely to delay their care, and thus their diseases are detected at a much later stage. Thus, the differences in patterns of disease partly reflect lack of access to services, or sociocultural barriers which contribute to fragmented and poor quality of care. Health status has also more recently been linked to social and public health problems that influence women's lives. There are a set of sociomedical problems such as substance abuse and domestic violence that recently have been recognized as contributing to adverse health consequences for women. These issues are integrally related to women becoming the fastest growing population with AIDS.

AIDS/HIV: A Woman's Health Issue

Early AIDS/HIV investigations and prevention efforts centered on male homosexuals. While many large cohort studies of the natural

history of HIV have been conducted, these studies focused on homo-
sexual men and individuals with hemophilia. Reliable information
about HIV infection in women is far less available. Without an understanding of the special characteristics and sexual practices of women,
effective strategies to prevent the spread of HIV infection in women
will continue to be ineffective. Questions regarding whether or not
there are gender-specific differences between men's and women's
immune systems, response to HIV infection, and rate of disease progression need to be addressed with well-designed research studies. The
outcomes of these studies will have important implications for what
constitutes appropriate treatment for women.

Recent data provide evidence that certain diseases occur in HIV-
infected women. These include vaginal candidiasis, dysplasia, carcinoma
of the cervix, pelvic inflammatory disease, and other sexually transmitted diseases (DHHS, 1991).

AIDS is escalating among females (Corea, 1992; Mosher, 1993).
Of particular concern is the incidence of AIDS in adolescents and ethnic
and racial minority groups, many of whom live in economically and
socially adverse situations. Women with AIDS have few resources, are
hard to reach, and often experience sociocultural and economic barriers in accessing medical care. For any treatment approach to be successful, it will be necessary to realistically consider the situations in
which AIDS-infected women live. Many female AIDS victims not only
deal with their own disease but also care for infected children and
partners.

Changing behavior patterns is always challenging, and perhaps even
more so with women. Their lives are often dominated by the males
with whom they have relationships and the communities in which they
live. If their partners are infected, women may not have the power to
prevent sexual transmission in the absence of male cooperation. Failure to address AIDS as an interpersonal problem within the context
of community is to perpetuate the victimization of women that is
commonplace in society today.

Heterosexual contact is the principal mode of AIDS transmission
to women. Of the 12,881 adult-adolescent cases reported to the Centers for Disease Control and Prevention through March 1992, women
constituted about 60 percent of all persons whose only exposure was
heterosexual contact with a person at risk for AIDS. Among this group,
62 percent had contact with an injecting drug user.

The impact of AIDS on minority groups is especially significant.
For example, as of 1992, Hispanic women represented 21 percent of
all women diagnosed with AIDS, and Hispanic men accounted for 16

percent of all men diagnosed with AIDS. Among children, 25 percent of all children with AIDS are Hispanic. As of 1991, AIDS was the fifth leading cause of death among Hispanics (DHHS, 1991).

These data on women suggest a cluster of behavioral and psychosocial risk factors that contribute to excess mortality and morbidity, including less than 12 years of education, unemployment, partner using drugs, high-risk sexual activities, history of sexual abuse, and the likelihood of experiencing violence. This set of risk characteristics, also referred to as *psychosocial morbidity*, is compounded by the lack of comprehensive services available for women who use substances, by legal and social sanctions which inhibit women from seeking help, by lack of health insurance, and by other sociocultural and institutional barriers that contribute to lack of access and delays in seeking care.

The limited knowledge on the health of women is a serious concern in the scientific community. As we approach the end of the 20th century, there is a dearth of clinical evidence on risk factors for major chronic diseases that affect women, such as cardiovascular diseases, arthritic conditions, and menopausal symptoms, as a result of the exclusion of women from clinical research. The Institute of Medicine has completed a major study of the issues related to the inclusion of women in clinical studies. The report presents scientific evidence of gender differences in biological and psychosocial risk factors that can affect disease risk, treatment, and prevention. The authors also provide compelling scientific reasons for expanding current federal policy to assure sufficient numbers of women, including racial and ethnic minorities, are represented in research studies to advance knowledge in women's health (Mastroianni, Faden, & Federman, 1994).

Future work on women's health must depart from a multidimensional conceptual paradigm and include interdisciplinary team work. Lastly, there is sufficient evidence to unequivocally state that the health of women, especially poor women and women of color, cannot be improved without attention to the social, environmental, and psychosocial factors that exist within their communities and society. Most importantly, it has become clear that knowledge of the culture, poverty, and community resources are key to the development of appropriate and relevant interventions. Future research needs to build on the scientific evidence which demonstrates that women are at higher risk for a significant number of diseases, and thus resources must be allocated to increase our knowledge in this area. Further, lifestyle behaviors and social and environmental factors also significantly contribute to morbidity and mortality. Thus, policies that influence the performance of women's roles must be formulated to enhance their physical and mental functioning.

Violence

The United States Department of Commerce (1989) reported that women are physically and sexually abused at least 10 times more frequently than men. An expert panel convened by the Alcohol, Drug Abuse, and Mental Health Administration (ADAMHA) highlighted the mental health effects of violence (Public Health Service, 1985). In addition, the National Institute of Mental Health, the National Coalition for Women's Mental Health, and the National Black Women's Health project all identified violence as a significant public health issue.

The pervasive pattern of violence is tolerated by various male-dominated institutions. In data collected from 70 countries, Morgan (1984) found that there was widespread acceptance of beating women. Profit in pornography further reinforces the objectification of women and the acceptance of violence against women (MacKinnon, 1982). Sherwin (1992) reports that in the United States, 93 percent of women experience sexual assault or harassment; 44 percent of women experience rape or attempted rape; 43 percent of girls are sexually abused; 16 percent of sexually abused girls are abused by a male family member; 30 percent of women experience systematic battering in their homes; and 70 percent of women are beaten at some time in their married lives. There is a consensus that higher levels of violence exist than are reflected in official statistics. This is due to nonreporting and to crime survey instruments that do not ask the right questions. Koss (1985) found that only 5 percent to 8 percent of women who were assaulted reported the crime and noted that the crime survey instruments were flawed. Sampselle (1992) described a marked increase in forcible rape, up 35 percent, from 1978 to 1987. Finklehor (1984) and Russell (1983) reported that 15 percent to 38 percent of women experienced childhood sexual assault. Investigators generally acknowledge that the official statistics are low. It is astonishing to note that based on the data from the literature, about one third of women will experience violence at some time in their lives. Violence against women persists and continues to be a global problem.

Domestic Violence

Domestic violence is a public health concern that disproportionately affects women, particularly low-income women, in our society. Effort to assist women who are victims of domestic violence have been viewed as antifamily when they encourage women to leave the spouse or mate. Societal values maintain a bias in favor of two-parent families, and thus there are limited economic support programs to assist women who are without a partner. For example, the absence of affordable housing combined with poor child support enforcement leaves many women with the all-too-accurate belief that they cannot make it on their own. Any attempt to assert themselves by obtaining protection from a spouse's physical or emotional abuse is not met with sympathy, but rather a mixture of contempt and indifference. Our society is willing to protect children from abuse, and all states now have mandatory reporting and response to child victimization, but such protections have not been extended to women in abusive domestic situations.

Recent data suggest a link between child abuse and spousal abuse (McKay, 1994). The concurrence of both is more common than believed, suggesting that child abuse may need to be investigated when spouse abuse is present. Even if child abuse is not present, there may be neglect when marital abuse reduces the mother's capacity to care for her children. Our unwillingness to institute punitive measures against spouse abusers is rooted in our views of women as property, and our determination to maintain the family within the private domain. As a result, the law enforcement system has been reluctant to intervene, complaining when women drop charges against their assaultive mate. They have not recognized the problems that a women is confronted with when she takes legal action. She usually fears retaliation from her mate, but often has no alternative other than to remain with him, and recognizes that legal action will make it even more difficult to stay. Other types of assault are not handled in the same manner, nor do victims of assault from strangers face the kind of censorship that has been inflicted on victims of spousal abuse.

Recently some jurisdictions have begun to implement pro-arrest policies, which instruct police officers to arrest the abuser when they have probable cause to believe an assault has occurred or is imminent. Pro-arrest policies have not been uniformly adopted, and many jurisdictions continue to arrest only when they are confident that the victim will follow through and testify. It is often presumed that she will not testify, and women find it difficult to secure arrest warrants when this presumption exists.

Domestic violence is considered a less significant crime in our society inasmuch as it is prosecuted as a misdemeanor. The impact of arrest is minimal and usually results in no more than one night in jail. Nonetheless, jurisdictions that have begun arresting find that it is an effective intervention, because it sends a message that society will not tolerate wife abuse. When combined with counselling, studies have demonstrated that recidivism rates can be reduced (Buzawa & Buzawa, 1990).

The reluctance of many jurisdictions to adopt pro-arrest policies or provide adequate counselling services is reflective of the gender politics that pervade decision making in many communities. The decision makers (in law enforcement and local politics) are predominantly male, and there are no national guidelines or policy that exists to guide local decision makers on the handling of domestic cases. The result is that the extent to which women who are abused can expect societal protection varies considerably from one jurisdiction to the next.

Women who use hospital emergency rooms (ERs), as a consequence of their battering, also experience institutional indifference. ERs have no responsibility either for reporting this victimization or for referring or assisting the patient in securing alternative housing; in other words, they "patch them up" and send them home. Staff in ERs receive no training to identify domestic violence victims, nor are data maintained to enable planners to assess the extent of the problem. If a woman has the economic means to see a private physician, her experience is likely to be the same. In 1994, the American College of Obstetrics and Gynecology (ACOG) issued clinical guidelines for the identification and reporting of domestic violence in emergency rooms (ACOG, 1995). The key issue remains as to how ER staff will be trained to use the guidelines, and how systematically will they be implemented in all medical care settings.

The evidence is clear that failure to intervene in domestic violence situations usually results in additional and often more severe abuse (Anderson, 1988). Twenty-four percent of all homicide victims die at the hands of a family member, and half of the time, this relative is a spouse (Buzawa & Buzawa, 1990).

Historically, wife and child abuse have been ways for men to assert their authority in the family. In 1976, Rubin portrayed the "worlds of pain" experienced by working class women, in which men view the family as the only place where they can exercise power and demand obedience. Middle class women, she suggests, have it easier because the professional middle class man is more secure and has more status and prestige than the working class man—factors which enable him to assume a less overtly authoritarian role within the family. However, domestic violence occurs across the socioeconomic spectrum. Reducing violence requires socioeducational experiences that convey society's expectation that women have a right to safety from assault, both within and outside of the home.

Advocacy and Policy for Women

Work-Related Policy

Public policy has not kept pace with the changing expectations and roles of women in our society. Adequate support systems do not exist to enable women to fulfill their work, family, and community responsibilities. The pressure to work and maintain the family has increased the stress experienced by women, and the gap in the frequency of stress-related illnesses is closing between men and women. Women who work experience not only the same job pressures encountered by men, but they also must assume responsibility for arranging child care and elderly parent care when they are away from home. In addition to working outside the home, it is generally assumed that the female, not the male in the household, will assume responsibility for all family-related matters.

Child care, family leave, flextime, flexible benefits, and job sharing are not earned rights or linked to our employment benefits in the United States. There is no public policy commitment to facilitate the economic roles of women in United States society. Family leave only recently became a reality (in 1993 when President Clinton signed into law the Family and Medical Leave Act), but it is unpaid leave, requiring a woman to choose between her responsibility for her family and her financial needs in deciding whether to take time off to stay home with a baby or elderly parent.

Quality child day care is very expensive, requiring many working mothers to depend instead on relatives or friends, or shift work if they have a spouse who can adjust his work schedule to allow him to babysit. Job sharing is useful in accommodating mothers to whom at least a part day program is available, but these arrangements tend to be informal and limited in availability, depending as they do on the good will of the employer to make the necessary adjustments (The Conference Board, 1991). There is currently no incentive for employers to accommodate job sharing or flextime arrangements.

Women are returning to work sooner after childbirth than in the past, in part out of economic necessity as well as the growing expectation that new mothers will continue to work outside the home. Six months is now the norm; no longer do most women stay home until the child starts school, as they did in the past. In fact, it is predicted that by the year 2000, 75 percent of the mothers with children under 1 year of age will be in the labor force (Caruso, 1992). One consequence of this is that there is a growing crisis in the availability of quality infant child care. Infant care is labor intensive, which has discouraged some providers from expanding to meet the need. As a result, many women rely on relatives and friends to provide infant care, but often this is done out of necessity, not as the plan of choice. In effect, there is no assurance that the child will receive quality care when friends or relatives are the provider.

The Family Support Act of 1988 established minimum provisions so that all states have licensing standards for child care centers, but there is no regulatory mechanism that applies to relative care, and some nonrelative care also does not have to be licensed. Currently, licensing regulations in most states exclude family homes serving four or fewer children, church-operated day care programs, and most camps. According to the Children's Defense Fund (CDF; 1994), only 37.9 percent of child care (other than parents) is provided through center-based care, leaving most children in care situations where there are no clear health or safety standards or routine inspections. In addition, licensing regulations are written to include as many programs as possible. More stringent licensing regulations would make a short supply even smaller, which discourages most states from upgrading their standards. Additionally, enforcement is minimal, and there is virtually no system in most states for inspecting family day care homes, and most are exempt from licensing (CDF, 1994). This leaves the working mother with no assurance in many instances that her child is being well cared for. Studies have documented that concerns about children's well-being detract from a mother's performance on the job and contribute to her absenteeism. Some of the more progressive companies, consequently, are providing on-site child care programs as well as referral services, as part of an effort to improve worker productivity. However, few government incentives exist to encourage companies to provide day care service. In some instances, referral services associated with Employee Assistance Programs (EAPs) include day care information and referral.

Inadequate licensing standards are a major issue relative to infant care due to risk for injury, accidents, and the spread of infectious diseases when infants are housed together. Yet in 19 states, child care centers are permitted to operate with five or more infants per adult, and some states permit a ratio of 8–12 infants per adult. Preventing the spread of a disease such as measles is extremely difficult under these conditions. Recently, the incidence of AIDS among children has highlighted the need to upgrade health standards in licensing to assure that children are properly protected while their parents are working (CDF, 1994).

Today about one in three of the children of working mothers are cared for in nursery schools, preschools, and other organized child care facilities, making the regulation and funding of child care programs issues that should command more attention than they presently receive. Little or no attention has been given, for example, to the chronic problem of inadequate salaries resulting in high turnover among staff. Many child care workers barely earn minimum wage, and most states have no mandatory training for staff. Increasing salaries for staff means higher child care costs, which get passed on to working mothers, who are already struggling to make ends meet. The only solution to these rising costs is some form of government subsidy. Yet there is no consensus that child care subsidies are a legitimate public responsibility. We have middle class child care subsidies in the form of child care tax credits for middle-income families, as we have direct vouchers for low-income families through the Child Care and Development Block Grants. However, many single mothers fit into neither category and are on their own with no assistance or benefits to defray their child care costs.

Attorney General Reno has suggested that child care is an important crime prevention effort (CDF, 1994). Publically supported child care is commonplace in other industrialized countries. In Sweden, it is regarded as essential for full-time work and women's career development (Gustafsson & Stafford, 1991). Child care subsidies in the United States are means tested and available only to low-income families.

In addition to subsidized child care, Head Start programs are an important resource for low-income mothers, and presumably these will expand because President Clinton made a commitment in his 1992 campaign to serve all eligible 3–4-year-olds in Head Start by 1996. Head Start has the advantage over other preschool and child care programs of operating as a "two-generational" program (Collins, 1994); that is, Head Start has traditionally offered a range of medical, dental, and nutritional services as part of its services to both parents and children. Parents are an integral part of the planning and operation of Head Start programs. But many Head Start programs traditionally operate on a part-day and seasonal basis which does not by itself accommodate the full-time working mother.

Facilitating Work and Family Responsibilities

To facilitate women's labor force participation, public policy makers must examine ways in which a woman's family responsibilities limit her work participation as well as the ways in which inequities in job opportunities and pay have limited her ability to support herself and her family. We blame the welfare mother for her inability to support herself, in spite of the failure of our society to commit to a full employment policy or to make funds available so that she can reach the minimal educational level required for work.

One of the ways that economic inequality was approached during the War on Poverty was to make available small business loans to encourage the development of minority-owned firms. In order for women to become major players in economic growth, they will have to become corporate owners, and this same kind of encouragement needs to be extended to all women, whether or not they are members of cultural minority groups.

One of the businesses in which women should be economically invested is the day care business. Corporate involvement in day care is growing, and large franchises are springing up (e.g., Kinder Care). These are largely male-owned corporations, however. They have been shown to be no less generous in staff salaries, and in fact, pay less than most, and their prices tend to be higher than the average. Grants to build or develop day care centers for children have been almost nonexistent, which has been especially problematic for centers located in inner cities where structures available to house day care (churches, schools, and leased buildings) are dilapidated, jeopardizing the program's ability to meet licensing codes.

Promoting women's corporate ownership will not be easy for the same reasons that protecting small businesses presents hazards. Many benefits, such as health insurance, are not affordable to small businesses, which represents a barrier in obtaining support for universal health coverage.

Social programs need not threaten the existing economic power base, and mechanisms must be found for improving social conditions and economic opportunities. Parental leave was a viable social policy provision because it was responsive to family needs without creating additional governmental expenditures. While very few benefits have no fiscal impact, corporate tax credits are preferable to direct payment programs because they minimize the economic impact. Loans are preferable to grants, and private sector training is preferable to public sector community service to increase employability. Unfortunately, the most disadvantaged minority women are less likely to be knowledgeable of how to take advantage of incentive programs. As more women fill the professional ranks and stop viewing their employment as supplemental, issues of pay equity should begin to gain greater attention. More "comparable worth" legislation and pay equity lawsuits should emerge. Serious problems of economic equity between women and men persist (Anderson, 1988).

Future Policy Directions

The political arena is changing and has changed significantly over the past 25 years. The years between 1970 and 1990 have been described by some historians as the era of "social retreat" as the federal government, especially during the Reagan years, reduced federal expenditures for social programs and returned decision making to the states. The reductions in social programs have meant that women in our society, who are the primary recipients of welfare benefits, have been told to do more with less public support. Under the guise of welfare "reform," states are now adopting plans to limit the amount of time that benefits may be given under the Aid to Families with Dependent Children (AFDC) program. If this trend toward forced employment continues without adequate provision for job training, educational remediation, or job placement, women and children will swell the ranks of the homeless, and more and more children will end up in foster care. Such policies are not only antifamily, they are antiwomen because AFDC recipients are predominantly women. Ambromovitz's (1994) arguments regarding the sexist and racist nature of the social welfare system are compelling. To propose cutting immigrants from the welfare rolls to fund welfare reform is to pit one disadvantaged population against another. Equity in social programs must be raised more vociferously as an issue, and punitive approaches must be protested.

Women who are welfare recipients have little or no voice in shaping the new reform proposals. Who, then, speaks on their behalf? Our ability to curtail further welfare reductions is hindered by the fact that cuts in social programs have been identified as essential to deficit reduction. In the male-dominated Congress, social reform issues that benefit mostly women are likely to take a back seat to "fiscal responsibility" unless we can be more convincing regarding society's social responsibilities to its most vulnerable and least powerful groups.

Adovocacy as a Strategy for Change

If women are to be effective advocates, they will need to be more cognizant of how to obtain and use power. Power, according to Hunter (1959), is contained in the hands of a few who are responsive to minority needs only when it suits their political purposes. Gaining power involves developing relationships with people in power as well as organizing large numbers of supporters/constituents who can be vocal and articulate about women's common concerns. What is not clear is who should do the organizing, and what organizational structure is likely to be effective in involving the greatest number of women possible. One of the major problems in organizing women is that they are not of one mind on economic, social, or political issues. For example, while all working women share a mutual interest in the availability of quality child care and affordable health care, these issues are far more pressing for the single working mother than for the woman in a two-parent household. Women who have a partner on whom to depend have different economic, social, and political priorities. Similarly, women who have remained homemakers and not joined the ranks of working women are not interested in issues like equal pay or quality day care. These differences must be negotiated as we work to arrive at priorities to which the majority of women can subscribe if advocacy is to be effective.

Lobbying by women in support of women's issues is less effective because it lacks the financial backing that is generally associated with corporate lobbying and special interests. It depends on the good will of legislators who are largely men, both at the local and national levels. Men currently outnumber women in the United States Senate 16 to 1 and in the House of Representatives 9 to 1. Local ratios are not dramatically different.

One of the strategies that traditionally has been advocated is to work to put into political positions those who can best represent the woman's point of view. Our success in electing women to Congress has improved, but we are still dependent on the good will of men to achieve change. Schram and Mandell (1994) suggest three methods of change—educating (including consciousness raising), persuading (lobbying), and pressuring (direct action, including sit-ins and pickets). Sometimes single-purpose groups can bring an issue to the forefront; other times coalitions are needed. The organizing tactics of the 1990s emphasize building healthy coalitions, identifying and promoting charismatic leadership, and finding ways to involve clients in decision making so that they can speak for themselves (Austin & Lowe, 1994).

Should women focus on building coalitions even if this means diluting attention to critical single issues? Who are the leaders who can represent the greatest number of concerned women? Can we bridge the political gaps between White middle class suburban housewives and inner-city minority single parents so that women can have a single agenda? These are the questions that must be answered if women's issues are to have the broad-based support that is essential for critical change to occur.

References

Ambromovitz, M. (1994). Is the social welfare system inherently sexist and racist? In H. J. Karger & J. Midgley (Eds.), *Controversial issues in social policy.* Boston: Allyn and Bacon.

American College of Obstetricians and Gynecologists. (1990). *Domestic violence.* Technical Bulletin #209. Washington, DC: Author.

Anderson, M. L. (1988). *Thinking about women: Sociological perspectives on sex and gender* (2nd ed.). New York: Macmillan.

Austen, M. J., & Lowe, J. I. (1994). *Controversial issues in communities and organizations.* Boston: Allyn and Bacon.

Baca-Zinn, M., & Dill, B. T. (1994). *Women of color in U.S. society.* Philadelphia: Temple University Press.

Buzawa, E. S., & Buzawa, C. G. (1990). *Domestic violence: The criminal justice response.* Newbury Park: Sage.

Caruso, G. L. (1992). Patterns of maternal employment and child care for a sample of two-year olds. *Journal of Family Issues, 13*(3), 297–31.

Center for Women Policy Studies. (1993). *Defining work and family issues: Listening to the voices of women of color.* Final report. Washington, DC: Author.

Cherlin, A. J. (1988). *The changing American family and public policy.* Washington, DC: The Urban Institute Press.

Children's Defense Fund. (1994). *The state of America's children.* Washington, DC: Author.

Collins, R. C. (1994). Head Start: Steps toward a two-generation program strategy. *Young Children, 48*(2), 25–33.

The Conference Board. (1991). Work-family roundtable: Flexibility. *The Conference Board, 1*(1), 5–22.

Corea, G. (1992). *The invisible epidemic.* New York: HarperCollins.

Fee, E. (1983). *Women and health: The politics of sex in medicine.* Amityville, NY: Baywood.

Finkelhor, D. (1984). *Child sexual abuse: New theory and research.* New York: Free Press.

Gimenez, M. E. (1994). The feminization of poverty: Myth or reality? In E. Fee & N. Krieger (Eds.), *Women's health, politics and power: Essays on sex/gender, medicine, and public health* (pp. 287–305). New York: Baywood.

Gustafsson, S., & Stafford, F. (1991). Child care subsidies and labor supply in Sweden. *The Journal of Human Resources, 28,* 224–29.

Hunter, F. G. (1959). Top leaders and planning. In E. Harper & A. Dunham (Eds.), *Community organization in action* (pp. 37–50). New York: Association Press.

Jordanova, L. (1989). *Sexual visions: Images of gender in science and medicine between the eighteenth and twentieth centuries.* Madison: University of Wisconsin Press.

Koss, M. P. (1985). The hidden rape victim: Personality, attitudinal, and situational characteristics. *Psychology of Women Quarterly, 9,* 193–212.

Kreiger, N., & Fee E. (1994). Man-made medicine and women's health: The biopolitics of sex/gender and race/ethnicity. In E. Fee & N. Krieger (Eds.), *Women's health, politics, and power: Essays on sex/gender, medicine, and public health* (pp. 11–29). New York: Baywood.

Leigh, W. (1994). The health status of women of color. In C. Costello & A. Stone (Eds.), *The American woman (1994–1995): A status report: Women and health.* New York: W. W. Norton.

Mastroianni, A., Faden, R., & Federman, D. (1994). *Women and health research.* Washington, DC: National Academy Press.

MacKinnon, C. (1982). Feminism, Marxism, method and the state: An agenda for theory. *Signs, 7*(3), 515–44.

Martin, E. (1994). Medical metaphors of women's bodies: Menstruation and menopause. In E. Fee & N. Krieger (Eds.), *Women's health, politics, and power: Essays on sex/gender, medicine, and public health* (pp. 213–232). New York: Baywood.

McKay, M. M. (1994). The link between domestic violence and child abuse. *Child Welfare, 73,* 31–38.

Miles, S. H., & August, A. (1990). Courts, gender, and "the right to die." *Law, Medicine and Health Care, 18*(1,2), 85–95.

Mosher, W. D. (1993). AIDS-related behavior among women 15–44 years of age: United States, 1988–1990. Washington, DC: U.S. Department of Health and Human Services, Public Health Service, Center for Disease Control, National Center for Health Statistics.

Public Health Service. (1985). *Women's health,* Vol. 2. Report of the PHS Task Force on Women's Health Issues (Publication No. 85-50206). Washington, DC: Department of Health and Human Services.

National Institutes of Health. (1991). *Opportunities for research on women's health.* Bethesda, MD: National Institutes of Health, Office of Research on Women's Health.

Rubin, L. B. (1976). *Worlds of pain: Life in the working-class family.* New York: Basic Books.

Russell, D. (1983). The incidence and prevalence of intrafamilial and extrafamilial sexual abuse of female children. *Child Abuse & Neglect, 7,* 133–146.

Russett, C. E. (1989). *Sexual science: The Victorian construction of womanhood.* Cambridge, MA: Harvard University Press.

Sampselle, C. (1992). *Violence against women: Nursing research education and practice issues.* New York: Hemisphere.

Schram, B., & Mandell, B. R. (1994). *An introduction to human services policy and practice* (2nd ed.). New York: Macmillan.

Seager, J., Olson, A., Kidron, M. (1986). *Women in the world: An international atlas.* New York: Simon & Schuster.

Sherwin, S. (1992). *No longer patient: Feminist ethics and health care.* Philadelphia: Temple University.

Stevens, C. (1992). How women get bad medicine. *The Washingtonian, 27,* 74–77.

U.S. Department of Commerce. (1989). *Statistical abstract of the United States.* Washington, DC: Author.

U.S. Department of Health and Human Services. (1991). *Action plan for women's health.* Washington, DC: Office on Women's Health.

United Nations. (1991). The world's women 1970–1990; Trends and statistics. In *Social statistics and indicators,* Series K, No. 8, Sales No. E. 90.XVII.3. Washington, DC: Author.

12

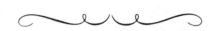

The Global Context
of Women's Health Care

Martha Neff-Smith
Andrew D. Lacatell
Allen F. Moore

Introduction

There have been many explanations over the centuries for the influence of gender and race on the different health risks experienced by men and women in different parts of the world, most of them based on popular beliefs about the inferiority of non-Caucasians, "ethnic" Europeans, and women. Phrenologists studied skulls to document a biologic basis for the supposed lesser intelligence of African Americans (Haller, 1971). Early geneticists used Mendelian laws and Morgan's fruit fly experiments to explain the high rate of tuberculosis and other infectious disease among immigrants from Ireland, Italy, and Eastern Europe, who they characterized as "inferior and sickly stock" (Krieger & Fee, 1994, p. 14). Social Darwinists, who provided the philosophic justification for the development of capitalism and the extension of colonialism, predicted the extinction of Negroes based on natural laws and the process of evolutionary selection (Degler, 1991); in the meantime, they said, very little could be done for "such an inherently degenerate, syphilitic and tubercular race" (Allen, 1915, p. 194). Scientific developments in the early 1900s, particularly the discovery of sex hormones and genes for gender, gave credence to the idea that the health of women was predetermined to be inferior (Jordanova, 1989).

The last three decades have seen a massive shift in philosophic and scientific paradigms from a determinist view of biology to an understanding that the real determinants of globally occurring racial, ethnic, socioeconomic, and gender differences in health are primarily *social*, not biological. Women in developing countries have poor access to health care, educational, and occupational opportunities. In developed countries, unplanned teen pregnancies, low levels of primary care, lack of inclusion of women in medical research, low levels of public funding for prevention and treatment of diseases that particularly affect women or affect women differently, and a lack of appropriate chronic disease care are indications that women are still second class citizens.

Throughout the world, the survival of women and the quality of their lives are determined primarily by their social and economic status. The traditional roles of women as bearers of children, family care givers, and subsistence gatherers have limited women's opportunities for education and better health care, while at the same time their importance to domestic survival remains undervalued.

International public health agencies have long recognized that the health of women is an excellent indicator of the health of a nation or a society. Women face a range of health hazards from complications in childbirth to the stress of domestic violence and war. Raising the status of women—through literacy, legal protection, economic opportunity, reproductive choice, and the valuing of women's work in the domestic setting—will improve the health of women across the globe.

It is important, in studying the health needs of women throughout the world, to acknowledge the legacy of 19th century pseudoscientific ideas about race, gender, and biological determinism. Their influence persists today in subtle and not so subtle stereotypes and forms of ethnocentrism that limit our ability to gather and interpret data accurately. It is common, for example, to assume that the "developed" nations are necessarily "advanced" over less industrialized nations. You will see, however, that the tiny country of Panama, with limited resources, committed itself long ago to a public health approach and universal access to health care—goals that the United States has failed to achieve in its latest round of health care reform debate. And you will see also, in the Panamanian and South African case studies, that women are not just passive victims of discrimination, who endure and persevere under oppressive conditions, but survivors and activists who can organize effectively to improve their access to health care. The goal of this chapter is to recognize the dignity and strength of women, while accurately, candidly, and bluntly reporting the effects of discrimination on their social status and health conditions.

The Elements of Health in the Global Community

The World Health Organization (WHO) definition of health as a state of complete physical, mental, and social well-being and not just the absence of disease has become the standard against which attempts to raise the level of health of the global community are measured. Health workers in all countries face fundamental problems. Health is determined by the interaction of economic, political, and social forces, yet across the globe women have been denied an effective economic and political voice, and in some regions of the world they have no voice at all. Social status, which is almost universally related to education and family position, has been low for women internationally. Lack of access to health care has contributed to the high levels of morbidity and mortality among women. Around the world, millions of people are denied life-sustaining resources because of extreme poverty.

Women and the Disease of Poverty

Jacobson (1993) describes a debilitating disease of poverty which affects two out of three women around the world. More than 62 percent of the world's women live in countries classified by the United Nations as having *very low GNP* or gross national product (equivalent to <$1000 U.S. per capita annually), and an additional 13 percent live in countries where the per capita income is, by United Nations' definitions, *low* ($1000–3,000 per capita annually). Common symptoms of this fast-spreading ailment include chronic anemia, malnutrition, severe fatigue, increased susceptibility to respiratory and reproductive tract infections, and premature death.

Poverty affects women disproportionately. In India, for example, caloric intake among females relative to males has declined since 1980, despite improvements in the availability of food and health care (Crossette, 1991). When resources are scarce, decisions about allocation are critical factors in subsequent morbidity and mortality.

Gender Bias, Resource Allocation, and Health Status

Within all societies, the majority of poor people are women (Last & Guidotti, 1990). When resources are limited, women are inequitably affected through the devastating cycles of devaluation, deprivation, and poor health. The poor have limited access to health care services in the developing world. In many regions, except for traditional healers, few health care providers are available. Even in areas where services are available, the poor cannot afford basic health care.

Gender bias exists in every country, at virtually every income level, and in every stratum of society; this bias is compounded by discrimination based on income, social class, and race, and is especially pervasive in the poorest areas of Africa, Asia, and Latin America (Jacobson, 1992). We see its manifestation in the unequal allocation of resources (Jacobson, 1992). Gender differences in mortality and morbidity in the developing world, as compared with the developed world, present a vivid picture of gender discrimination and abuse of women as manual laborers. Women everywhere work longer hours but earn less income, despite the fact that they are responsible for meeting 40–100 percent of a family's basic needs (United Nations Department of International Economic and Social Affairs [UNDIESA], 1991).

Unlike industrialized societies where women have longer life expectancies, in developing countries female life expectancies range from 54 years in Africa, to 64 years in Asia, and 70 years in Latin America. Women in developed countries have an average life expectancy at birth of 77 years (WHO, 1992). The world total of maternal deaths each year has been estimated to be 500,000 (out of 2.6 billion women worldwide), but experts consider the real total to be much greater, especially because many women who die in childbirth are poor and live in remote areas where deaths are not recorded. In 1986, in absolute numbers, Asia (308,000) and Africa (150,000) recorded the largest numbers of maternal deaths. Latin America and Oceania joined Asia and Africa with 34,000 and 2,000 maternal deaths, respectively, among the developing countries. The developed countries accounted for only 6,000 maternal deaths (WHO, 1986). Women in developing countries are 100 to 200 times more likely to die from pregnancy and childbirth than women living in more industrialized nations. In the rural Jamalpur region of Bangladesh, the maternal mortality rate is 623 per 100,000, compared to 2 in Sweden and 8 in the United States. Table 12-1 illustrates differences in selected regions of the world.

TABLE 12-1 Maternal Deaths as a Proportion of all Deaths of Women of Reproductive Age—Selected Countries, 1980–1985

Country	% of deaths from maternal causes	Maternal mortality rate[a]	Year
Bangladesh (Rural Tangail)	45	874	1984–1985
India (Urban Andhra Pradesh)	33	566	1982–1983
Paraguay	28	545	1984–1985
Indonesia (Bali)	26	510	1983
Egypt (South)	23	718	1980–1982
Ecuador	23	190	1981–1983
Romania	21	300	1984–1985
Mexico	15	190	1980
El Salvador	10	88	1984
Costa Rica	8	70	1984
Cuba	6	103	1985
Japan	5	26	1983
United States	3	45	1983
Hong Kong	1	16	1985

[a]Rate per 100,000 live births.

Source: World Health Organization, 1988.

In developing countries, the rate of population growth is influenced by a number of complex social and cultural factors, religious beliefs, and literacy rates. The latter factor is a result of women's status within the society. Literacy offers an opportunity to control one's destiny, especially where reproductive choices are concerned. As a result, health education opportunities are also an important factor in the prevention of disease and premature death.

The Sociohistorical Background to Women's Health

Throughout history, women have been denied access to the same opportunities as their male counterparts. These opportunities include health care and health education. Women have unequal access to education and constitute the majority of illiterate adults throughout history (Carmack, 1992). Women's status has been influenced by two forces: the ownership of society's means of production and the sexually defined status and roles of women.

The means of production, or the economic base of a society, has historically been controlled by males. The ownership of the means of production is also intimately related to the control of the ruling ideologies of the society; those in power make decisions which support their agendas and best interests. The ruling ideology in most societies has been patriarchal in nature, holding the belief that women are suited to take care of their husbands, children, and kindred (Stromquist, 1990) and that men are endowed by nature to control the economic means of the society. The uniformity of this sexual division of labor across all cultures is striking. The sexual division of labor has succeeded in limiting women's access to occupations that are not "feminine." Women have been denied the educational opportunities afforded men, because an education has not held a value within the home. In parts of Africa, women neither own land nor have rights to resources such as trees and crops on the land they cultivate. In Latin America, agrarian land reform laws have largely failed to benefit women, primarily because females are not considered full-time producers or heads of households (World Resources Institute, 1994).

Men have also controlled women's sexuality, from making the decisions as to when to have children and how many, to creating social stigmas of contraception and promiscuity, to physical violence and forced sexual relations. These controls have been largely institutionalized in the religious and social arenas. In war, as we have seen in the case of Bosnia, women's status as second class citizens is vividly illustrated in reports of gang rapes and other acts of violence mainly attributed to Serbian forces (Jones, 1994).

Literacy

Although women make up more than one half of the world's population, they constitute more than two thirds of the world's illiterate population (World Resources Institute, 1994). In 1990, an estimated 601.6 million adult women were illiterate, as compared with 346.5 million men (33.6 percent of all adult women, 19.4 percent of all adult men). The importance of literacy in the discussion of women's health cannot be understated. As a result of centuries of sexual and gender subordination, women have not had equal opportunity for educational and occupational development. Literacy is essential to the process of gaining legal and socioeconomic rights, including good health care and health education. In Costa Rica, for example, the emphasis on literacy among women from the early 1950s to the present resulted in a decrease in the infant mortality rate. In 1910, the infant mortality rate stood at 200 per 1000 live births, with approximately 10 percent of women having access to primary education. In 1980, the infant mortality rate was just above 5 per 1000 with over 70 percent of all women attaining a primary school education (Hammad & Mulholland, 1992).

This success is the exception and not the rule. Women have lower levels of literacy than men; in some of the developing world there is an average difference in literacy of 21 percent (Hammad & Mulholland, 1992, p. 105). Sadly, the proportion of illiterate women is growing. From 1960 to 1985, of the 154 million new illiterates, 133 million were women. The greatest absolute number, 109 million, was in Asia. The greatest rate of increase was found in Africa, a 44 percent increase (Stromquist, 1990). Literacy is only part of a larger problem, which is the unequal distribution of resources among men and women.

Moreover, because literacy is seen as a potential challenge to patriarchy, literacy programs are not systematically encouraged by the state. If programs are implemented, they mainly consist of material that reaffirms the existing sexual division of labor, emphasizing skills for subsistence gathering, child care, and family planning. Women are not developing the necessary awareness and collective consciousness of their historical subordination, most especially in developing countries. As Stromquist (1990) put it, "Women need knowledge not so much to read and understand the world, but to read, understand and control their world" (p. 107). Illiteracy is found primarily among poor and socially disadvantaged women of rural areas. Gender discrimination in literacy and other access issues is an institutionalized expression of the power structure in a particular society. Women's social status within these societies is influenced by a number of elements including parental socioeconomic status, religion, distance to schools, cultural attitudes, poverty, availability of schools, parental illiteracy, and proper curricula. Not only will literacy help women to redefine and expand their roles, but it will assist them in making solid family health and planning choices. According to the United Nations Population Fund, there would be 27 to 35 percent fewer births in developing countries if women were able to have the number of children they wanted (World Resources Institute, 1994). Those concerned about population growth contend that reductions in infant mortality and improved access to education combine to naturally reduce the number of children a woman chooses to have, as she seeks expanded roles for herself and has greater hopes of seeing the children she bears survive to maturity ("Life Expectancy," 1992).

Literacy correlates strongly with increased life expectancy and lower infant mortality rates (Hammad, 1992). Yet, literacy is only one contributing element in women's status and access to health and educational opportunities. Along with the cultural and social barriers of women's status, the distribution of financial and nutritional resources is a critical factor.

Depriving women of education is a form of social and physical isolation. Orubuloye, Cleland, Caldwell, and Caldwell (1993) indicate that maternal survival is improved in countries where education for women has been introduced. A study of 15 developing countries conducted by the United Nations concluded that "an additional year of mother's schooling reduces child mortality by 6.8%" (WHO, 1992). In Asia, the mortality of children among uneducated Nepali women is almost 15 times greater than it is among Malaysian women with 7 or more years of schooling. The education of young women has the potential, within 2 decades, to bring mortality rates of the third world close to those of industrialized countries (WHO, 1992).

Income and literacy correlate inversely with infant mortality rates. In an international study, countries with low income and with low literacy rates among women (0 to 35 percent of women literate) had an infant mortality rate of approximately 125 per 1000 live births. Poor families tend to reproduce early and have many children, with little time in between births. A primary reason for having many children concerns economics: offspring provide labor for basic survival and household income, as well as insurance against solitary old age. In numerous cultures, larger numbers of children equate with higher socioeconomic status (World Resources Institute, 1994). In countries with high income and high literacy rates among women (91 to 100 percent of women literate), the infant mortality rate is approximately 15 per 1000 live births. The trend is consistent: as income levels and literacy rates among women increase, infant mortality rates decrease. Problems are compounded when childbearing begins at puberty.

Women's Status and the Sexual Division of Labor

Mazur (1994) noted that women are behind men in each established social and economic indicator. Socially, the early marriage of daughters has greatly affected women's aspirations for future education, as the level of education necessary for marriage and motherhood is considered quite low. The sexual division of labor has therefore manifested itself in the everyday activities of motherhood and homemaking. "Studies of time use by rural African women reveal that approximately 67% of their day is spent cleaning, in family care, and in wood and water procurement, and subsistence agricultural work . . . women average more than twice as much time on production-supply-distribution tasks as men" (Hammad and Mulholland, 1992). Women in industrial countries spend 16 percent of their time in cleaning and family care. Women perform more housework, food preparation, and family health care than men. Yet, they are unequally represented in landownership, credit attainment, and lack access to technology, education, employment, and political power. These inequities are transferred to the health of the family, where women continue to be less healthy.

In India, the gender differences in domestic work and subsistence agriculture affect female literacy to the point that female literacy is suppressed. In rural areas female literacy is 18 percent compared to 48 percent in urban areas. The percentages for males are 41 percent in rural areas and 66 percent in urban areas (Stromquist, 1990).

Women in developing countries today marry much younger and have children for a much longer period of time than in industrialized countries. Inability to control the spacing and number of children has affected the availability of women's time for education and social activities. Reproductive health services are available to approximately 95 percent of east Asian people, but only to 57 percent in southeast Asia and Latin America, 54 percent in south Asia, 13–25 percent in the Arab states, and in sub-Saharan Africa, 9 percent (World Resources Institute, 1994).

Women's Health Issues

The poor health of women and mothers is one of the most preventable tragedies of this century. In some countries, the process begins with female infanticide (and, with the availability of ultrasound, increased abortions of female fetuses). It continues with the preferential feeding of male infants and the neglect of female children. The preference for male babies is an almost universal phenomenon, closely linked with the perception of women's poor economic potential. In Pakistan, males are preferred to females at a rate of almost five to one. Countries that have stronger preferences for male children are found mainly in Africa and in the Middle East (WHO, 1992). From birth, females generally receive less and poorer quality food than males. Female babies are breast fed for a shorter time, and receive less cereal, fat, milk, sugar, and total calories than boys until the age of 4 and beyond (World Resources Institute, 1994). As a result, half of all pregnant women in the world and 40 percent of all nonpregnant women were anemic as of 1985 (DeMaeyer & Adiels-Tegman, 1985).

Access to Health Care

Despite the fact that women are primary providers of household health care, they often lack access to outside health care for themselves. Data show, for example, that in India fewer women than men survive common diseases, are treated in hospitals, are prescribed medication, or receive qualified, timely treatment (World Resources Institute, 1994). The gender of health care professionals is a barrier in the health prospects of women. Because females have diminished educational opportunities, most physicians are male. In Muslim countries, for example, this has had a profound effect on health care access, since women are prohibited by their beliefs from seeking the advice and care of male physicians (World Resources Institute, 1994, p. 51). Only about one third of all births are assisted by trained attendants in Africa and south Asia, as opposed to 64 percent in Latin America, 93 percent in east Asia, and virtually 100 percent in North America (Jacobson, 1991). Many mothers of young children in developing countries are chronically ill due to a high prevalence of infectious disease, a life of chronically poor nutrition, overwork, and giving birth too often. Within this context, threats to life and physical well-being occur sporadically and are eclipsed by the more pressing concerns associated with managing daily living. Other critical stages during a woman's life process prior to pregnancy and after the reproductive years have been ignored.

Nutrition

Of the 1.1 billion women over age 15 in 1985, 500 million were stunted in growth because of protein-energy malnutrition, and 2 million were blind because of vitamin A deficiency. A cycle of suboptimal growth is perpetuated across generations. Infrequent feeding, low energy density of food, high exposure to infection with reduced immunocompetence as a result of inadequate nutrition, and anemia due to illness (Marchant & Kurz, 1993) all contribute to growth retardation and skeletal stunting.

Compromised growth at early life stages is difficult to make up for at later stages. Although the health of adolescent girls benefits from improved nutrition, the optimal time for breaking the cycle is in the earliest years (gestation through 3 years of age). Common indicators for measuring the nutritional status of women are body mass index (BMI), arm circumference, and height.

Reproductive System Health

Complications in pregnancy, childbirth, and delivery; reproductive tract infections; lack of access to safe contraceptive methods; and lack of appropriate diagnosis of or treatment for reproductive tract cancers are some of the most common threats to women's reproductive health. At least 100 million women will die of reproductive system problems this year, and more than 100 million others will suffer from disabling diseases. The causes of this excessive mortality and morbidity can be found primarily in the low status of women globally and the accompanying factors of illiteracy; poverty; malnutrition; lack of access to prenatal and postnatal care and safe abortion services; and governmental policies that limit access to health resources. Regionally, the risk of dying from pregnancy-related causes is highest in Africa (1 in 21), Asia (1 in 54), and South America (1 in 73), and lowest in northern Europe (1 in 9,850) and North America (1 in 6,366; Starrs, 1987). Hemorrhage, obstructed labor, toxemia, and infection are the main culprits in maternal deaths.

Some of the common barriers to care are based on patient-related factors. There may be a lack of awareness of the seriousness of a problem. Studies in India, for example, identified several situations in which women would have been brought to a hospital for care if family members had been aware of major danger signals (Sundary, 1994). It can also be difficult for women to be spared from the work of family survival. A study in Zaire demonstrated that the majority of maternal deaths occurs in the first five months of planting and harvest, seasons when the work of women is critical to maintenance of the community. Structural problems such as lack of transportation, poor patient management, lack of equipment and facilities, and shortage of trained personnel, however, account for the majority of avoidable maternal complications and deaths.

Moreover, one third of the population of the developing world (over 1 billion people) live in nations where abortion is illegal or access is highly restricted, and there is an appalling waste of women's lives from unsafe abortions (100,000–200,000 deaths every year). In Latin America, unsafe abortion is responsible for one fourth to one half of all maternal deaths. In Brazil where abortion is legal only to save a woman's life or in rape or incest cases, social security data covering about 70 percent of the population report over 200,000 women hospitalized each year for complications of illegal abortions. And even in nations that have liberalized their laws, safe services are sometimes unavailable to the majority of women. In India, where abortion has been allowed since 1971, there were 160 million women of reproductive age in 1979, 4,600 medical facilities and 15,000 physicians that perform abortions, and an illegal abortion rate of 4 to 6 million per year (Liskin, 1980). Safe abortion services could prevent 20–25 percent of the half a million deaths each year from pregnancy-related causes (Whiticoff & Sullivan, 1980).

Many women in the developing world, and some in the industrialized nations, lack the opportunity and resources to manage their reproductive lives through family planning. In Africa, 23 percent of women who do not want additional children are practicing contraception, 43 percent in Asia, and 57 percent in Latin America (Eschen & Whittaker, 1993). In most developing countries, less than one third of women are within range of family planning services. In addition to location of services, there are many barriers to obtaining contraception: cost, requirements for spousal consent, and problems and side effects from available methods are all important deterrents.

All current methods have major drawbacks. Oral contraceptives disrupt normal cycling, which is very disturbing to many women around the world who equate good health with having an adequate and regular flow. Long acting progesterone injections and Norplant can also produce irregular bleeding that interferes with intercourse. The T-shaped IUD, which is more easily tolerated, can cause amenorrhea. Sterilization is all too permanent for many women. New techniques—the contraceptive ring, which can be removed at will, transdermal patches, and antifertility vaccines (anti-hCG)—are currently in trial phase, but much work has yet to be done to find methods that are inexpensive and culturally acceptable. In general, women prefer to use family planning services that are linked with postpartum, postabortion, or primary care, and report better rates of compliance with the methods they have chosen through these integrated programs. Planning for new programs should be based on users' perspectives on health, contraceptive use, and sexuality.

Women and Violence

The issue of domestic violence has recently become the focus of public health efforts in the United States. One United States study revealed that 1 of every 10 women has suffered physical abuse from a partner or spouse. In the global context, violence against women is a particularly salient issue. In Peru, 70 percent of all crimes reported to police involve women beaten by their husbands. A study of female mortality in Bangladesh reveals 12.3 percent of the female mortality in that country is due to intentional injury. In Norway, 25 percent of female gynecology patients have been physically or sexually abused by their mates. In Kenya, a detailed family planning survey reported that 42 percent of women said they were beaten regularly by their husbands (WHO, 1992).

Unsafe Female Circumcision

Recently, international health providers have become concerned about female circumcision, often performed by untrained individuals in unsanitary conditions. Genital surgical procedures range from clitoridectomy to infibulation, in which the outer labia are removed and the vaginal opening is sutured almost closed, leaving a tiny opening through which to menstruate. If infibulation has occurred, the entrance to the vagina must be enlarged by tearing at the time of marriage to permit coitus, and surgical revision is necessary with each delivery to permit passage through the birth canal, after which the vaginal opening is resewn.

Female circumcision and/or infibulation is practiced in more than 20 African countries, with a wide variety of rates among African regions. According to WHO, more than 84 million women have undergone sexual surgery in Africa alone (Rushwan, 1990). The procedure is most common in countries with the highest child mortality rates among children aged 1 to 4 (>30 percent). The usual age for circumcision is 4 to 8 years, but there has been a recent increase in the numbers of girls circumcised at less than 3 years of age, because it is thought that a young child can tolerate more pain (Arbesman, Koller, & Buck, 1993). Some of the documented health risks of circumcision and infibulation are bleeding, infection, shock, difficult menstruation, urinary retention, painful urination, painful intercourse, prolonged labor, and chronic pelvic pain.

While female circumcision may have its origin in the male desire to control female sexuality (akin to the chastity belt of the European Middle

Ages), it is sustained today by a host of religious and cultural beliefs strongly subscribed to by many women themselves. In addition, women believe that the operation will increase fertility, affirm their femininity, and prevent stillbirth. Many others do not want to have themselves or their daughters seen as promiscuous, unclean, or sexually untrustworthy. The Inter-African Committee on Traditional Practices Affecting the Health of Women and Children was formed in Senegal, in 1984, representing 22 national committees, in an effort to sort out issues of safety for women in a context of respect for cultural diversity.

In recent years, feminist organizations in the United States have initiated campaigns against sexual surgery. Many of these expressions of horror at traditional African and Middle Eastern practices, despite the positive aspect of their advocacy for women, have also carried horrified overtones reminiscent of colonialist outrage against the savagery of primitive peoples. It is important to recognize that surgical abuse of women is found in both undeveloped and developed nations; medically unnecessary hysterectomy, common in the United States until recently for cosmetic reasons, as punishment for women who overstepped their bounds, or for reproductive control of those deemed mentally unstable, is not very different in principle from African traditional practices. Those who advocate for women in both developed and undeveloped nations must join together in mutual respect for women's safety *and* diversity if the goal of reducing mortality and morbidity from sexual surgery is to be reached.

Infection

Women are extensively affected by a wide range of infections from endemic diseases such as tuberculosis, parasites, and malaria to reproductive tract infections (RTIs) and human immunodeficiency virus (HIV). Consequences include not just mortality and morbidity but quality of life issues such as incontinence, painful intercourse, skin lesions that cause social ostracism, and fatigue that makes it difficult for women to work and meet basic survival needs for themselves and their families (McDermott, Bangser, Ngugi, & Sandvold, 1993). The poor nutritional status and anemia that also accompany poverty contribute to an increased vulnerability to infection.

The prevalence of RTIs is staggering. WHO estimates that 20 percent of maternal deaths are caused by tetanus or sepsis. In countries such as India and Indonesia, as many as 50 percent of women presenting for medical care may have RTIs. In Africa the incidence of maternal syphilis ranges from 4–15 percent, and gonorrhea is estimated to be present in at least 10 percent of women. HIV is heterosexually transmitted in Africa, Asia, and Latin America, and in sub-Saharan Africa it is the leading cause of death for women 20–40 years old. Dixon-Mueller, Gasse, and Wasserheit (1991) reported that in some central African cities, up to 40 percent of women aged 30–34 were found to be infected with AIDS. Cervical cancer, linked to RTIs, is a leading cause of cancer death in developing countries, and liver cancer, associated with Hepatitis B, is common. Access to and availability of culturally acceptable health care services is critical for prevention, diagnosis, and treatment, yet few programs address women's perspectives of causality and severity, despite the often wide gap between lay and medical world views (Brems & Griffiths, 1993).

Poverty and War

Extreme poverty, perpetuated by constant political and military conflict, undermines the lives of Northern Irish working class women. Women must often bear the total responsibility for managing households and rearing children because their husbands are imprisoned or in hiding. Many women are widows. Women represent the most deprived group in this six-county European country that is most affected by the massive military occupation by the British. Bomb strikes in the heavily populated areas of Londonderry and Belfast are a constant cause of fear for both children and women. Both in Northern Ireland and Bosnia, the presence of military tanks and armed soldiers serves as a reminder that home is not a safe haven. Socially constructed gender differences in fear of war and the stress related to real conflict have been documented (Conover & Sapiro, 1993).

Moreover, hundreds of thousands of women have been raped in this century's wars. In World War I, Japanese soldiers abducted 100,000 to 200,000 Korean women and sent them to the front lines where they were forced into sexual slavery. The United Nations High Commission for Refugees reported that 39 percent of Vietnamese boat women between the ages of 11 and 40 were abducted and/or raped at sea in 1985 (Swiss & Giller, 1993). Health workers in Uganda describe a situation in which approximately 70 percent of the women in a single community had been gang-raped by soldiers in the early 1980s. War presents particularly terrifying aspects of violence against women.

Environmental and Occupational Health Hazards

Lead poisoning is an international issue. Lead has been used in many occupations and industries, from plumbing to the manufacturing of ammunition. Lead is known to have adverse health effects at even low levels of exposure. In one region of Poland, in close proximity to a number of lead smelters, children had mean blood levels between 12.3 and 26.7 μg/dL (WHO, 1992). The Centers for Disease Control and Prevention have set a level of concern at 10 μg/dL, because values greater than and equal to 10 μg/dL have shown discernible health effects, but it should also be noted that there is no safe level of lead exposure. In certain places within the Katowiec region, 10 to 21 percent of the children had blood lead levels above 35 μg/dL. Mothers in these places had mean blood levels from 10.6 μg/dL to 21.6 μg/dL. Up to 14.7 percent of these women had blood lead levels greater than 35 μg/dL. Blood levels for pregnant women are of particular concern because of the ease with which lead is transferred to the fetus. Exposures from poorly maintained drinking water systems, peeling and cracking lead paint, living near high traffic areas in regions where leaded fuel is still used in automobile gasoline, and residential and/or recreational exposure to stationary sources of lead (i.e., lead smelters) are environmental hazards that affect both men and women, and more significantly children. In developing countries such as India, gasoline still contains lead; internationally, leaded gasoline emissions are second only to lead paint as a pathway of lead exposure (WHO, 1992).

Deforestation makes fuel gathering more difficult and time consuming, requiring the gatherer to walk longer distances and carry heavier loads. In the foothills of the Himalayas, for example, the gathering of firewood and fodder took no more than 2 hours a generation ago; now it takes a full day of walking through mountainous terrain. Over a 10-year period in the Sudan, the time it takes to gather fuelwood increased more than fourfold. When fuelwood is not available at all, women in some countries such as Bangladesh shift to alternative and sometimes inferior fuel, such as animal dung and crop residue. These take longer to burn and produce hazardous fumes. Lack of fuel may also reduce the number of hot meals a family can receive. Water collection is also becoming more difficult. Women may spend up to 4 hours a day retrieving water for the home and the farm, often carrying up to 20 kilograms or more in containers on their backs, shoulders, or heads (World Resources Institute, 1994).

In the United States, in 1993, the leading cause of occupation-related death for women was murder (homicide is the third leading cause of occupation-related death for men). Forty percent of women who died on the job were homicide victims as contrasted to 15 percent of men. The reason for the disparity between men and women has been credited to the fact that a large number of women are exposed to crime while working late at night in all-night convenience stores ("High Murder Rate," 1993). Women are disproportionately represented in these high-risk sales positions, and their health is therefore disproportionately affected. Appropriate measures to ensure the safety of all employees in these positions must be taken.

Global Implications

The World Bank recognizes that development is necessary for the health of people throughout the world. International organizations have long agreed on the necessary elements for improving standards of health for women: environmental protection; stable government with citizen participation; increasing levels of education; adequate food supply; safe water and sanitation; and the empowerment of women to free themselves from unwanted childbearing and domestic labor. Equality of opportunity is the goal toward which successfully developed countries strive. Women are today virtually absent from decision-making positions in all realms of development and environmental management; only 3.5 percent of the world's cabinet ministers are women, and in 93 countries women hold no ministerial positions. Only 6 of 159 United Nations member countries were headed by women at the end of 1990. Women represent less than 5 percent of management-level staff at bilateral and multilateral development agencies (World Resources Institute, 1994).

Poverty is directly linked to the status of women. In order to survive, women in developing countries must perform the most menial of tasks. Documentaries call attention to the plight of women in Asia and Africa who must collect and sell kindling for food. In many rural agrarian societies, women's lives are still determined by elders of the family or tribe; most of them are destined to spend their lives in a combination of childbearing and heavy manual labor. They will work crops, carry food and water long distances, crouch over cooking fires in ill-ventilated huts, and inhale toxic fumes in greater amounts than if they smoked two packages of cigarettes a day.

In addition to poor manual working conditions, women's health is affected by their domestic workload. In Gambia, female working hours are 213 percent of male working hours. In Uganda, women work 163 percent as many hours as men (WHO, 1992). In addition to manual labor, domestic labor can pose a disproportionate strain on women's health (WHO, 1992). Technology development aimed at giving women more time could have a powerful effect on their productivity and their well-being, thus giving women more opportunities for educational and income-generating activities (World Resources Institute, 1994). In some developing countries, poverty among women is intensified where men have migrated and left the village or countryside (Turshen, 1993), indicating that economic and political conditions must be improved for both men and women.

Summary

For centuries, world politics has focused on territory and economic interests. Human rights, equality of opportunity, and the subordination of women have been lesser concerns. Only when media attention exposes the atrocities of war or famine and natural disaster does the international community cry out against the daily situation of women in developing countries. As a result of such publicity, attention has recently been focused upon child labor and slavery, the better distribution of food and other resources to minority ethnic groups, and the treatment of women as property to be used as the dominant community determines.

The status of women in China, parts of Africa, and New Zealand has been prominently featured in international journals. Discussion of the social and health needs of women by international agencies is the first step toward essential action. Specific programs resulting from international outrage have been focused on reducing infant and child mortality. The lives of women have improved as a side effect of food and resource allocation, educational programs, and surveillance of labor rules. Nevertheless, the campaign for "health for all by the year 2000" has not yet produced major changes in the lives of hundreds of thousands of women throughout the world's regions.

The time has come for educated, articulate women to use their influence on behalf of all women throughout the world. Women's status in the home and in the marketplace has traditionally and universally been below that of men. Subsequently, women's health in general has suffered. The sexual division of labor has dictated a male-dominated economic structure and a female-dominated domestic structure. Domestic work, primarily performed by women and thus devalued, has not proven a viable economic pathway for equality. Women must be allowed to participate equally in educational and occupational programs. Literacy is essential to educated health choices and family planning decisions. International studies of time use among men and women reveal that women consistently spend more hours in food gathering, family care, and economic-survival activity. Men spend the majority of their time in economic-gain activities. For women, participation in the work force and fewer hours spent in parenting and family care responsibilities would result in better access to good health education and health care. The health of women is inextricably linked to their status in the home and the marketplace. As a result, women's health has been detrimentally affected by their low social status in the global context. As long as women are not considered equals, there can be no world unity or harmony.

References

Allen, L. C. (1915). The Negro health problem. *American Journal of Public Health*, 5, 194.

Arbesman, M., Koller, H., & Buck, G. M. (1993). Assessment of the impact of female circumcision on the gynecological, genitourinary and obstetrical health problems of women from Somalia to Poland: Literature review and case series. *Women's Health*, 20(3); 27–42.

Brems, S. & Griffiths, M. (1993). Health women's way: Learning to listen. In M. Koblinsky, J. Timyan, & J. Gay (Eds.), *The health of women: A global perspective* (pp. 255–273). San Francisco: Westview Press.

Carmack, N. A. (1992). Women and illiteracy: The need for gender specific programming in literacy education. *Adult Basic Education*, 2(3) 176–194.

Conover, P. J., & Sapiro, V. (1993). Gender, feminist consciousness and war. *American Journal of Political Science*, 37, 1079–1099.

Degler, C. N. (1991). *In search of human nature: The decline and revival of Darwinism in American social thought*. Oxford: Oxford University Press.

DeMaeyer, E., & Adiels-Tegman, M. (1985). The prevalence of anemia in the world. *World Health Statistics Quarterly*, 38, 302–16.

Dixon-Mueller, R., Gasse, F., & Wasserheit, J. (1991). *The culture of silence: Reproductive tract infections among women in the third world.* New York: International Women's Health Coalition.

Eschen, A., & Whittaker, M. (1993). Family planning: A base to build on for women's reproductive health services. In M. Koblinsky, J. Timyan, & J. Gay (Eds.), *The health of women: A global perspective* (pp. 105–131). San Francisco: Westview Press.

Haller, J. S. Jr. (1971). *Outcasts from evolution: Scientific attitudes of racial inferiority 1859–1900.* Urbana: University of Illinois Press.

Hammad, A. E. B., & Mulholland, C. (1992). Functional literacy: Health, and quality of life. *The Annals of the American Academy of Political and Social Sciences, 520,* 103–120.

High murder rate for women on job. (1993, October 3). *New York Times,* Section 1, p. 29.

Jacobson, J. L. (1991). *Worldwatch paper 102, women's reproductive health: The silent emergency.* Washington, DC: Worldwatch Institute.

Jacobson, J. L. (1992). *Worldwatch paper 110, gender bias: Roadblock to sustainable development.* Washington, DC: Worldwatch Institute.

Jacobson, J. L. (1993). Women's health: The price of poverty. In M. Koblinsky, J. Timyan, & J. Gay (Eds.), *The health of women: A global perspective* (pp. 3–31). San Francisco: Westview Press.

Jones, A. (1994). Gender and ethnic conflict in ex-Yugoslavia. *Ethnic and Racial Studies, 17,* 115–134.

Jordanova, L. L. (1989). *Sexual visions: Images of gender in science and medicine between the eighteenth and twentieth centuries.* Madison: University of Wisconsin Press.

Krieger, N., & Fee, E. (1994). Man made medicine and women's health: The biopolitics of sex/gender and race/ethnicity. In E. Fee & N. Krieger (Eds.), *Women's health: Politics and power: Essays on sex/gender, medicine and public health* (pp. 11–29). Amityille, NY: Baywood Publishing.

Last, J., & Guidotti, L. (1990, 1991). Implications of human health of global ecological changes. *Public Health Review, 18*(1), 49–67; discussion, pp. 69–72.

Life expectancy: How some low-income nations beat the odds. (1992, April 13). *Business Week, 3261,* p. 22.

Liskin, L. S. (1980). Complications of abortion in developing countries. *Population Reports,* July 7.

Mazur, L. A. (Ed.). (1994). Women's Voices '94. *Beyond the numbers: A reader on population, consumption, and the environment,* (pp. 267–280). Washington, DC: Island Press.

McDermott, J., Bangser, M., Ngugi, E., & Sandvold, I. (1993). Infection: Social and medical realities. In M. Koblinsky, J. Timyan, & J. Gay (Eds.), *The health of women: A global perspective.* San Francisco: Westview Press.

Orubuloye, I. O., Cleland, J., Caldwell, J. C., & Caldwell, P. (1993). African women's control over their sexuality in an era of AIDS: A study of the Yoruba of Nigeria. *Social Science Medicine, 37*(7), 859–72.

Rushwan, H. (1990). Female circumcision. *World Health,* April–May. pp. 24–25.

Starrs, A. (1987). *Preventing the tragedy of maternal deaths: A report on the International Safe Motherhood Conference.* Nairobi, Kenya: World Health Organization.

Stromquist, N. P. (1990). Women and illiteracy: The interplay of gender subordination and poverty. *Comparative Education Review, 34*(1), 95–111.

Swiss, S., & Giller, J. E. (1993). Rape as a crime of war: A medical perspective. *Journal of the American Medical Association* [*JAMA*], *270*(5), 612–615.

Turshen, M. (1993). The impact of sexism on women's health and health care. *Journal of Public Health Policy, 14*(2), 164–173.

United Nations Department of International Economic and Social Affairs (UNDIESA). (1991). *The world's women: Trends and statistics, 1970–1990.* New York: United Nations.

Whitcoff, B., & Sullivan, M. (1980). Assessing the role of family planning in reducing maternal mortality. *Studies in Family Planning, 18,* 128–143.

World Health Organization. (1992). *Women's health: Across age and frontier.* Geneva: Author.

World Health Organization. (1988). *World development charts.* Geneva: Author.

World Health Organization. (1986). *Maternal mortality rates: A tabulation of available information.* Geneva: Author.

World Resources Institute. (1994). *World resources 1994–1995.* New York: Oxford University Press.

Case Study
in International
Health Issues for Women

Changing Trends
in Health Policies in Panama

Amelia Marquez de Perez

Editors' Note: This case study is presented to provide an opportunity to reflect on the concepts presented in this chapter, and suggest a method of analysis for understanding the basis of specific situations you may encounter in research and practice in international health. As you read, think about the following questions:

1. How does the health care system in Panama compare with situations in other developing nations? With Europe and the United States?

2. What relationship exists between the economic situation in Panama and the health of women?

3. What are the implications for women's health of each of the health care delivery systems described?

4. What are the new criteria that give impetus to privatization, and how will women fare under the new private-sector system?

5. In what way do improvements or deterioration in both the availability of health services and the status of women parallel the development and resolution of political conflicts within a country and internationally?

6. If you were a nurse practicing in a community health center in Panama today, what would you expect your daily practice to be like, and what problems might you be likely to face?

Panama is located in the narrowest part of Central America, facilitating world communications and trade through the Panama Canal. Its population is a little over 2 million, and it is one of the Latin American countries that performs well on standard health indicators. At the beginning of the 1990s, the gross birth rate per 1,000 was 21.4, the gross mortality rate per 1,000 was 3.4, and life expectancy was 67.8 for males and 74.1 for females. According to data furnished by the General Controller of the Republic of Panama, there were 670 health institutions and centers, and 87.7 percent of women were assisted in childbirth by professionals. The average number of children was three, demonstrating a trend toward decrease, and average family size was 4.4 members. Accidents and violence were the main causes of death for the population as a whole, but for women the highest contributor to mortality was cancer. There were almost 12 physicians and 11 nurses per 10,000 persons, and 3.3 hospital beds per 1,000 persons.

These statistics compare very favorably with other nations in Central and South America, but in the last 7 years, Panama has experienced increased poverty, unemployment, and violent crime, and health levels have begun to deteriorate (Comision Economica para America Latina y projecto regionale para la Superacion de la Pofreza, 1990). For instance, while the fertility rate is decreasing overall, it is increasing among young adolescents (10–12 years old), and there is a higher incidence of diseases such as malnutrition, tuberculosis, and diarrheal illnesses that are associated with poverty. Sexually transmitted infections have also increased, and AIDS continues as a black box, despite governmental efforts. The violent crime rate is actually higher than the official figures because domestic violence against women and children is rarely reported (Moreno de Rivera, Marques de Perez & De Leonde Bernel, 1993).

In order to understand the development of health resources in Panama, their allocation patterns, the evolution of recent problems, and the choices facing the Panamanian people, it is important to look first at the health care system models that have been employed and the methods of financing them (Programa de Las Naciones Unidas para el Desarollo, 1991; Katzman & Gerstenfeld, 1990).

The Original Public Health Model

Since the beginning of the Republic (1903), health services were considered entirely the responsibility of the Panamanian government. There were few private clinics, and physicians provided care as a social obligation. Community services were offered through visiting nurses, local children's clinics, prevention programs to improve nutrition and increase vaccination rates, and public health campaigns against infectious diseases. Civic organizations devoted their efforts to raising funds for the blind and for tuberculosis patients, but communities were spectators rather than actors. Health issues related to the environment were always ascribed to the governmental domain.

The Creation of the Social Security System

The Panamanian Constitution of the 1940s established social rights, including a right to health care, parallel to individual rights. In accordance with this principle, the Social Security System was developed to offer health services as well as retirement pensions to the working population. At this time, women were also granted a 14-week paid leave of absence for pregnancy (6 weeks before delivery and 8 weeks after).

Since the beginning, participation has been both a right and a duty for employers and employees, and there is a strong private contribution, with the system maintained by deductions from earnings (10.75 percent for employers and 7.25 percent for employees). Money also accrues to the fund from investment in the commercial housing market.

The introduction of the Social Security System marked a change from the prior orientation of sole public responsibility. A two-tiered health care system evolved, with sophisticated services provided for workers, and a poorly funded public health sector, which could not meet the demands of the poor, nonworking people and those relatives of workers who were not eligible under the Social Security System.

This inequality in health care was contradictory to the spirit of the Panamanian Constitution. Private investment in health centers and hospitals created services that were only accessible to upper and upper middle class families. There was not much of an insurance market to

fill in the gap, because the wide coverage available under the Social
Security System removed the potential for insurance industry profit.
For example, Mutual of Omaha covered the workers of the Panama
Canal Company, but offered no national program. By the end of the
1960s the Panamanian health care system had evolved a tripartite structure: a public sector, covering the majority of the population, that
provided a low level of care; a mid-level Social Security System to attend
to the needs of the working population, and a developing private sector to permit the upper and upper middle classes access to advanced
modern technology (Esping-Andersen, 1990).

The Community Health Model

The Panamanian Constitution of 1972, based on a welfare state philosophy, resulted in a revised health policy with the slogan, "Equal
health for everybody!" The Ministry of Health, which had been a
subsection of Work and Social Welfare, gained independent status. The
concept of health as an absence of disease (a remedial approach) was
transformed to a definition that envisions communities as producers
of health through preventive interventions.

Communities were organized around health issues in local district,
province, and national networks, and even in remote areas, there were
local health committees that coordinated activities with professionals
and paramedics from the health center and subcenters or hospitals.
The responsibility of the local organizations was to motivate community and professional participation, while the networks served to link
community people and health services, diffuse programs and specific
activities, and oversee the quality of care. Women played an important role as leaders of a significant number of local health committees,
but not in national leadership.

With this new focus, nontraditional preventive programs were
developed. Some of the most outstanding were the development
of rural aqueducts, massive construction of latrines in rural and
ghetto areas, training and technical assistance for producing vegetables and fruits in community gardens, and breeding fish in artificial lakes. Seeds, animals, and equipment were donated, and
volunteer labor and time were dedicated to intensive community
campaigns on a massive scale for vaccination and neighborhood
cleanup.

There were concomitant gains in the employment and upgrading of health workers. New careers such as community nursery worker and health educator were created. Paramedical professions improved in status and wages, and scholarships were made available for masters' level education, especially in public health.

During the 1970s, even with this intense effort, governmental health expenditures represented less than 3 percent of the gross national product (GNP) at the 1990 price index. Although a great part of the resources came from the Social Security System, the style of work and community participation were what made the difference.

Within the Social Security System itself, coverage was broadened. Each worker, male or female, could register spouse, parents, and children up to 18 years of age. Services were expanded to include health services, medicines, laboratory testing, treatments, and hospitalizations. In addition to the standard maternity benefits, women were protected by labor laws to the extent that they could not be fired in the year following the birth of a child.

The health integration system was developed as a financial policy to correct maldistribution of resources, the concentration of services and health centers in the nation's capital. The Social Security System and the public health system were combined as a resource pool, thus dividing functions and extending services to the majority of the population, even the poor, and providing access to all in any governmental health center, subcenter, or hospital.

The 1980s—Testing the Universal Access Public Model

During the period after introduction of this integrated system, there were political conflicts between those who favored universal, government-sponsored health care and those who pushed for privatization of health services. Panama was one of the few Latin American countries that experienced an increase in the GNP between 1980 and 1986. Along with economic growth, there was a corresponding increase in health expenditures, representing around 5–6 percent of the GNP (Marquez de Perez, 1994). Unlike the experience of the 1970s, the increased health expenditures of the 1980s, especially the crisis period of 1987–1992, did not mean better health care (Esquivel, 1989). On the contrary, health services deteriorated, and there was a lack of equipment and equipment maintenance, creating a lack of confidence and dissatisfaction among the population.

Analysis suggests that three factors appear to have contributed to this deterioration. First, physicians' salaries were increased as a result of effective labor organization and several strong strikes on their part. These salary increases drained off money that was needed by other parts of the medical care system. Second, there was intense lobbying from international financial organizations to privatize health services and discontinue the wide coverage available under the Social Security System, coupled with an internal political crisis that began in 1987. Third, there was pressure from the growing insurance industry, newly interested in health insurance marketing, who benefited from neglect and deterioration in the public sector.

Transition to a Privatized Model

The United States Army invasion of Panama in 1990 broke the status quo. The new government that was subsequently established mainly represented private enterprise interests. It signed agreements with international financial organizations to privatize several governmental services and change the Social Security law in order to permit reductions in coverage. Drastic changes were proposed, but moderated to some degree after workers' and women's organizations exercised political pressure and organized popular protests in the streets on behalf of those most negatively affected by the shift in public policy.

Several types of problems have resulted. Privatization was supposed to save money, but the end result has been the highest expenditures of GNP in the last 20 years (10 percent at 1990 prices), combined with a continued deterioration in services. Moreover, the oversupply of physicians and nurses that began in the 1980s intensified. Because wage increases for physicians have cut into other available funds, the government has not been able to provide enough public service positions for all graduating nurses and doctors, who are required by law to serve 2 years before being employed in the private sector or going on for specialty training. As a result, there is both an oversupply and a bottleneck of health care practitioners.

Meanwhile, the private health sector continues to develop along the lines of the United States health industry, creating a competitive market of health services. Insurance companies have designed a variety of proposals for working and middle class families who used to be the backbone of the Social Security System. Private health insurance is no longer the privilege of higher-income people.

On the other hand, the costs of rapidly changing and expensive sophisticated medical technology have now been transferred to patients. Health services in communities have been reduced to a pilot project in 11 areas, called the Localized Health System or SILOS (Ministerio de Salud, 1990). This program is actually a restricted reproduction of the original community model of the 1970s.

Current Realities and Dilemmas

Although the Panamanian government has formally adopted privatization, the road from policy adoption to model implementation is a long one. Pressures from international financial organizations are countered by a long and strong historical tradition of reliance on a public health approach. But there is not only the problem of competing philosophical trends and political controversy. The new government that took office in September of 1994 will have to confront many competing interests.

There is the newly established but sizeable and powerful private health sector, which has replaced the former missionary approach to medical care with an economic perspective in which the main criteria are not service, but competency, free market principles, and efficiency. They want government to support the private health care sector, not compete with it. On the other hand, the people expect the government health services to recover the high standards they had in the past and make the new technologies widely available. Physicians want job security and high wages. These competing needs do not appear to be compatible.

The choices confronting policy makers will have implications for the health of the Panamanian people, and especially women, for a long time to come. The debate today focuses on 10 central questions (Annis, 1991; Anderson, 1990; Interamerican Development Bank, 1990; Conferencia Regional sobre la Pobreza en America Latina y el Caribe, 1991):

1. Should the main costs of health services be assumed by the private or public sector?

2. Should social class be a determinant of the quality of health care?

3. Are the people and government still committed to equity and health as a social right?

4. Is it possible for government to assure equity for health services?

5. Can the public sector achieve levels of efficiency and technology to parallel private efforts?

6. What is the real distribution of health expenditures if increased spending results in decreased quality?

7. What roles could be assumed by communities as part of civil society?

8. Must there be a return to the traditional definition of health as the absence of sickness?

9. All over the world countries are being pressured in contrary directions. WHO, on the one hand, demands higher levels of health care accessible to the entire population, while international financial organizations, on the other hand, demand reductions in levels of social services, including health care. How can Panama and other nations reconcile these competing interests?

10. What effects will the growth in the private insurance industry have on the Social Security System in the long run?

Choices made by the new government will certainly affect the health status of Panama's population. One can but hope that innovative models for health care delivery will be developed in response to the competing demands of the different interest groups. It is also to be hoped that Panamanian women who developed community organizing skills in the public health campaigns of the 1970s, who have entered the workforce in record numbers and developed leadership skills in the process, will be able to use those skills to advocate for their own health needs.

References

Anderson, J. (1990). *Economic policy alternatives for the Latin American crisis.* New York: Taylor and Francis.

Annis, S. (Ed.). (1991). *Poverty, natural resources and public policy in Central America*. New Jersey: Transaction Publishers.

Comision Economica para America Latina (CEPAL) y AProyecto Regional para la Superacion de la Pobreza. (1990). Magnitud de la pobreza en America Latina en los anos 80. LC/L, *533*, 31 de mayo.

Conferencia Regional sobre la Pobreza en America Latina y el Caribe (1991). *Hacia un desarrollo sin pobreza*. Bogata, Colombia: PNOD.

Esping-Andersen, G. (1990). *The three worlds of welfare capitalism*. New Jersey: Princeton University Press.

Esquivel, J. R. (1989). Marco conceptual de la salud integral de la comunidad: El caso de Panama. En Grupo Editor Latinomexicano, Editores. *Como Enfrentar la Pobreza*. Buenos Aires, Argentina: SRL.

Interamerican Development Bank. (1990). *Economic and social progress in Latin America*. Washington, DC: Author.

Katzman, R., Gerstenfeld, P. (1990). The complexity of evaluating social development. *Cepal Review, 40*.

Marquez de Perez, A. (1994). Social expenditures in Panama: The seventies and the eighties. Unpublished manuscript.

Ministerio de Salud. (1990). *Politica nacional de salud*. Cuidad, Panama: MINSAL.

Moreno de Rivera, A., Marquez de Perez, A., DeLeon de Bernal, A. (1992). *Perfil de la situacion de la mujer en Panama y lineamentos de acciones prioritarias*. Cuidad, Panama: UNIFEM-PNUD-MIPPE-CEDEM.

Organizacion de la Salud. (1990). *Salud de las Americas*. Washington, DC: OPS.

Programa de las Naciones Unidas para el Desarrollo. (1991). *Desarollo humano: Informe 1991*. Bogota: Tercer Mundo Editores.

Case Study in the Social Determinants of Health
Women in South Africa

Snowy Molosankwe

"Her wings are clipped and it is found deplorable she does not fly"
(Simone de Beauvoir;
quoted in Genovese, 1993, p. 1)

1. As you read, consider: what are the similarities and differences between Panama and South Africa?

2. What parts of the American health care system might provide useful models for the women of South Africa?

3. A health care system designed to detect and treat illness might be quite different from a system based on the definition of health described in this study. What would those differences look like?

4. If you were Minister of Health for Women in South Africa, what would be your order of priorities? What would you use as indicators to measure the effectiveness of your new orientation, programs, and campaigns?

Women in South Africa: Past and Present

Health refers not only to the absence of physical pain, sickness, and disease; health means that people develop and function in accordance with their innate physical, intellectual, emotional, and social potential; that their inherent constructive, developmental energy is unfolding freely and spontaneously, and is not being blocked and transformed into destructive and self-destructive expressions; and that their talents and capabilities are not wasted or lost, but are actualized toward their own fulfillment and their society's enrichment (Gil, 1993a, p. 4). This type of health reflects the extent to which people are able to satisfy their basic human needs in the context of the social, economic, and political institutions of their societies. This type of health also recognizes health consequences arising from the cultural, social, political, and economic environments in which women live and work (Year of Woman, 1993).

As is the case in most countries, the position of women in society has undoubtedly negatively affected the health of women in South Africa. In understanding the history of South Africa and the health status of women in that society, Thompson (1990) suggests that we derive approximations, probabilities, and informed conjecture from the available evidence. Precolonial and colonial history provide a background for viewing the constraining and enabling factors that affect the health of women in South Africa.

According to Thompson (1990), for thousands of years during the precolonial era, communities lived by hunting, fishing, and collecting edible plants. The basic social unit was the nuclear family, but several families usually formed bands numbering between 20 and 80 people. As in other preindustrial societies, there was division of labor between men and women. Men were responsible for clearing the land for agricultural purposes, cattle keeping, and building huts. Men also engaged in many crafts, including making clothes of cowhides and pelts of wild animals. Women were responsible for raising the children, and planting, weeding, and harvesting the crops. Women were also responsible for maintaining the home, making clay pots, and serving the food. With all this work, humans in these societies, especially women, managed to meet their basic needs within the context of their social, economic, and political institutions. These in turn provided good health and thus long life.

The economic power of women in these early societies was directly related to their health status. Guy (1990), for example, argues that in the precapitalist societies women exercised control over the agricultural process, and by virtue of the central importance of their fertility to society, enjoyed considerable status and a degree of autonomy not appreciated or replicated within the colonial society (Walker, 1990). Women were presumed to possess superior powers. They were also accorded leading social and political responsibilities. As Gil (1993b) adds, many societies revered women as the source of life.

The root cause of the health conflicts, constraints, problems, and challenges facing South Africa today lies in the origins and processes of colonization. The South African colonial state had, from the time the first Dutch settlers set foot on South African soil until May 1994 when the Mandela regime took office, both covertly and overtly instigated and maintained measures geared toward apartheid and the injustice which perpetuated the oppression and degradation of women in general, and the African woman in particular. A range of factors emanated from apartheid or what Gil (1993b) refers to as "oppression" and "injustice." According to him, oppression refers to "relations of domination and exploitation—economic, social, and psychologic—between individuals; between social groups and classes within and beyond societies; and, globally, between entire societies" (p. 4). He sees injustice as "discriminatory, dehumanizing, and development-inhibiting conditions of living (e.g., unemployment, poverty, homelessness, and lack of health care), imposed by the oppressors upon dominated and exploited individuals, social groups, classes, and peoples" (p. 4).

Oppression and injustice as experienced by women in South Africa included the allocation of jobs on the basis of gender; unequal pay; discrimination in hiring, promotion, and firing; and failure to provide work-related safety in regard to women's reproduction systems, child care, and flexible hours. Other acute gender questions pertained to societal attitudes toward women's physical health and control of their bodies and reproductive capacity; violence against women, both physically and mentally, direct and indirect, including rape, domestic violence, and sexual harassment in its various forms; the demeaning use of women in advertising; and the degradation of women in pornography, the media, and advertising. Gil (1992) argues that "differentiations within the society by occupation, location, rights, life style, social class, consciousness, and perceptions of interests . . ." affect the health of women. Support for Gil's argument can be seen in the policies derived from the Roman-Dutch Law (for example, the New Matrimonial Act, the Black Administration Act, and the Natal Code). These policies served as ex post facto ratification and legitimation of these intrasocietal differentiations, and resulted in an absurd and very painful situation for women.

Regardless of their economic means, education, or the fact that approximately 1.9 million households are for all practical purposes headed by females (due to the migrant labor system and other colonial practices), women were denied comprehensive health coverage. Most of these female-headed families, even today, are bringing up their children in conditions of extreme deprivation and squalor.

South African society is profoundly patriarchal. Women in South Africa constitute the majority population (54 percent of the total population according to the 1991 census); yet, their status is one of powerlessness. The past constitutions of South Africa have been based on discrimination, thereby denying the majority of people, especially women, their fundamental rights. In this day and age of advanced education and technology, most women, especially Africans, are illiterate. Thousands occupy the lowest ranks in employment and are grossly underpaid. All of this was perpetuated by the denial of people's fundamental human rights to satisfy their intrinsic human needs.

As the 1991 census revealed, women constitute more than half of the South African population. They make up 39.4 percent of the country's economically active people. Women are 54 percent of the voting population; however, they constitute only 2 percent of those in power, and they represent only 19.2 percent of managerial, executive, and administrative occupations (Year of Woman, 1993). South African women face one of the highest rates of rape in the world: a woman is raped every 83 seconds, and she is more likely to be Black than White ("South Africa," 1993). Maternal mortality ranks high in South Africa, approximately 80 times higher than for women in the United States. Women who become pregnant, especially in the rural areas, face a risk of death due to lack of health service facilities and personnel, births not being attended by trained personnel, availability of few backup services for high-risk pregnancies, poor transportation networks, lack of treatment for complications, and malnutrition. Abortion has been and still is a major cause of maternal mortality, especially illegal or street abortions. As reported in *The World's Women: 1970–1990: Trends and Statistics* (United Nations, 1991), maternal mortality rates in South Africa stand at 83 per 100,000 births, compared to 45 per 100,000 births in the United States. According to the World Health Organization, acquired immunodeficiency syndrome (AIDS) is now the leading cause of death among women ages 20–40. Sexually transmitted diseases (STDs) render millions of women subfertile or infertile. These diseases also cause women to suffer with recurrent infections. AIDS and STDs account for maternal deaths in South Africa as well. Until recently, the social, economic, and political impact of AIDS and STDs on women in South Africa was neglected, and these diseases are spreading at alarming rates.

Women in South Africa are no different from other women around the world. The United Nations (1991) indicates that around the globe there are gaps in policy (integration of women in mainstream development policies and counting women's work), investment (education, health services, and productivity), and earnings (lower pay or no pay) which perpetuate women's inequality; everywhere in the world the work place is segregated by sex. Women around the globe are translating their struggle against discrimination into political action.

The Conditions and Tasks for the New South Africa

Apartheid in South Africa today has been officially abolished and replaced with the new nonracial, nonsexist democratic government. However, as reported in the *Human Development Report 1993*, the country's African people (or *Blacks*, as used in this report) still live in a world apart. According to the report, the richest 5 percent of the population, mostly White, owns 88 percent of all private property. Half the population, mostly Black, lives below the poverty line. Many poor Black children, about 40 percent in the rural and 15 percent in the urban areas, suffer from malnutrition. One third of the Black population over 15 (some 3 million people) is illiterate. Three quarters of the Black teachers are either unqualified, or underqualified, for their jobs. The education system therefore perpetuates a vicious circle of deprivation and discrimination.

Although the people of South Africa are faced with the difficult and complex task of unravelling apartheid completely, the new government, in an attempt to meet this challenge, came up with a policy document called The Reconstruction and Development Programme (RDP). This RDP of president Nelson Mandela is an integrated, coherent, socioeconomic policy framework. The RDP seeks to mobilize all people of South Africa and the resources of the country toward a final eradication of apartheid and the building of a democratic, nonracial, and nonsexist future (*The African National Congress's Reconstruction and Development Programme Document, 1994*). In meeting basic needs, the RDP aims at eliminating hunger by providing land and housing to all people, providing access to safe water and sanitation for all, ensuring the availability of affordable and sustainable energy sources, eliminating illiteracy, raising the quality of education and training for children and adults, protecting the environment, and improving the country's health services and making them accessible to all.

As stated in Mandela's RDP document, the history of South Africa has been a bitter one dominated by colonialism, racism, apartheid, sexism, and repressive labor policies. The economy was built on systematic enforced racial division in every sphere of the society. Segregation in education, health, welfare, transportation, and employment left scars of inequality and economic inefficiency. In its dying years, apartheid unleashed a vicious wave of violence. Poverty is the number one major problem. Millions are affected, the majority of whom live in the rural areas and are women. The new South Africa must struggle to improve lives, to restore peace, and to bring about a more just society.

The Role of Women in Improving Their Health in South Africa Today

Meeting the goals of the RDP will not be possible if women are not involved in the decision-making processes. Women in South Africa have achieved success and made invaluable contributions to society despite widespread gender discrimination. The RDP has in place mechanisms to address the disempowerment of women and boost their role within the development process and economy. Existing gender inequalities as they affect access to jobs, land, and housing, for example, are being addressed. A passage from the South African *Women's Charter for Effective Equality*, adopted at the National Convention convened by the Women's National Coalition, 25–27 February 1994, states that women are breaking their silence, claiming respect and recognition of their human rights and dignity, and requiring effective change in their status and material conditions in the new South Africa ("Extracts from the Women's Charter," 1994). In improving their health, women of South Africa claimed their right to full and equal participation in the creation of a nonsexist, nonracial, democratic society. The women's coalition drew from their diverse experiences and defined what changes are required within the new political, legal, economic, and social systems. They set out programs designed to achieve equality in all spheres of public and private life, including the law and the administration of justice; the economy; education and training; development of infrastructure and the environment; social services; political and civic life; family life and partnerships; custom, culture, and religion; violence against women; health; and the media. The roles that women have played and will play to satisfy these needs cannot be underestimated. Women, particularly African women, are members of Mandela's cabinet today. There is, for example, Nkosazana Dlamini Zuma, Minister of Health; Stella Sigcau, Minister of Public Enterprises; and Frene Gincwala, Speaker of the House. At the provincial level there are women occupying prominent roles as well.

As men and women take their seats on the green benches of the House of Assembly to close the chapter of apartheid in its manifold forms in South African politics, women in particular know that there is more work ahead of them. Most women are proud of their past and confident of the future. For women to play a prominent role in improving their health requires clear goals and a workable plan. In an attempt to encourage women to engage in the struggle for health, Sackey (1993), in her presentation of a paper on African women's struggles, quoted the following passage from a poem whose author is unknown: "O ye daughters of Africa, Awake! Awake! Arise!/No longer sleep nor slumber, but distinguish yourselves,/show forth to the world that ye are endowed noble/and exalted faculties" (p. 1384).

References

The African National Congress's Reconstruction and Development Programme Document. (1994).

Extracts from the Women's Charter for Effective Equality, SA. (1994, August 12). *The Mail.*

Genovese, M. A. (1993). *Women as national leaders.* Newbury Park, CA: Sage.

Gil, D. G. (1992). *Unravelling social policy.* Rochester: Schenkman Books.

Gil, D. G. (1993a). Beyond access to medical care: Pursuit of health and prevention of ill. *Evaluation and the Health Professionals, 16,* 1–42.

Gil, D. G. (1993b). Confronting oppression and social injustice. In F. Reamer (Ed.), *The foundations of social work knowledge* (pp. 231–263). New York: Columbia University Press.

Guy, F. (1990). Gender oppression in Southern Africa's precapitalist societies. In C. Walker (Ed.), *Women and gender in Southern Africa*. Cape Town, SA: David Philip.

Human Development Report. (1993). New York: Oxford University Press.

Sackey, C. (1993, August 9–15). African women fight on. *West Africa*, 1384–1486.

South Africa through women's eyes. (1993, September/October). *MS*, 11–15.

Thompson, L. A. (1990). *A South African history*. New Haven: Yale University Press.

United Nations. (1991). *The world's women 1970–1990: Trends and statistics*. New York: Author.

Walker, C. (1990). *Women and gender in South Africa*. Cape Town, SA: David Phillip.

Year of women in South Africa. (1993, March). *Prodder newsletter: Programme for Development Research*. 5(1), 1–32.

13

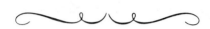

Developing a New Model for the Care of Women

Martha Neff-Smith

For all of recorded history, women have experienced health care that has been largely restricted to that required by pregnancy and childbirth. Indeed, to examine the historical scholarship on women and health raises questions of control, oppression, reform, belief, and the meaning of health (Lynaugh, 1994).

There is, in fact, no mystery about why the needs of women have been neglected by the health care system. Although there are some examples of females as shamen, the first professional class in the evolution of societies were the "medicine men" who assumed ritual masks and language. Over time their role evolved into the institution of sacred kinship. The parallels between these ancient forms of treatment and the hegemony of male physician "father figures" in contemporary health care delivery are inescapable.

Although the health care system evolved over the past 4 centuries in response to human need for the alleviation of suffering, there were other, equally important causal factors, including the social need to isolate persons with contagious disease, and the desire to appear humane and moral. Hospitals developed as places where the sick poor went to die out of the view of the masses. Devastation by waves of epidemics, namely smallpox, diphtheria, and bubonic plague, underscored the need for quarantine of infected persons. During the Middle Ages, hospitals were established by charitable groups in small houses where nursing care was provided by monks and nuns. When care was not focused on infectious disease, however, it centered around the needs of men—namely soldiers and specific occupational groups. Social position had everything to do with the diagnosis and treatment of disease (Rosen, 1974).

Women have always assumed roles as both healer and keeper of the sick. The role of wives and mothers as *health servant* is documented in the Old Testament. An example is found in the writing about Ruth and her strong bond with her mother-in-law, Naomi. Ruth was a tireless friend and nurse. History is rich with examples of women who sacrificed their own health or, indeed, their lives to care for others. Sister Kinney and her decades of work among polio victims inspired others. One of the most important figures in the history of nursing, Florence Nightingale, risked her life to save the lives of soldiers in the Crimea. There are many remarkable contemporary women, such as Mother Teresa, who work among the poorest of the poor in developing countries. Most of the visible and enduring stories of self-sacrifice have been related about women and few about men. Generally, these famous persons have been quite ordinary in their backgrounds and training. Daily newspapers provide us with modern-day examples of the women who sacrifice to promote the health of their children or the poor and homeless. These women refer to themselves as ordinary.

From the earliest times, women have shared care-giving roles with socially designated providers of healing, and for the last 500 years, access to care has been largely through communication with women. In various places of the world today, female family members are entrusted to intuitively discern the presence of illness and take the appropriate steps to restore health to the ill person. For example, in the Gypsy culture of Eastern Europe, very young women are often assigned the role of diagnostician and *gatekeeper* in deciding whether family members should be sent to traditional Gypsy healers or to trained providers. Because these women healers lacked opportunities for education and depended on the oral tradition to pass on their learning, a great part of the historical record has disappeared and much of the tradition of natural healing has been lost.

Many health care providers have received little training in the care of women apart from a specific specialty—the medical practice of obstetrics and gynecology (OB/GYN). Many OB/GYN nurse practitioners have been educated into this medical model, which treats symptoms rather than people, focuses on illness instead of health, and favors the specifics of reproductive pathology over broad assessment of health needs. The largest number of nurse practitioners who continue to be educated and practice without an advanced degree in nursing are in the OB/GYN field, and their certification examination is administered by the only certification corporation that does not require a minimum of a master of science in nursing degree. It is only recently that women's health practitioner programs, which educate advanced practice nurses in a more comprehensive approach to women's health, have begun replacing the more traditional programs.

Contemporary health care reflects social questions of autonomy, gender issues, and the conflicts between personal and professional survival. The most salient women's health problems in the United States today cause us, as sentient human beings, to reexamine the public policy of reliance on volunteerism and altruism espoused by state and federal agencies.

Most health providers will state unequivocally that they are satisfied with their professions because of the humanitarian service they provide. Historian Susan Reverby (1987) raises disturbing questions about the implications of assigning the work of caring solely to women, in effect ordering women to care without assigning fair economic value to that caring effort. Thus the health care providers most likely to care are those at the bottom of the wage scale, nurses and allied health professionals who are financially unable to provide unpaid or volunteer service. Homeless and women's shelters, for example, are so poorly staffed that clients must wait for hours to be served. In the hierarchy of American medicine, technological sophistication is far more monetarily rewarding than the typical concerns of nursing intervention that are characterized as women's work: pain relief, amelioration of chronic conditions, prevention, and improvement in quality of life (Lynaugh, 1994).

Although technology is perceived to have positive social value, most medical technologies are developed and diffused without an evaluation of the ultimate price society pays or the establishment of priorities. Women consumers are seldom queried about the necessity or acceptability of particular technologies used in the diagnosis of simple health problems (Stauning, 1994). Technologies for the care of women have often served to complicate care and increase its cost without making major differences in outcome. A perfect example of this can be found in the widespread use of mammography for women aged 40–50, who experience the least risk, and the low rates of use among women 60 and older, who are at the greatest risk of breast cancer and could benefit the most from this technology.

Due to the focus on reproductive health, women have been forced to become experts in order to receive comprehensive care. All too often they have found themselves to be the victims of astute marketing strategies that lure them to ambulatory care centers and hospitals that promise a range of women's specialty services, but in reality offer the same fragmented approach with only geographic, not conceptual, unity. Recent media marketing strategies have used encouraging female actors with "success stories." The disappointing services received in response to such advertisements retain the same reproductive focus and are directed only at increasing profits for medical conglomerates.

As a result, women often seek advice from family, friends, and, sometimes, a trusted health care professional about a nonreproductive health problem. Unfortunately, time is on the side of the disease process, and existing disease can progress substantially while the person is trying to find effective care. Preventive, restorative, and palliative services for women are simply not based on women-centered epidemiologic and clinical research. A new paradigm for the care of women is in order, and many nursing leaders such as Claire Fagin (1994) argue that as the focus of health care delivery switches from cure to care, nurses who have developed knowledge, interest, and skill in the caring mode will at last be able to realize their potential in an expanded role.

Clinical investigations of problems affecting women have been a long time in coming. In the United States, women's groups are encouraged by the Women's Health Initiative, a study by the National Institutes of Health. The thrust of this study initiated in 1991 is to examine the major causes of death, disability, and frailty in women of all races and socioeconomic groups. The hope of advocates for women is that this research will identify women's needs and result in a new mode and model of care which considers both mortality and morbidity as important issues.

Current Barriers to Care

Time, resources, access, social neglect, infantilization, and misdiagnosis are barriers that prevent women from receiving consistent, appropriate health care in what has been called the best health care system in the world. The United States has yet to establish affordable, high quality, appropriate, primary and secondary care access to women of all races and means. An examination of some of these barriers will assist us in the development of a new health care model.

In addition to the expanded *bill of rights* that has been proposed by ethicists to protect the autonomy of all patients, women need attention to issues that specifically affect them:

1. Access to care for women should not be related to status as child-bearer or to marital status. Aside from seeking care for a few episodes of acute disease, most young women see a primary care provider for contraception and issues related to pregnancy. They receive the most intense attention when they are pregnant. When the services requested are related to the termination of a pregnancy, the technology is less developed and the care is often less safe, available, and humane. When not pregnant, the woman who seeks ongoing care for a chronic disease is far less likely to find appropriate diagnosis, treatment, and care. Because of male dominance of medicine, she is not likely to find a primary care provider who can empathize. Female physicians trained in the male model also are unable to empathize. As a result, the health care experience adds to women's already unequal burden of pain and disability.

2. Providers should avoid the often routine attachment of a sexual diagnosis to routine visits for young women. In particular, lesbian women should never be forced by embarrassment to accept unnecessary prescriptions for contraception.

3. The orientation of the medical model toward acute disease episodes should be shifted to accommodate the illness patterns experienced by women, who have more chronic disease than men. Rehabilitation units, which were developed to meet the needs of stroke patients who had short life expectancies and were not expected to return to the work place, need to focus more interest on the long-term needs of women. Osteoarthritis and other musculoskeletal conditions, cancer, and circulatory disease are major sources of disability in women over 50 years of age, and three times as many women as men have rheumatoid arthritis (Byyny & Speroff, 1990). Unfortunately, the continuing stereotype is that women just stay home, so disability can be tolerated. This prejudicial thinking may affect the type and level of treatment, and, of course, outcome.

4. Both undertreatment for serious illnesses (e.g., lung cancer and hip fracture) and overtreatment (hysterectomy) have been established as serious problems for women, and in this era of cost cutting, females are particularly vulnerable to being either undertested and undertreated in order to save money for hospitals and insurance companies, or overtested to make money through lucrative procedures. In a study out of University of

California San Diego (Fisher, 1986), for example, an equal number of men and women presented with the same symptoms; in *every case* the men received more thorough workups than the women. Research money must be allocated to the needs of women to determine guidelines for an appropriate level of diagnosis and treatment.

5. The particularity of the ways that certain health problems manifest themselves in women must receive adequate attention. Obesity, for example, is a problem for 26 percent of the American population. Because obesity is considered by the present health care system to be a behavioral problem, a treatment of choice by the provider is a prescribed behavioral regimen. This knee-jerk reaction to an overweight patient does not take into account the issues related to body image that are associated with bias against women, and all too often results in a failure to conduct a complete clinical evaluation that might uncover potentially life-threatening health problems.

6. Practitioners need to become more aware of the epidemiology of disease in women. More women than men are hospitalized, but the average length of stay of men (6.9 days) exceeds that of women (6.2 days) until after age 65. The longest average stay was for cerebrovascular disease, which occurs more frequently in women aged 65 and older. Fractures accounted for an average of 9.4 days, malignant neoplasms 8.3 days, and diseases of the heart for 7.2 days (U.S. Bureau of the Census, 1990). There is growing evidence that the severity of women's illnesses is improperly assessed in both physicians' offices and emergency departments. A glaring example is *undertriage* of women over 65 who have sustained a hip fracture. Although this is a very serious injury and carries a high injury severity score (ISS), the individual is frequently admitted to a community hospital rather than a trauma center where more appropriate care is available. As a result, a majority of the oldest women with hip fracture suffer from long-term complications and are institutionalized, or die within the year.

7. There is a need to develop systematic screening programs to identify women at risk for suicide or malignancies, and develop interventions that are acceptable to women. Women are continuing to smoke, for example, in greater numbers than men because of the metabolic properties of nicotine. More teenage girls than

at any time in the last two decades are beginning to smoke (American Cancer Society [ACS], 1994). Poorly educated women who may have little understanding of biochemistry or physiology do understand that the nicotine in cigarettes helps control weight. Virtually all of the leading causes of death among women are related to smoking, except traumatic injury. Lung cancer deaths have surpassed breast cancer as a leading cause of cancer death in women (ACS, 1994). Chronic obstructive pulmonary disease is a prominent problem for women, beginning in the third decade of life. The social ecology of smoking needs consideration and action.

8. The delivery of health care services must be altered to reflect the realities of women's lives. In Western countries it has become necessary for women to work outside of the home because of social norms and financial need, leaving them little time in which to seek care for themselves and members of their families. When there are children involved, their needs generally take precedence over the needs of mothers. For these mothers, access to care for their own health needs becomes an issue of time and energy. Health care delivery in the form of *care as a business with business hours* presents serious barriers to access.

9. The economics of health care must be adjusted to reflect the needs of women. For members of the female population, employment does not necessarily improve access to health care. It has been estimated that three fourths of the uninsured are employed persons and their dependents (Wilensky, 1987). Because of family responsibilities, many women choose to work part-time, and as a result they have no health insurance. The average pay for women is far less than that of men (U.S. Department of Labor Statistics, 1994). Affordability is especially a concern when health services related to prevention and health promotion are required. The care provided to women without health insurance generally takes the form of crisis intervention. Work injuries carry very low Worker's Compensation benefits for women. A common scenario is the woman injured at work becoming a welfare recipient when her low worker's compensation (two thirds of her already low wages) is not sufficient to pay her rent and utilities. Recently, a 60-year-old widow working as a nurse's aide ruptured a lumbar disk while moving a patient. Four weeks later, the company physician for the nursing

home where she worked referred her to an orthopedist and she was finally x-rayed. Since her injury, this person has received $142 each week in compensation. She may never return to work and may soon lose the home which represents her only security. She is still in pain and has no hope that the future will be better financially or physically.

10. Women need mental health benefits. As described in earlier chapters, women have more depression than men. Depression and affective/mood disorders, which affect at least 4 percent of the American population at any given time, are major risk factors for suicide (Regier, 1988). In fact, depression is the most frequently occurring mental health problem. There appears to be a strong environmental link. Women who have low incomes and live alone with children are overrepresented compared with more affluent women with stronger support and access to care. In the context of causes of death, the symptoms of depression cannot be ignored any longer. Mental health services are basic components of care models for women and yet are seldom considered in routine evaluations of a woman's health.

11. The diversity of women must be respected. Black women are more vulnerable to arteriosclerotic heart disease than White women. They suffer from congestive heart failure and angina more often (Byyny & Speroff, 1990). Hypertension affects more African Americans than Whites. The diseases of obesity afflict more African American women than others. Hypertension, diabetes, arthritis, gallbladder disease, and coronary disease cause women of color to die earlier than their White counterparts because of access and quality of care issues. Only recently have scientific studies begun to evaluate potential physical and cultural determinants that may be associated with obesity (Bowen, Tomoyasu, & Cause, 1991). Mexican American women experience more diabetes and more serious complications from the disease. HIV is unequally opportunistic for all women of color. Providers need to be aware of differences in epidemiologic patterns of disease among women of color, and should work to eliminate the substantial differences in health outcomes that currently exist.

12. Women must be permitted to be equal partners in their care, and must be treated with respect in provider-patient communication.

Women's Health Groups

Beginning in the 1960s, strong networks began to be constructed by and for women who have physiological and emotional needs not met by official and voluntary agencies. This has been a phenomenon emerging naturally from the power of women to care for and nurture others. It has been noted by group members that women also have the psychological willingness to accept help from other women. The group model has provided a structure in which women have been able to collectively identify common problems and risks and begin to construct methods for providing care. Although these groups began as unofficial social groups, they have evolved into highly informative, professional bodies. Groups of women have come together around issues of alcoholism (for themselves and their family members), spouse abuse, depression, cancer recovery, injury rehabilitation, and a variety of other concerns. The model provides emotional support, education, and a way to discuss very personal problems in a creative, nonjudgmental forum.

The women's health group also facilitates the resolution of these same problems without assuming the prescribed role of *patient*. Participation in a women's group as a part of diagnosis and therapy assists individuals in avoiding labels such as *menopausal*, *PMS*, *hysterical female*, *neurotic*, or *hypochondriac*. The collective experience and wisdom provide a time-tested method of problem solving. When women are able to question prescribed medical protocols openly, they are more likely to adhere to a regimen.

Developments within Health Care: A New Ecological Model of Women's Health

Women around the world have some powerful leaders to thank for the tremendous strides made in women's health care in the last 20 years. These women have proposed that we abandon the paternalistic obstetrical model for the delivery of care (Boston Women's Health Collective, 1984) and replace it with a specific new ecological model. This model will be based on the known health risks and knowledge of specific problems gained from new research initiatives. The environmental context of a woman's life will be considered. Women cannot succeed in obtaining a high level of health if they are so busy caring for others that they are not getting care for themselves. Primary prevention will be supported for children, men, AND women.

A shift of this magnitude requires partnership between women as workers—those who provide the bulk of health care, especially at the lower levels of the system—and women as patients—advocates for their own health needs and the health of their communities. Special attention should be paid to the role of women of color, who have major deficits in their own health care, yet have labored for centuries to improve the health care of others. The legacy of slave medicine and segregated health care is with us yet, in barriers to care for patients and in the positioning of women of color for the most part at the bottom of the health care delivery pyramid—as housekeepers, nurses' aides, and technicians. Despite progress in admissions to medical schools, the rate of growth for minority physicians lags behind the growth of minority populations. In 1988, fewer than 5 percent of new admissions to nursing schools were African American (National Center for Health Statistics, 1990).

The ecological model proposes additional changes in the delivery of care. For the last two decades, the women's movement has promoted an upheaval in health care delivery. Since 1970 there has been a reemergence of the use of traditional healers, the identification of high-risk groups by women investigators, and home births and birthing centers. Women are encouraged to become strong advocates as consumers and voices in the establishment of health policy. Several concerned women are now in the political arena and stand willing to speak out. It is vital that a new paradigm be developed and an agenda be set immediately in order to save women from death, disability, and suffering.

The time has come for a new covenant between women and their health care providers and the health care system. The agreement will be constructed on the following tenets:

1. Women represent a unique collective of individuals with varying strengths and requirements for health care.

2. Women have the responsibility and the privilege of making decisions about their bodies and minds.

3. Women have a right to the most current knowledge and the most appropriate technology.

4. Given all available knowledge, women have the right to seek any type of care from any person of their choice.

5. There will be no punishment in the form of denial of services if traditional healing is sought as a part of care.

6. When presented with medical test findings, women will be given viable alternatives.

7. Women are entitled to care by an individual who respects them and is educated and specifically trained in women's health and disease.

8. Care given to women will be based on specific scientific epidemiologic research.

9. The ecological context of each woman's life will be considered.

10. The rights and needs of women as health care providers will be respected.

In 1985, Choi called for a new paradigm for women's health care that includes injury and disease prevention, health promotion, and education for self-care and responsibility. Extensive collaboration and self-care are critical elements of her proposed paradigm. The education of women about specific risks and established disease prevalence (including mental health problems) is long overdue. Given complete information, women can manage their own prevention programs. For centuries women have been given the responsibility to care for others. The time has come for them to care for themselves.

The collaboration called for by leadership in the women's movement, especially Judy Norsigian and members of the Boston Women's Health Collective, requires broad training (Boston Women's Health Collective, 1984). Physicians and nurse practitioners trained in the medical model betray women when they place system values ahead of human and professional values, and replace the mission of service with new goals of advancing careers and gaining financial rewards. The present bureaucratic systems of health care delivery and practitioner education should be challenged and replaced rather than supported; the role models of Margaret Sanger (family planning pioneer), Lillian Wald (public health reformer), and Mabel Staupers (crusader for the rights of African American nurses) will stand us in good stead as we forge a new path forward.

The ecological model includes care by groups as an integral element. Women sharing knowledge and experience in groups as a method of promoting and protecting health will welcome a new class of nurse practitioners who are specialists in and advocates for women. The model of care will be ecological in assessment, prescription, and treatment. Environmental risk will be considered a basic science. The United States health care system can no longer be forgiven for neglecting the prevention, protection, and health promotion needs of women.

References

American Cancer Society. (1994). *Facts about smoking.* Atlanta: Author.

Boston Women's Health Collective. (1984). *The new our bodies, ourselves: A book by and for women.* New York: Simon and Schuster.

Bowen, D., Tomoyasu, N., & Cause, A. (1991). The triple threat: A discussion of gender, class, and race differences in weight. *Women and health, 17*(4), 123–143.

Byyny, R. L., & Speroff, L. (1990). A clinical guide for the care of older women. Baltimore: Williams and Wilkins.

Choi, M. (1985). Preamble to a new paradigm for women's health. *Image, 17,* 14–16.

Fagin, C. (1994). Women in nursing, today and tomorrow. In E. Friedman (Ed.), *An unfinished revolution: Women and health care in America* (pp. 159–176). New York: United Hospital Fund.

Fisher, S. (1986). *In the patient's best interest: Women and the politics of medical difference.* New Brunswick, NJ: Rutgers University Press.

Hart-Brothers, E. (1994). Contributions of women of color. In E. Friedman (Ed.), *An unfinished revolution: Women and health care in America* (p. 136). New York: United Hospital Fund.

Lynaugh, J. (1994). Women and nursing: A historical perspective. In E. Friedman (Ed.), *An unfinished revolution: Women and health care in America* (pp. 143–157). New York: United Hospital Fund.

National Health Interview Survey. (1990). Hyattsville, MD: U.S. Department of Health and Human Services.

Regier, D. A. (1988). One month prevalence of mental disorders in the United States: Based on five epidemiologic catchment sites. *Archives of General Psychiatry, 45,* 972–986.

Reverby, S. (1989). *Ordered to care: The dilemma of American nursing 1850–1945.* Cambridge, England: Cambridge University Press.

Rosen, G. (1974). *From medical police to social medicine: Essays on the history of health care.* New York: Science History.

Stauning, I. (1994). Women, health and medical technology. *International Journal of Technological Assessment in Health Care, 10*(2), 273–81.

Wilensky, G. (1987). Viable strategies for dealing with the uninsured. *Health Affairs, 16*(2), 33.

Index

Relationships
  enduring, 112
  with parents, 112–114
Religions
  founding of new patriarchal, 4–5
  sex-role differentiation promoted by, 249
Reproductive disorders
  in older women, 206–210
  in reproductive years, 120–131, 136
Reproductive system health, global context of, 294–295
Reproductive tract infections (RTIs), 297–298
Reproductive years, 107, 140
  accepting responsibility in, 108–110
  decision to parent in, 114–115
  defined, 107
  health promotion and illness prevention in, 136–140
  lifestyle-related disorders of, 131–134
  marriage and enduring relationships in, 112
  physical health maintenance during, 107–108
  psychiatric illness of, 134–136
  psychosocial domain of, 108–115
  relations with parents in, 112–114
  reproductive disorders of, 120–131
  systemic illness in, 115–120
  work and career identity in, 110–112
Responsibility
  accepting, 108–110
  facilitating work and family, 277–278
Retirement, 198
  early, 227
  views on, 228
Rheumatoid arthritis, 50, 116, 204–205, 269, 326
Risk-taking behavior, 75
Ritalin, 94
Roe v. Wade, 124
Role binding, 82–83
Role blocking, 82, 83
Role changes, aging and, 198–199
Roles, multiple, of women, 12, 13, 265
  See also "Sandwich generation"
Role sharing, 82, 83
Role strain, 133–134
RU-486, 160

Safe sex, 97, 139–140
Safety tips, for older women, 227
"Sandwich generation," 108–109, 114, 164–165, 178
Schizophrenia, 135
Screening, health, for older women, 220–221
Seatbelts, use of, 140
Self
  in adolescence, 72
  emergent, 257–258
  woman's search for, 241–243

Self abuse, 132–133
  in adolescence, 83–87
Self-esteem, 257
  male vs. female levels of, 244, 245
Sepsis, 297
Sexism, 46, 110, 197, 245, 251
Sexual abuse/assault, 87, 88–89, 272
Sexual and reproductive problems, in adolescence, 75–83
Sexual division of labor, 289
  women's status and, 291–292
Sexual harassment, 116, 267, 272
Sexual intercourse, in adolescence, 78, 79
Sexuality
  at menopause, 157–158
  power of female, 23–24
Sexually transmitted diseases (STDs), 50, 118–120, 131, 317–318
  in adolescence, 75, 78, 79–80, 87, 88, 101
  condoms to prevent, 139, 160, 251–252
Sexual Maturation Rate (SMR), 77
Sexual needs, meeting, of older women, 229
Silence, 37–38, 40
Single parents, 48, 249
Skin cancer, 117
  risk factors for, 118
Sleep changes, in menopause, 168–169
Small-for-gestational-weight fetuses, 129
Smoking, 52, 250, 251, 327–328
  in adolescence, 83–84
  cessation, 138–139
Social network
  aging and, 199–200
  strengthening, 228–229
Social Security benefits, 110, 199, 227
Society
  position of women in early, 3–4
  women in context of community and, 266
Sociohistorical background to women's health, 288–289
South Africa, 285, 314
  conditions and tasks for new, 318–319
  role of women in improving their health in present day, 319–320
  women in, 315–318
Spastic colon, 50, 268
Spermicides, 123, 125, 160
Spiritual support, 225
Sponge, contraceptive, 123, 160
Stereotypes, 45
  about aging, 196–198
Sterilization, 9, 124, 295
Stress, 133–134, 164–165, 172
  reduction, 138
Stroke, 50
Substance abuse, 131–132
  legal, 250–252
Subzonal insertion of sperm by microinjection (SUZI), 126

GAYLORD

PRINTED IN U.S.A.